Intellectual Disability

April 2o,

To NILDA

With best wishes
for your success

Best Personal regards

DEVELOPMENTAL PERSPECTIVES IN PSYCHIATRY

SERIES EDITOR
James C. Harris, M.D., Johns Hopkins University

Tuberous Sclerosis Complex, 3rd Edition
Manuel Rodríguez Gómez, M.D.
Julian R. Sampson, D.M.
Vicky Holets Whittemore, Ph.D.

Neurodevelopmental Disorders: Recognition and Treatment
Randi Hagerman, M.D.

Demystifying Anorexia Nervosa: An Optimistic Guide to Understanding and Healing
Alexander R. Lucas, M.D.

Intellectual Disability:Understanding Its Development, Causes, Classification, Evaluation, and Treatment
James C. Harris, M.D.

INTELLECTUAL DISABILITY

Understanding Its Development, Causes, Classification, Evaluation, and Treatment

James C. Harris, M.D.

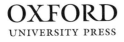

OXFORD
UNIVERSITY PRESS

2006

OXFORD
UNIVERSITY PRESS

Oxford University Press, Inc., publishes works that further
Oxford University's objective of excellence
in research, scholarship, and education.

Oxford   New York
Auckland   Cape Town   Dar es Salaam   Hong Kong   Karachi
Kuala Lumpur   Madrid   Melbourne   Mexico City   Nairobi
New Delhi   Shanghai   Taipei   Toronto

With offices in
Argentina   Austria   Brazil   Chile   Czech Republic   France   Greece
Guatemala   Hungary   Italy   Japan   Poland   Portugal   Singapore
South Korea   Switzerland   Thailand   Turkey   Ukraine   Vietnam

Copyright © 2006 by Oxford University Press, Inc.

Published by Oxford University Press, Inc.
198 Madison Avenue, New York, New York 10016

www.oup.com

Oxford is a registered trademark of Oxford University Press

Library of Congress Cataloging-in-Publication Data
Harris, James C.
Intellectual disability : understanding its development, causes, classification, evaluation,
and treatment / James C. Harris.
p. ; cm.—(Developmental perspectives in psychiatry)
Includes bibliographical references and index.
ISBN-13: 978-0-19-517885-2
ISBN-10: 0-19-517885-8
1. Mental retardation. 2. Developmental disabilities.
[DNLM: 1. Mental Retardation. 2. Developmental Disabilities. WM 300 H314i 2005]
I. Title. II. Series.
RC570.H373 2005
616.85'88—dc22 2004024148

9 8 7 6 5 4 3 2 1

Printed in the United States of America
on acid-free paper

Foreword

When the original President's Panel on Mental Retardation was established in 1961 by President John F. Kennedy at the urging of his sister Eunice Kennedy Shriver, there was a deep divide between biomedical scientists and educators. This dichotomy almost destroyed the excellent work of the panel until the differences were reconciled by the Chairman, Leonard Mayo, and honorary advisor, Eunice Shriver. At that time most leading educators espoused the position that mental retardation was an educational problem and should be treated as such through adequate funding. They criticized the "medical model," which was identified with the low quality of institutional care under the supervision of psychiatrists. Unfortunately many psychiatrists and other physicians showed little interest in persons with mental retardation who were considered untreatable and incurable.

This was not the case with Leo Kanner, the head of Child Psychiatry in the 1930s, 1940s, and 1950s at Johns Hopkins University School of Medicine and a member of my department there, who awakened interest in the field of mental retardation. One of his disciples, James Harris, has expanded that tradition. Although there still remain differences, there is more recognition by leading special educators that there are important medical needs of persons with mental retardation and by enlightened physicians that there are educational and social needs as well.

The enormous change in societal attitudes toward the subjects of this book, aided greatly by the Special Olympics, has been followed by changes in terminology—no longer is a person with Down syndrome a "Mongolian idiot" or "Mongol." "Retards" is now a denigrating term used only by insensitive teenagers. As a less stigmatizing general diagnosis, "intellectual disability" has replaced "mental retardation," just as "physical disability" has replaced "physical handicap."

The author of this text, James Harris, M.D., has had a distinguished career capped by a full professorship in psychiatry and pediatrics at Johns Hopkins University School of Medicine. His strength has been his meticulous pursuit of a wide range of clinical research on the etiology, pathogenesis, clinical features, developmental aspects, and educational and social needs of persons with intellectual disability. His training in both pediatrics and psychiatry provides a broad perspective to his work and to the present publication.

Dr. Harris emphasizes that intellectual disability is not a static condition; that change occurs over time; that treatment, care, training, and education are a lifetime problem. My own bias is similar, as described by the term "reduced efficiency of learning." This description emphasizes that the greater the input (care and education), the greater the output (progress in behavior and adaptive skills). Modern diagnostic manuals emphasize multiaxial criteria leading to treatment plans focused on intellect, social progress, and societal needs and emphasize future planning.

Those persons with higher levels of functioning, the so-called mildly retarded ("slow learners" in some countries), make up the largest number of persons with intellectual disability. Progress is being made in identifying some etiologies— fetal alcohol syndrome, fragile X syndrome, lead poisoning. The strongest correlation remains with low economic status based on parental limitations, genetic or acquired. Much remains to be learned. Although inadequate stimulation early in life is no longer considered an adequate explanation for all of these children, early intervention remains as an essential modality in their care.

The most important contribution by Dr. Harris is his emphasis that intellectual disability is a "developmental" problem, meaning change with time. Infancy, childhood, adulthood, and even senescence are life stages in persons with intellectual disability, just as they are in persons with normal intellect. Finally the author, unlike most scientists, addresses the spiritual and religious needs of the intellectually disabled, and I applaud him for that. This is a text for many disciplines, certainly not for psychiatrists or pediatricians alone. Whether it is read from cover to cover (which I recommend) or used for specific reference, it adds substantially to the academic field of intellectual disability.

In closing, let me say that I am very proud to have had Dr. Harris as one of my residents in the Department of Pediatrics and Fellow in Developmental Pediatrics and Psychiatry at the Kennedy Institute at Johns Hopkins University School of Medicine.

Robert E. Cooke, M.D.
Medical Director
Joseph P. Kennedy, Jr. Foundation,
formerly Chairman, Department of Pediatrics,
Johns Hopkins University School of Medicine
and Vice Chancellor for Health Affairs
University of Wisconsin

Acknowledgments

Intellectual Disability provides a comprehensive summary of knowledge acquired through my work with children, adolescents, and adults with intellectual disability for the past 30 years. It is the result of long-term contact with intellectually disabled persons and their families and discussions with faculty members, residents, and medical students and nonmedical professionals at the Johns Hopkins Medical Institutions and the Kennedy-Krieger Institute. Gratitude is expressed to the many authors whose publications that I have referenced and that have enhanced my understanding. I assume full responsibility for my synthesis of their work. I thank Eunice Kennedy Shriver, director of the Joseph P. Kennedy, Jr. Foundation, for her inspiration and example of dedication to intellectually disabled persons all over the world. My teachers and colleagues, Robert E. Cooke, medical director of the Joseph P. Kennedy, Jr. Foundation, and Hugo Moser, past president of the Kennedy-Krieger Institute, have instilled their scientific passion for understanding the etiologies of intellectual disability. Appreciation is expressed to Bryan King and Ludwik Syzmanski, who reviewed the draft manuscript and provided valuable recommendations for its improvement, and to my wife, Catherine DeAngelis, for her infinite patience.

I particularly thank Irving B. Harris of the Irving B. Harris Foundation for financial support that allowed me to complete this book. Special thanks are due to Joan Bossert, my editor at Oxford University Press, who provided continuing support and insightful suggestions regarding the publication of this book. Finally, without the unfailing efforts and diligence of Joan Bendall, this book could not have been completed.

J.C.H.
Baltimore, MD

Contents

Intellectual Disability

1

Introduction

The aim of this book is to provide professionals with the latest and most reliable information on intellectual disability and associated impairments. It utilizes a developmental perspective and reviews the various types of intellectual disability, discusses approaches to classification, diagnosis, and appropriate interventions, and provides information on resources that may offer additional help.

The term "intellectual disability" is used throughout this book instead of "mental retardation" to reflect current perspectives. Intellectual disability refers to impairments in both cognitive functioning and adaptive skills whose onset is during the developmental period. It is a developmental, intellectual, and cognitive disability. Although the term "mental retardation" continues to be used in the International Classification of Diseases (ICD-10) and DSM-IVTR, the continued use of this designation has been questioned because it implies a static, unchanging condition rather than one that can change over time. Other terms, such as "mental handicap" and "learning disability," have also been used. These variations in terminology are derived from long-standing concerns about the stigma of applying the term "mental retardation" to individuals.

A more general term applied to individuals with intellectual disability is "mental disability." The World Health Organization and the United Nations generally use the term "mental disability" as a broad descriptor, and the U.S. Supreme Court, in the Olmstead decision emphasizing the importance of community living, also used the term "mental disability."

The definition of "mental retardation" has changed nine times over the past 100 hundred years in the United States. Such changes in nomenclature come about with the acquisition of new knowledge regarding causes and efforts to preserve the dignity of persons who are intellectually disabled. Reflecting this new knowledge and concerns about the stigma sometimes associated with the term, on July 25, 2003, the name of the federal advisory committee, the President's Committee on Mental Retardation (PCMR), was changed to the President's Committee for People with Intellectual Disabilities (PCPID). Because the name designates the committee that advises the Secretary of Health and Human Services and the President on federal policy regarding programs and services, the change is noteworthy. It is expected that "intellectual disability" instead of "mental retardation" will gradually become the preferred designation in the United States. The term "intellectual disability" is used by the International Association for the Scientific Study of Intellectual Disability (IASSID) and the major research journal *The Journal of Intellectual Disability Research (JIDR)*.

In this book, the focus is on development, intellectual disability, and associated cognitive disabilities. Emphasis is placed on human development and the impact of impaired cognition on individuals throughout their lives. In persons with intellectual disability, both intellect and cognitive processes are affected. Indeed, the national association for families, The Arc of the United States, in its mission statement, focuses on the needs of those with cognitive, intellectual, and developmental disability. Other organizations, such as the Special Olympics, use descriptive language to describe the disability that is culturally appropriate, depending on the country where the Special Olympics program is located. Still, the critical issue is a comprehensive assessment and individualized case formulation rather than simply relying on the diagnostic category that is applied. Historically, the names used to categorize individuals with intellectual disability have frequently become stigmatizing. Witness the demise of the terms "moron," "imbecile," and "idiot" that were once part of a formal classification. Those who object to the term "mental retardation" point out that those so designated and referred to as "retarded" are diminished as people by this label. They suggest that mental retardation is a term that emphasizes what a person is not—not functioning normally—rather than simply describing the type of disability. By emphasizing development and designating intellectual disability as a developmental problem that starts in early life, the focus shifts to the individual who is adapting and growing as a person.

There is concern that a change in the use or definition of the term "mental retardation" may affect federal and state policy in regard to the termination of program eligibility, citizenship, legal status, and criminal justice. This issue has been addressed through an in-depth study, commissioned by the Resource Network International to the Kansas University Center for the Study of Family, Neighborhood, and Community Policy. The study investigated past and current use of the term "mental retardation" in the context of federal and state government programs. They found that "few Federal or State policies [were] affected by the term 'mental retardation' during the past 20 years" (Schroeder et al., 2002). They did indicate that within federal programs, a diagnosis of "mental retardation" is used for determination of disability under IDEA, SSI, SSDI, and Medicaid HCBS Waiver programs. No alternative terms for determining eligibility have been mandated within any of the state and federal programs studied, but use of alternative terms has been permitted within state special education programs receiving IDEA financial support. The most widely used alternative term is "mental disability" (32%). Currently, 36 states have adopted the term "developmentally delayed" as a new special education eligibility category as permitted by the IDEA legislation. Thus, in the past 20 years, there has been a shift in special education programs away from the use of the term "mental retardation" and toward a focus on "developmentally delayed," as described in the IDEA legislation. Overall, the study demonstrated that federal and state programs are generally based on functional assessments along with IQ measurements rather than emphasizing the specific name used to designate the disability.

In 2002, the American Association on Mental Retardation (AAMR) voted to continue with the name "mental retardation" for now, although the previous year their Board of Directors had recommended that the name be changed. It is expected that eventually the name of this organization will change, too. This process has already begun through the AAMR's efforts regarding functional classification. This paradigm shift to functional classification is consistent with the use of the term "intellectual disability." Mental retardation, in the AAMR definition, is not a trait existing in an individual, but rather an expression of the interaction between a person with limited intellectual and adaptive skills and that individual's environment. The AAMR definition also focuses on the person's individual needs rather than emphasizing their deficits (Schalock et al., 1994). This emphasis on interaction with the environment is a developmental one. Development occurs as a consequence of an individual's engaging in and mastering experiences in their environment. Thus, using the term "intellectually disabled" to describe a person who is challenged by environmental demands and masters them may be more appropriate from a developmental perspective than "mentally retarded." "Intellectual disability" should be a term that anticipates habilitation or rehabilitation.

In summary, at a time of transition in nomenclature, the most objective designation must be applied to individuals who are in need of services. The developmental perspective may be a helpful orientation when the type of impairment that exists is intellectual and cognitive. The developmental perspective may provide a framework for appropriate interpersonal and appropriate developmental intervention plans designated to assist the individual in attaining a sense of self-efficacy and confidence.

The emphasis in this book is on the development of the person, the provision of interventions for associated behavioral and emotional problems, and the needed positive supports for self-determination. It includes detailed discussions of the diagnosis, classification, epidemiology, etiology, and interventions. It also discusses the facilitation of transitions throughout the life course from infancy to maturity and old age. Evaluation for associated behavioral and emotional problems, as well as discussions of genetic factors, appropriate psychosocial, medical, and pharmacological interventions, and family and community supports, are reviewed. Case examples are provided to highlight specific diagnostic and treatment issues of concern to parents and professionals and issues related to community integration. The appendices contain a detailed listing and description of where to go for information on intellectual disability (appendix A), as well as information on the Special Olympics (appendix B), the Report of the

Surgeon General's Conference on Health Disparities and Mental Retardation (appendix C), Research Issues Involving People with Intellectual Disability (appendix D), the NIH workshop Emotional and Behavioral Health in Persons with Mental Retardation/Developmental Disabilities: Research Challenges and Opportunities (appendix E), Keeping the Promises: National Goals, State of Knowledge, and Research Agenda for Persons with Intellectual and Developmental Disabilities (appendix F), and information on The President's Committee for People with Intellectual Disabilities (appendix G).

During the past three decades, enormous progress has been made in providing educational services for children with intellectual disability and associated impairments and community programs and supportive employment for adults. Parents, teachers, and professionals have struggled to develop the most innovative psychoeducational and treatment programs. As a result of these efforts, we have educational services for intellectual disability that are required by law. However, behavioral and emotional problems in affected children and adults often prevent full participation in these programs. In many states, intellectual disability (mental retardation) services are separate from mental health services. Thus, persons with intellectual disability who have behavioral and emotional problems may not have access to appropriate services. It is not widely recognized that persons with intellectual disability may be doubly handicapped and require the dual diagnosis of both intellectual disability and behavioral or emotional disorder. The lack of recognition of dual diagnosis is emphasized in the Report of the Surgeon General's Conference on Health Disparities and Mental Retardation (2002).

The provision of services requires background knowledge from genetics, the neurosciences (especially social neuroscience), general medicine, pediatrics, neurology, psychiatry, psychology, education, and social sciences. An understanding of the developmental course of the various intellectual disability syndromes is essential. Knowledge in these areas is proceeding at a rapid pace. Three conferences have been held to highlight the needs of intellectually disabled persons for services and research. These are the Surgeon General's Conference on Health Disparities and Mental Retardation (December 5–6, 2001), the NIH workshop Emotional and Behavioral Health in Persons with Mental Retardation and Developmental Disabilities (November 29–December 1, 2001), and the Keeping the Promises Conference (January 6–8, 2003) organized by The Arc of the United States and the American Association on Mental Retardation (AAMR). The next steps in dealing with research for intellectual disability and mental illness are outlined in the NIH workshop report.

The following chapters review history, classification, epidemiology, etiology, assessment, associated features, behavioral phenotypes, lifespan development, interventions, ethics, and spirituality.

Chapter 2 reviews the early history of intellectual disability and provides an overview of changing concepts and legal safeguards. Although recognized since antiquity, explanations of the nature, causes, and treatment of intellectual disability have varied over time. This chapter traces the origins of intellectual disability and emphasizes how definitions of disability have changed as a result of psychosocial influences and cultural attitudes. The origins of intellectual testing are reviewed, as are the beginnings of our understanding of intellectual disability as a developmental disorder of cognitive and adaptive abilities. Finally, the legal rights of persons with intellectual disability are discussed in the context of landmark legal decisions.

Chapter 3 discusses how intellectual disability is recognized and classified. Diagnostic criteria and current classification systems are critically reviewed. This chapter includes a comprehensive description of the evolution of current diagnostic systems. The DSM-IVTR, ICD-10, and AAMR definitions of mental retardation are described and their criteria are compared, and the International Classification of Functioning (ICF) is reviewed. Although each of these definitions is of mental retardation, the term "intellectual disability" is used in this text. A detailed summary of the dimensional approach used in the AAMR Multidimensional Classification that focuses on the needs of the individual is provided. A developmental perspective that reflects the extent of intellectual and adaptive impairment is proposed for various levels of intellectual disability. Finally, the issue of adapting the diagnostic criteria for classifying mental, emotional, and behavioral disorders is discussed. The Royal College of Psychiatrists' Diagnostic Criteria for Psychiatric Disorders for Use with Adults with Learning Disabilities/Mental Retardation (DC-LD) and the progress on the National Association for the Dually Diagnosed (NADD) in association with the American Psychiatric Association Supplemental Classification that provides detailed instructions on how to apply DSM-IV criteria to persons with intellectional disability are reviewed.

Chapter 4 discusses the epidemiology of intellectual disability. Epidemiology provides a basis for the understanding and dynamics of health and disease. It can provide information about the nature and scope of intellectual disability and associated general medical, behavioral, and emotional disorders. One aspect of epidemiology involves providing estimates of the number of persons with intellectual disability as required by national and state planning agencies for the purpose of treatment planning and determining the impact of interventions. Both the occurrence of intellectual disability in the general population and information on the occurrence of specific intellectual disability syndromes is required. This chapter reviews how definitions of intellectual disability have influenced occurrence estimates. It discusses risk and protective factors and such characteristics of persons with intellectual disability as age, sex, socioeconomic level, variations in prevalence between urban and rural populations, and associated features. Three approaches to case identification are considered: statistical models, pathological models, and social systems models. Factors that impact prevalence, such as early diagnosis, normalization, inclusion, and improved interventions, are discussed. Finally, the life span occurrence of intellectual disability is reviewed, and the importance of the developmental trajectory of specific neurogenetic syndromes is reviewed.

Chapter 5 discusses the etiology and assessment of intellectual disability. There are multiple causes of intellectual disability, so the specific etiology must be determined. The many etiologies of intellectual disability may be classified in several ways, based on the identification of a causative agent or a specific mechanism. Advances in biomedical technology allow identification of a biological basis for an increasing number of intellectual disability syndromes. This chapter discusses multiple causes, etiologic assessment, and the interface between neurobiology and the environment. Prenatal causes (chromosomal disorders, syndrome disorders, inborn errors of metabolism, developmental disorders of brain formation, and environmental influences); perinatal causes (intrauterine disorders and neonatal disorders); and postnatal causes (head injuries, infections, demyelinating disorders, degenerative disorders, seizure disorders, toxic metabolic disorders, malnutrition, and environmental deprivation) are reviewed. The chapter discusses the most severe forms of intellectual disability, in which specific causes are most likely to be found and milder forms of intellectual disability, in which the cause may be less certain. It highlights the etiology of more common forms of intellectual disability, such as Down syndrome and fragile X syndrome. Finally, the components of a comprehensive evaluation are outlined, along with specific guidelines for clinical and genetic assessment.

Chapter 6 reviews behavioral problems and mental disorders in persons with intellectual disability. Historically, intellectual disability and mental disorders have been regarded as mutually exclusive. However, it is now clear that they are commonly linked. How frequent is emotional and behavioral impairment, and how is it diagnosed? Mental disorders and behavioral disturbances in persons with intellectual disability are not only expressions of maladaptive learning and adverse psychosocial experiences but also are indications of mental disorder. It is not uncommon for professionals to fail to consider mental disorder in an individual with intellectual disability. This chapter reviews the prevalence of behavioral, emotional, and mental disorders in persons with intellectual disability. The evaluation of emotional and behavioral impairment in persons with intellectual disability is described, and the elements of a comprehensive assessment that involve the intellectually disabled person and caregiver are discussed. The assessment includes evaluation of disorders of interpersonal functioning, communication, emotion, and behavior. The chapter begins with a discussion of difficulties in applying diagnostic criteria and reviews the frequency of mental and behavior disorder in persons with intellectual disability. Both institutional and community surveys are included. This is followed by a discussion of the spectrum of mental and behavior disorders in persons with intellectual disability, such as depression, attention deficit/hyperactivity disorder, conduct disorder, anxiety disorders, schizophrenia, and personality disorders. Rating scales for psychopathology in persons with intellectual disability are summarized. Assessment and diagnostic interviewing of persons with mild and moderate intellectual disability involve the same types of assessment that are used for emotional and behavioral problems in nondisabled individuals, with some modification. The chapter emphasizes how assessment takes into account the individual's cognitive and adaptive limitations. Tests of adaptive functioning are reviewed.

Chapter 7 describes genetics and genetic mechanisms in specific neurogenetic disorders. A growing body of evidence suggests that specific intellectual disability syndromes may be associated with particular patterns of behavior, temperament, and psychopathology. The term "behavioral phenotype" has been introduced to describe outwardly observable behaviors that are so characteristic of children with the syndrome that they suggest the underlying condition. These patterns have been studied most extensively in fragile X syndrome, Down syndrome, Rett's disorder, Williams syndrome, Prader-Willi syndrome, Lesch-Nyhan disease, Velocardiofacial syndrome, Smith-Magenis syndrome, and fetal alcohol syndrome. This chapter reviews advances in genetics that have furthered the understanding of intellectual disability. In addition to discussing the definition of behavioral phenotype, it provides a detailed description of the features in several disorders. The natural history of the behavioral phenotype throughout the life cycle of several disorders is also discussed.

Chapter 8 discusses intellectual disability over the life span. When intellectual disability is considered from a developmental perspective, the emphasis is on progression from one cognitive developmental stage to the next. This approach must be distinguished from a statistical approach that places intellectual disability on a continuum and does not consider the various etiologies that result in different cognitive profiles. A developmental approach emphasizes the impact of the disorder on the mastery of age-appropriate developmental tasks and differences in reasoning associated with different cognitive levels. A developmental model acknowledges the capacity for growth and emphasizes how adaptive behavior may improve with habilitation. This chapter initially reviews intellectual disability from the traditional developmental delay/developmental difference viewpoint and moves on to discuss the similar sequence and multiple pathways hypotheses. It suggests that "failure in cognitive progression" may be preferable to the term "developmental delay." There is a discussion of the importance of normalization, self-determination, and inclusion programs in facilitating developmental progression intellectually and socially. Issues of aging are discussed.

Chapter 9 discusses appropriate interventions and positive supports—family, behavioral, interpersonal, psychoeducational, pharmacologic, and community—that may facilitate self-determination. Treatment programs for children, adolescents, and adults with intellectual disability must consider the complex interplay of neurobiological and psychosocial factors. A comprehensive interdisciplinary approach is required, and consideration must be given to the full range of treatments that are used with non–intellectually disabled persons. Most commonly, multiple treatment modalities are required. This chapter discusses preventive interventions, environmental provisions (living conditions, vocational opportunities, and leisure time activities), psychoeducational interventions, skill development, behavioral interventions, pharmacotherapy, interpersonal psychotherapy (individual, group, family) and methods for fostering self-determination. Case vignettes of persons with intellectual disability and emotional and behavioral impairment are used to highlight these interventions. The experience of the person with intellectual disability and that of their family as they are engaged in the treatment process are reviewed.

Chapter 10 deals with ethics, spirituality, and intellectual disability. To assess a person with intellectual disability, developmental cognitive disabilities, and adaptive limitations from a spiritual point of view requires consideration of fundamental concerns about what it means to be human and the role of the sacred both in the life of that person, as well as in the life of the parent, the family, and the community. Parents must consider whether there is a difference between their own religious practice and a practice in which their child or adult family member can participate. To consider spirituality raises questions about the meaning of suffering experienced by a person with intellectual disability and the purpose of that individual's life. It also raises questions about how family and community are connected in a spiritual sense to those with intellectual disability. The AAMR definition of mental retardation (intellectual disability) asks questions that are linked to values in regard to the independence, productivity, and the role in, and meaning of, life for persons with intellectual disability. To consider the spiritual life of a person with intellectual disability is to reflect on the nature of human experience and to plan for means to organize support to facilitate growth toward their further spiritual development.

Thus, spiritual awareness as an aspect of human life and the need for spiritual supports is discussed. In consideration of the functional life of a person with intellectual disability, one must, from this perspective, look upon spirituality as a basic dimension of human life and an essential consideration when establishing systems of support. Gaventa (2000) proposed that spiritual considerations be included as an additional dimension in the AAMR multidimensional approach to diagnosis, classification, and supports.

References

Gaventa, W.C. (2000). Defining and assessing spirituality and spiritual supports: Moving from benediction to invocation. In S. Greenspan and H. Switzky (eds.), *What is mental retardation: Ideas for the new century.* AAMR Books, Washington, DC.

NIH Workshop. *Emotional and behavioral health in persons with mental retardation and developmental disabilities: Research challenges and opportunities.* Nov. 29–Dec. 1, 2001. Rockville, MD. http://ord.aspensys.com/asp/workshops/search.asp

Schalock, R., Coulter, D., Polloway, E., Reiss, S., Snell, M., Spitalnik, D., and Stark, J. (1994). The changing conception of mental retardation: Implications for the field. *Mental Retardation,* 39:181–193.

Schroeder, S.R., Gerry, M., Gertz, G., and Velazquez, F. (2002). Final Project Report. Usage of the term "mental retardation": Language, image and public education, p. 1. Center for the Study of Family, Neighborhood and Community Policy, University of Kansas, Lawrence, KS.

Turnbull, A., and Lakin, C.K. (eds.). (2005). *National goals and research for people with intellectual and developmental disabilities.* American Association on Mental Retardation, Washington, DC.

U.S. Department of Health and Human Services (2002). *Report of the Surgeon General's conference on health disparities and mental retardation. Closing the gap: A national blueprint to improve the health of persons with mental retardation.* Office of the Surgeon General, Rockville, MD.

2

Origins, Changing Concepts, and Legal Safeguards

When a health care professional becomes engaged in diagnosing and treating or supporting a person with intellectual disability, the complexities of the disorder become apparent. To provide the best care and the best support, knowledge about neurogenetic syndromes, management of biomedical and behavior features, psychosocial interventions, and the natural history of the disorder are critical. Background knowledge and sensitivity to the needs and life challenges of the affected person are especially important. With new knowledge in genetics, the neurosciences, and social sciences, and the utilization of the richness of family, school, and community resources for these individuals as they develop, the historical stigma of the diagnosis can be reduced and hopefully eliminated. Professionals, families, and community support personnel must join forces so that all available resources are fully utilized, thus allowing the person with intellectual disability to be appropriately treated for his condition and to begin to make choices and become a self-advocate to the extent possible.

This chapter will review changing concepts of intellectual disability over the centuries to provide a context for current diagnostic and treatment approaches. An awareness of this history provides perspective on the centuries-long struggle to recognize the needs of and to provide support to persons with intellectual disability. Legal safeguards are now in effect and are continuing to emerge as services are established that use a developmental model and emphasize a developmental perspective. This model emphasizes how comprehensive evaluation and positive supports at home and in the community can make a difference in the lives of persons with disabilities. The starting point is a definition of the term "intellectual disability." This will be followed by a brief historical survey of origins and attitudes that are changing after centuries of stigmatization and separation. National and international efforts, which began in the 1970s, are continuing to encourage community placement of and self-determination by persons with intellectual disability.

INTELLECTUAL DISABILITY DEFINED

Although "mental retardation" is the term used in both the International Classification of Diseases (ICD-10) (World Health Organization, 1992) and the Diagnostic and Statistical Manual (DSM-IV, DSM-IVTR) (American Psychiatric Association, 1994, 2000) systems that describe an intellectual and adaptive cognitive disability that begins in early life during the developmental period, the preferred term is "intellectual disability" internationally, especially in English-speaking countries.

What is meant by disability? Disability is socially defined and refers to the interpretation of an impairment by others (Braddock and Parish, 2002). Thus, disability is viewed in its cultural and societal context, while impairment designates a known biological condition. Davis (2000) wrote:

> Disability is not so much . . . the presence of a physical or mental impairment as it is the reception and construction of that difference. . . . An impairment is a physical fact, but a disability is a social construction. For example, lack of motility is an impairment, but an environment without ramps turns that impairment into a disability . . . a disability must be socially constructed; there must be an analysis of what it means to have or lack certain functions. (p. 56)

Intellectual disability is a developmental disability, but it is not one specific disease or illness (Clarke, Clarke, and Berg, 1985); rather, it refers to cognition and adaptive functioning. There is no single cause, mechanism, clinical course, or prognosis for the general category "intellectual disability." Intellectual disability is not a static disorder, but it is rather a dynamic condition with a variable course that depends on its etiology and the available environmental supports. Multiple etiologies result in intellectual disability, and these must be considered in treatment planning. In intellectual disability, thinking is not characteristically disordered and perception is not distorted unless there is another concurrent developmental or mental disorder. Intellectual disability includes a heterogeneous group of conditions that range from genetic and metabolic disorders to functional changes in cognition following trauma to the nervous system at birth or trauma to the brain occurring later in the developmental period. Because of its diagnostic heterogeneity, each person with intellectual disability must be considered individually according to whether or not there is an associated syndrome, for example, Down syndrome, or an associated etiology, for example, head trauma. In Down syndrome, genetic background, medical, psychological, and environmental factors interact to determine the degree of cognitive and adaptive disability. An understanding of such factors can be translated into a specific treatment program for an individual.

Persons with intellectual disability may be diagnosed with a full range of behavioral and mental disorders. The prevalence of associated mental disorders is three to four times greater in persons with intellectual disability than in the general population. Moreover, persons with intellectual disability are at greater risk for exploitation and physical or sexual abuse. Because their adaptive behavior is impaired, social stressors are of particular concern. Still, in protected social environments where adequate supports are available, such impairments may not be obvious; this is particularly the case for those with mild intellectual disability.

ORIGINS AND ATTITUDES

The earliest reference to intellectual disability may be in the Egyptian Papyrus of Thebes (1552 B.C.) (Bryan, 1930). Over the centuries, attitudes have ranged from humane concern to ostracism and abusive treatment. Traditionally, the major religions have taught that people with intellectual disability should be treated with kindness, yet humane education for persons with intellectual disability and educating the community about their needs are recent developments. In some countries, persons with intellectual disability were viewed as harmless innocents who were allowed to wander at will. In England, Henry II showed a humane view and promulgated legislation to make persons with intellectual disability wards of the king.

Ancient Greeks and Romans (1300 B.C. to A.D. 476)

Infanticide

Attitudes toward intellectual disability have varied considerably. The ancient Greeks and Romans proposed that a congenital anomaly was a sign that the parents had displeased the gods. In some instances, the Greeks practiced infanticide by exposure to the elements, although this practice was not as common as once believed (Garland, 1995). Aristotle (384–322 B.C.) supported this practice and in his *Politics* wrote: "As to exposing [to the elements to die] or rearing the children born, let there be a law that no deformed child shall be reared . . . if the regular customs hinder any of those born being exposed, then there must be a limit fixed to the procreation of offspring. . . ." Infanticide also was practiced for economic reasons when there were too many children.

Legal Rights: Guardians

Care for people with deformities was primarily available to those who were wealthy and could afford treatment. For the most part, those who were impaired were marginalized and excluded from societal activity. Despite this marginalization, early Roman law did protect property rights of people with disabilities. Moreover, some of those who were intellectually deficient were provided with guardians to assist in management of their affairs (Winzer, 1993). Deaf people who had speech were given authority to discharge legal obligations, such as marriage and property ownership. Those without speech and hearing were classified alongside people with intellectual disabilities, mental illness, and infants and could not perform legal acts (Hodgson, 1953). In the Roman Empire, slaves with intellectual disabilities were maintained by those with wealth for purposes of entertainment. It was thought that keeping such individuals brought good luck.

With the emergence of Christianity in the West, a more supportive attitude was expressed. The apostle Paul wrote: "Now we exhort you, brethren . . . comfort the feebleminded, be patient toward all men" (1 Thess. 5:14).

Eventually, Roman law outlined specific rights for people with disabilities. In the sixth century A.D., the Justinian Code classified people with disability. It delineated rights that were linked to different types and degrees of disability. For example, individuals with mental disabilities were not permitted to marry.

Middle Ages (A.D. 476 to A.D. 1500)

Religious Superstitions

During the early Middle Ages, some European countries held that intellectually disabled people were innocents and children of God who were to be cared for by religious sects. Later in Europe, intellectual disability, mental illness, deafness, and epilepsy, all disabling conditions, were considered to have supernatural or demonological causes. It was thought that the devil might cause epilepsy, and belief in demonic possession as a primary etiology for mental illness led to attempted cures based on religious ideas about exorcism. In addition, people with disabilities sought cures from the early Medieval times, reflecting supernatural beliefs in the abilities of the clergy. When witches were persecuted and heresy executions occurred in the Middle Ages, it was thought that disabled persons were among those persecuted, although the extent to which this occurred is not known.

Despite the impact of such superstitions about people with disabilities, there is evidence that other attitudes persisted during the Middle Ages. Kroll (1973) notes the absence of demonology in medical texts from the medieval era. There were advocates for the natural causes of mental illness. Moreover, the fact that towns assumed responsibility for people with mental disabilities is evidence that demonological beliefs were only one view of disability. Sympathetic attitudes toward people with disabilities led some towns to fund pilgrimages for people with epilepsy and mental illness, allowing them to visit religious sites to seek cures (Rosen, 1968). Thus, networks of people were concerned about those who were disabled. Such support involved family members, neighbors, employers, and charitable institutions (Farmer, 1998). In court records from the thirteenth to seventeenth centuries in England, beliefs about the origins of brain disorders are presented (Neugebauer, 1996). The Crown described legal incompetence, differentiating between persons with intellectual disability (termed "natural fools") and those with mental illness (lunacy).

Legal Rights and Property

In the second half of the thirteenth century, the *Prerogativia Regis* gave the Crown the responsibility of protecting property rights of people whose mental disabilities rendered them legally incompetent. In the *Prerogativia Regis,* intellectually disabled and mentally ill persons were distinguished, thus enabling the Crown to take custody of and profits from land owned by intellectually disabled persons. On the other hand, the Crown had the responsibility to ensure the safekeeping of lands held by those with mental illness. The Crown was not entitled to profits generated on lands owned by those with mental illness that it was supervising. Verbatim transcripts of medieval custody hearings show that mental disability was gauged by tests of literacy, numerical ability, general reasoning, knowledge as to place and kin, etc. Records of these examinations demonstrate that questions used to determine the presence of mental disability were essentially constant from the thirteenth through the seventeenth centuries, indicating a stable understanding of mental disability during this time period (Neugebauer, 1996).

Hospice Care

During the Middle Ages, monastically inspired hospices were established in several countries, including France, Syria, and Turkey. Such hospices were refuges for people with disabilities in religious enclaves (Winzer, 1993). Bishop Nicholas is reported to have cared for persons with intellectual disability in a hospice in southern Turkey as early as the fourth century, and the Belgian village of Gheel provided support and family care for people with mental disabilities in the thirteenth century (Roosens, 1979). The community at Gheel offered vocational opportunities in a community setting that included an infirmary and a church.

During the Middle Ages, Arab armies conquered Spain and southern France and occupied parts of the continent. They reintroduced Greek and Roman medical and philosophical traditions into Europe. Asylums for individuals with mental disabilities had been established by Arabs in Baghdad, Morocco, Damascus, and Cairo in the eighth century. The Arabs believed that mental disability was divinely inspired and was not demonic in origin. Thus, care in their institutions was generally benevolent. In keeping with this attitude, the Priory of St. Mary of Bethlehem was founded in London in 1247. The Order of Bethlehem began supporting physically ill persons as a hospital as early as 1330 and, subsequently, began caring for intellectually disabled persons, a role that gradually replaced that of caring for the physically sick. This hospital, the Bethlem Hospital (now Bethlem Royal Hospital), is still in operation and is the oldest mental hospital in Europe. Other mental hospitals were established in Spain, Germany, and other European countries.

During the fourteenth to sixteenth centuries, humanistic practices were initiated with better understanding of the anatomy and physiology of hearing, vision, and the human body. This led to new approaches to people with impairments, particularly those involving hearing and vision. Yet the view that mental disabilities were the consequence of demonic possession persisted, resulting in various treatments that included voluntary beatings of the head for individuals with depression, paralysis, and intellectual disability (Bromberg, 1975). Physicians used trepanning (making a hole in the skull) or purged people with mental disabilities of blood to release the black bile thought to cause mental disease. Such efforts to cure illness and disability were primitive, yet they resulted from a shift in attitude that emphasized biological causes and specific interventions. These attitudes signified a shift from believing that disabilities and illnesses were caused by supernatural beings to believing that they resulted from natural causes. Efforts to treat disabilities and illnesses were based on primitive understandings of biological functions.

Gradually, the appreciation that the impairment in intellectual disability arose in early life and was fixed gained currency. It was recognized that mental illness had an onset in later life and could be transitory. Differentiating intellectual disability from mental illness remained important because of property law rather than because of an emphasis on finding approaches to treatment.

Seventeenth and Eighteenth Centuries

Emergence of Science

The seventeenth century brought forth the Age of Reason, or the Enlightenment. Drawing on contributions from Francis Bacon (1605), Isaac Newton, and John Locke (1690), new approaches to care and treatment of people with disabilities began to emerge. De Condillac (1754) proposed a sensationalist theory of knowledge that lay the foundation for new psychological and intellectual intervention. He proposed that experience and reason were the primary sources of all knowledge and dismissed the innate ideas and biblical views of divine punishment as causes of disorders. Moreover, he taught that social and environmental modifications could improve human society. The Enlightenment supported a belief in the merits of natural science to advance the species (Edwards, 1996). Following the sensationalist school of philosophy, there were changes in attitudes and voluntary charitable societies, and new interest groups and institutions were formed. The sensationalist philosophies that arose during the Enlightenment and belief in the efficacy of natural science offered the moral imperative and new tools and interventions.

At the beginning of the seventeenth century, the scientific approach that emerged encouraged the systematic study of causes of intellectual disability. Bacon (1605) in England called for experiments based on the collection of empirical data. He proposed that the secrets of nature could be revealed by systematic observation of its regularities. In 1605, he published his *The Advancement of Learning, Divine and Humane* to refute the idea that divine punishment was a cause of mental illness and suggested lines of inquiry that would guide psychological research for the next three centuries. Studies involving the mental faculties, the interaction of mind and body, individual case studies, postmortem studies, anatomical investigations, and the investigation of the interface and interaction between the individual and society were proposed.

Legal Rights and Property

An emerging scientific consensus was accompanied by changes in attitudes toward poverty that impacted individuals with disabilities. The English Poor Law

provided needed relief for the community, yet, paradoxically, it also led to social stigma. England's Poor Law assigned responsibility for the poor and other
people unable to provide for themselves and for their condition. If a person
could not find a living for himself or herself, the first line of responsibility was
his or her family. If the family could not provide support, local communities
were charged with providing for him or her (Rushton, 1996). This tradition was
carried into the American colonies where local responsibility for people with
disabilities who were unable to care for themselves was a common practice.
Community support, religious, and medical institutions and family resources
were gradually linked. Thus, people with intellectual disability were commonly
supported through the Poor Law as relief for those unable to care for themselves was organized during the early modern period. The administration of
care or welfare had shifted from predominantly family provision, which was
the case in medieval times (Rushton, 1988), to community support. Most persons with intellectual disability stayed in the community with their families.
People with mental illness who were not intellectually disabled were treated
differently than those with intellectual disability and were more likely to be removed from their homes and placed in jails or houses of correction (Rushton,
1996). In 1637, Benoni Buck, a man with severe intellectual disability, was referred to the Court of Wards and Liveries in Jamestown, Virginia. This case
raised issues regarding the social obligation to protect the mentally disabled.
This is the first case of mental disability reported in the English colonies (Neugebauer, 1987).

Custodial care was ordinarily not used for people with intellectual disability
or mental illness; however, families would seek relief when their poverty was
linked to impairment of a family member. The first almshouse was established
in the United States in 1652 and served a heterogeneous population that included
those with physical and mental disabilities. In the United States, the development
of institutions for disabled persons occurred slowly over the next 180 years,
from that time until the 1820s.

Respect for the Individual

During the eighteenth century, emphasis on respect for the individual increased.
This enlightened attitude provided the impetus for the French and American
revolutions. The intellectual revolution that accompanied the Renaissance and
the Enlightenment resulted in essential changes in relationships between humans
in society and God. Now individuals were thought capable of intervening in
what previously was considered to be the natural order. This theme of the per-
fectibility of humans led to a new focus on treatment for individuals with disabilities. It resulted in the education of professionals, including physicians, educators, and care takers. Professional involvement and medical involvement with
disability led to the establishment of more schools and institutions in Europe
and in the United States. The trend toward institutionalization was particularly
striking.

Nineteenth Century

Special Education

There was greater recognition for the rights of slaves, persons with mental illness, the blind and deaf, and intellectually disabled persons (Kanner, 1964) in the nineteenth century. Early interventionists such as Jean-Marc-Gaspard Itard, despite the opinion of the experts of the time such as Pinel (1801), spent five years (1801–1806) (Lane, 1976) teaching a cognitively disabled boy, Victor, the so-called wild boy of Aveyron (Itard, 1802). Victor did not achieve normalization, but the methods that Itard developed in teaching him were recognized as highly meritorious by the French Academy of Sciences, which closely followed Victor's progress. Itard also focused on oral education of deaf persons and was a contributor to the medical specialty of otolaryngology. He used behavior treatments and special education approaches and rejected the general categorization of individuals as "idiots." Itard also distinguished between children with intellectual disability and those with pervasive developmental disorders and, in 1828, discussed these distinctions in the essay "Mutism Caused by a Lesion of the Intellectual Functions" (Carrey, 1995). Subsequently, an organized effort to educate intellectually disabled persons began in Switzerland and eventually moved to other parts of Europe and to the United States. Interest in intellectual disability at the time was stimulated by new, more hopeful ideas about humane interventions inspired by the philosophy of Rousseau, the encyclopedists, and Pestalozzi. Following Itard's example, Edouard Seguin devoted himself to the investigation and treatment of intellectually disabled persons. Itard was influenced not only by his scientific teachers, but also by his religious orientation. He was "striving for a social application of the principles of the Christian gospel, for the most rapid evolution of the lowest and poorest by all means and institutions, mostly by free education" (Kanner, 1960).

Like Itard, Seguin began with one boy with intellectual disability. Based on his success with this one individual, he began to work with other children at the Hospice for Incurables (Kanner, 1960). Seguin reported that his training of intellectually disabled persons embraced the muscular, imitative, nervous, and reflective functions. Seguin provided a more comprehensive approach than Itard did, describing his approach as the "physiological method." He emphasized sensory-motor, academic and speech, and moral training or socialization (Simpson, 1999). Seguin (1846) pointed out that intellectual disability, deafness, and congenital blindness shared the characteristics of an early age of onset and permanence of the condition. Seguin's approach became the standard worldwide and was recognized by the French Academy of Sciences in 1844. Later, he came to the United States where he made contact with Samuel Gridley Howe (1848), who was instrumental in establishing interventions for intellectually disabled persons in America. In 1866, Seguin's text *Idiocy and Its Treatment by the Physiological Method* advocated institutional training for the treatment of children who were too severely intellectually disabled to profit from normal classroom instruction. In 1876, Seguin was selected as the first president of the Association of Medical Officers of American Institutes for Idiotic and Feeble

Minded Persons, now the American Association on Mental Retardation (Scheerenberger, 1983).

Custodial Institutions

Institutional programs for individuals with intellectual disability increased in size and number in the mid-1800s. In the United States, the first distinct institution for intellectual disability opened in 1848. During that time, urbanization was increasing and the demographics were changing as more immigrants arrived. The institutional settings were a solution to social problems and social changes in the United States. Rothman (1990) proposes that the development of orphanages, asylums for people with mental illness, prisons, almshouses, and reformatories emerged to manage the social order at a time of change.

It is reported that many of the training efforts were successful, and children with intellectual disability were returned to their communities as "productive workers" (Trent, 1995). With the onset of the Civil War and the economic recessions that followed it, there was less employment available for those with intellectual disability trained in residential settings. In some instances, unpaid labor led to exploitation. By 1880, the training schools established by leaders such as Howe and Seguin had become custodial asylums with less emphasis on education and return to community life (Wolfensberger, 1976). Supportive social services, family support, and work opportunities in the community were lacking. Moreover, negative attitudes toward people with intellectual disability persisted in the general public, and Wilbur (1888) suggested that lifelong protective custodial care was appropriate.

Samuel Gridley Howe disputed the trend toward lifelong institutionalization and, in a speech in 1866 over 20 years before, stated that people with disabilities "should be kept diffused among sound and normal persons. Separation, and not congregation, should be the law of their treatment" (Wolfensberger, 1976). By this, he meant that they should not be separated from society, not congregated in groups away from society. He proposed that the states should gradually dispense with custodial institutions. However, the states did not do so; they continued to build them, to expand them, and to emphasize their economical management and self-sufficiency. By 1900, the census of intellectual disability institutions in the United States was 11,800 persons (Fernald, 1917). Often the institutions were located in remote areas. In their institutional settings, residents were given work in laundries, on farmlands, and in workshops, contributing to the self-sustaining economy of the institution. Seguin (1870) did not support the growth of large institutions, stating "Let us hope that the State institutions for idiots will escape that evil of excessive growth . . . in which patients are so numerous that the accomplished physicians who have them in charge cannot remember the name of each."

During the nineteenth century, interventions and the use of institutions increased. Schools and institutions for individuals with various types of disabilities including intellectual disability, deafness, blindness, and mental illness were established throughout both Europe and North America. Techniques used to diagnose various types of disability and develop treatment interventions and educational approaches improved. Those with similar disabilities and impairments began to identify with groups of others with similar handicaps.

Classification: Multiple Etiologies

The first medical periodical devoted to intellectual disability, *Observations on Cretinism,* was published in 1850. Due to the work of Thomas Curling in 1860 and Charles Fagge in 1870 (Scheerenberger, 1983), cretinism was linked to hypothyroidism. Wilhelm Griesinger (1876) made the important distinction, stating that although every cretin is intellectually disabled, every intellectually disabled person is not a cretin. In making this distinction, he insisted that intellectual disability is not a single entity but may have specific etiologies. The general trend at that time was not to make distinctions between the causes for intellectual disability. Etiologically, amentia, or idiocy, was considered to be a homogeneous category, and both "idiocy" and "insanity" were regarded as separate entities. However, in his classical essay, *Observations on an Ethnic Classification of Idiots* (1866), John Langdon Hayden Down clearly distinguished several types of intellectual disability and documented the heterogeneous nature of intellectual disability, suggesting Ethiopian, Malay, Negroid, Aztec, and Mongolian types. In 1880, Désiré-Magloire Bourneville described tuberous sclerosis complex as a cause of severe intellectual disability. Moreover, levels of intellectual disability were considered. In 1845, Jean-Etienne Dominique Esquirol, in his *Mental Maladies: A Treatise on Insanity,* had divided intellectual disability into two levels: the imbecile and the idiot and acknowledged degrees of variance in each of these categories. The first group, imbecile, was near normal in their intellectual faculties but never reach their expected knowledge for age, educational level, or social relations. In the second group, idiot, the intellectual and moral faculties are almost nil and never develop. "Incapable of attention, they cannot control their senses. They hear but do not understand; they see but do not regard. Having no ideas, and thinking not, they have nothing to desire; therefore, have no need of signs, or of speech" (Scheerenberger, 1983, p. 54). He distinguished amentia (intellectual disability) from dementia (mental illness).

Seguin (1846) considered four levels of intellectual disability: (1) idiocy (probably moderate, severe, and profound intellectual disability); (2) imbecility (mild-to-moderate intellectual disability with defects in social development); (3) backwardness or feeblemindedness; and (4) simpleness or superficial retardation with slowing of development.

Twentieth Century

Intellectual Testing

By the beginning of the twentieth century, institutions for persons with intellectual disabilities were firmly established throughout the world. The first textbook on intellectual disability was written by Barr (1904). Barr completed an international survey that found that 21 nations operated 171 institutions for persons with intellectual disability. Twenty-five of these were in the United States. Although he prepared a widely used educational classification of the feebleminded, it was not until the establishment of intelligence testing at the beginning of the twentieth century that classification was refined. In 1905, psychometric tests were developed in France by two physicians, Alfred Binet and Theodore Simon. They sought to find a way to select children for specialized education based on their abilities. When in 1912 Henry Goddard introduced these tests in the United States, they were used specifically to diagnose intellectual disability. The availability of the new tests in the United States led to the testing of large numbers of individuals at various ages. Intelligence quotients (IQs) that resulted from the tests were determined to be an adequate and accurate measure of intelligence. Intelligence was proposed to be a constant feature reflecting a permanent and inherent level of mental ability. Because they were considered objective and scientific, these intelligence tests gradually replaced the individualized clinical evaluation. Goddard proposed that an intellectually disabled person would perform at a mental age of 12 years or less and would have an IQ score lower than 75 or 80. In 1910, the Committee on Classification of the Feeble-minded of the American Association of Mental Deficiency proposed a tripartite classification: idiots (mental age <2 years), imbeciles (mental age <7 years), and morons (mental age <12 years).

Eugenics and Intelligence Testing

The development of intelligence testing and an interest in eugenics resulted in an emphasis on the study of the heredity of intellectual disability. During the decades between 1880 and 1925, persons with intellectual disability were seen to have incurable diseases and, in some quarters, thought to be socially deviant and a menace. The eugenics movement proposed that intellectual disability was inherited and downgraded the species (Fernald, 1915; Galton, 1883; Roberts, 1952). Intellectual disability was reported to be higher in studies of criminality and in those who were paupers. Intelligence tests were used in correctional institutions where substance abusers, criminals, prostitutes, and others showing antisocial behavior frequently tested in the mild range of intellectual disability. Unfortunately, some considered intellectual disability to be the source of the antisocial behavior rather than considering the interface between intelligence and life experience and appreciating the impact of neglect, poverty, early mistreatment, and limited cognitive capacity on socially maladaptive behavior.

Intelligence tests developed after 1900 were used to identify children with intellectual disability and place them in special classes to be better educated. Unfortunately, intelligence tests also were used to support class bias against immigrants coming to the United States. Intelligence tests were applied at points of entry, and deportations for intellectual disability increased. Their use in classifying immigrants and poor Americans as intellectually disabled became a concern. Social Darwinism, as proposed by Galton (1883), assumed prominence, resulting in the attitude that people with intellectual disability were burdens and a menace to society. Society should be protected and institutional care might achieve these goals. A corollary of the eugenics movement was the refusal to treat infants born with disabilities and birth defects, which resulted in their death (Pernick, 1996).

Barr (1904) reported evidence in support of the theory that "the transmission of imbecility is at once the most insidious and most aggressive of the degenerative forces; attacking alike the physical, mental, and moral nature, enfeebling the judgment and the will, while exaggerating the sexual impulses and the perpetuation of an evil growth . . . refusing to be shaken off; laying latent it must be, but sure to reappear . . . through a century to the fourth or fifth generation" (p. 102). Feebleminded women were said to be almost invariably immoral and carriers of venereal disease or to give birth to children who were defective themselves. Fernald wrote that there was "no other class of person in our wide population who, unit for unit, are so dangerous or expensive to the state" (Fernald, 1912). These judgments were supported by several genealogical investigations. The most famous of these is Goddard's study of the Kallikaks, published in 1912. Kallikak was a fictitious name derived from two Greek words: *kalos,* meaning pleasing or attractive, and *kakos,* meaning evil.

The *Kallikaks* study sought to document that intellectual disability and antisocial behavior were linked and genetically based rather than socially transmitted. Goddard's description of the Kallikaks presented intellectually disabled persons as a menace to society, a source of criminality and drug abuse, and the genetic source for even more intellectually disabled persons. Thus, the eugenics movement proposed that mildly intellectually disabled persons were a danger to society because of their "moral imbecility," indiscriminate sexual behavior, and excessive procreation. The eugenics movement promulgated the idea that their indiscriminate sexual behavior would increase the number of intellectually disabled persons and, therefore, the number of delinquents in the population. Propelled by eugenic considerations, a movement began to place intellectually disabled persons in institutions and to sterilize them. Such views resulted in an increase in not only the number of people in institutional settings but also the number of those admitted to psychiatric hospitals.

At the beginning of the twentieth century, it was not only the eugenics movement that was growing. Segregation and prohibitions on marriage and procreation by people with disabilities was common. Moreover, conditions in facilities for people with mental disabilities began to deteriorate. Sterilization of institutional residents with intellectual disability was utilized in some states. The 1927 Supreme Court decision on *Buck v. Bell* allowed states the right to sterilize people with intellectual disability (Reilly, 1991). In the 40 years between 1907 and 1949, more than 47,000 sterilizations of people with intellectual disabilities were recorded (Woodside, 1950). Legislation in Germany based on eugenics led to sterilization of between 300,000 and 400,000 individuals, the majority of whom were said to be "feebleminded"; most of these persons were in institutions.

Overcoming Misconceptions and Identifying Abuses

Despite the eugenics movement, evidence emerged that refuted assumptions of deviance in persons with intellectual disability. Fernald (1919) showed that, with proper support from their families, individuals with intellectual disability could function in the community. He concluded that only approximately 8% of a sample of 5,000 school children with intellectual disability showed behavioral problems of any kind. The link between intellectual disability and criminality also was disputed and discredited by Wallace (1929). Moreover, institutional discharge was possible, and a parole plan for those with milder forms of mental impairment was developed in the first decade of the twentieth century. Generally, those who were "paroled" were taken care of in the community by relatives, friends, or volunteers.

Still, abuses of individuals placed in institutional settings, which took various forms, occurred. At the Wrentham and Fernald facilities in Massachusetts, residents with intellectual disability participated in research with foods that contained radioactive elements, although neither the individuals who served as subjects nor their parents were aware of the nature of the foods they were ingesting. Residents at the Willowbrook Institution in New York were exposed to hepatitis B virus for research purposes without informed consent or their knowledge (Rothman and Rothman, 1984).

In the 1930s, owing to unemployment and poverty during the Depression, families frequently placed their relatives with intellectual disability in institutional settings (Noll, 1996), resulting in overcrowding. In 1935, Title X of the Social Security Act, which provided relief for blind people but not for those with other disabilities, was passed. With this aid, by 1940 approximately 50,000 blind people were receiving government support. In 1936, the National Advisory Committee for Crippled Children Services concluded that "Children with incurable blindness, deafness, or mental deficit . . . and those requiring custodial care" were beyond the scope of this new program (Social Security Board, 1946, p. 1). Ultimately, Title V of the Social Security Act authorized funds for services for crippled children (Braddock, 1986a).

Despite these deplorable institutional approaches and eugenic ideas, scientific research into the causes of intellectual disability continued. The first preventive intervention for an intellectual disability syndrome occurred in 1934 (Folling). That year, Folling clarified that phenylketonuria (PKU) is a metabolic disturbance that results in intellectual disability and that its impact on intelligence can be reversed by proper diet. The recognition of a biochemically based syndrome resulting in intellectual disability led to intellectual disability research as a legitimate focus in the biological sciences. Subsequently, the medical profession began to look more carefully for the etiology of other intellectual disability syndromes (Kanner, 1967).

During the Depression and World War II, there was little innovation in service delivery for people with intellectual disability (Noll, 1996). Still, some innovative programs did develop, including the foster family care system of New York State that began in the 1930s, which authorized payment for care of people with intellectual disability in family homes. Research on these placements indicated benefits of placement in foster or adoptive homes (Skeels and Harms, 1948), as well as benefits of preschool intervention programs. After World War II, there was a refocusing on the need for research in mental health, leading to the creation of the National Institute of Mental Health in 1946. The creation of the National Institute resulted in increased community services for people in the United States with mental illness (Braddock, 1986b) but not specifically for those with intellectual disability.

Following the Second World War, changes in community attitudes again emphasized the possibility of remediation of intellectual disability, as had been the case a century and a half before when Itard initiated the first remedial education program. Parents began to insist on improved remediation programs. The 1950s saw the organization of parent groups in the United States and other countries, culminating in the establishment of the National Association for Retarded Children, now The Arc of the United States. An advisory board with representatives of the various medical and nonmedical specialties who study the prevention of intellectual disability and care of intellectually disabled persons was established. In 1960, with the election of John F. Kennedy as president of the United States, the focus on intellectual disability services and services for those with mental illness expanded. In 1961, President Kennedy issued a statement calling for a national plan in the field of mental retardation: "We, as a nation, have too long postponed an intensive search for solutions to the problems of the mentally retarded. That failure should be corrected" (Kennedy, 1961). Kennedy subsequently appointed the President's Panel on Mental Retardation, which prepared 95 recommendations that addressed issues ranging from the need for scientific research on etiology and prevention to civil rights. A downsizing of institutional facilities and an increase in community services that would focus on the principle of normalization as a guide to service delivery were proposed (Nirje, 1969, 1985; Wolfensberger, 1972). Table 2.1 provides the guidelines for normalization.

The recommendations of the President's panel, in many instances, were included by Congress in Public Laws 88-156 and 88-174. Public Law 88-156, the Maternal and Child Health and Mental Retardation Planning Amendments of 1963, doubled spending for existing maternal and child health state grant programs. This legislation established new mental retardation planning grants in the various states. All 50 participating states were required to produce comprehensive plans for the development of better residential, community, and prevention services. Subsequently, the Community Mental Health Centers Act of 1963 became law and facilitated the development of such centers throughout the United States. These programs provided a basis for a network of community support for people with mental illnesses. Individuals with both intellectual disability and mental illnesses received limited services in these programs.

National programs brought medicine, education, psychology, sociology, genetics, and the various specialties that are pertinent to the needs of persons with intellectual disability together into special centers affiliated with universities, now the Association of University Centers for Disabilities (AUCD), to establish

Table 2.1 Guidelines for Normalization

1. Normalization means a normal rhythm of the day for the retarded.
2. Normalization implies a normal routine of life, that is, not always structured.
3. Normalization means to experience the normal rhythm of the year with holidays and family days of personal significance.
4. Normalization means an opportunity to undergo normal developmental experiences of the life cycle, that is, experiences and opportunities should be consistent with the appropriate life cycle whenever possible; adjustments and special provisions should be made for the mentally retarded adult and elderly.
5. Normalization means that choices, wishes, and desires of the mentally retarded themselves have to be taken into consideration as frequently as possible and respected.
6. Normalization means living in a world with both sexes.
7. Normalization means normal economic standards for the mentally retarded
8. Normalization means that the standards of the physical facility should be the same as those regularly applied in society to the same kind of facilities for ordinary citizens.

From Nirje (1969).

programs for intervention). Through federally funded mental retardation research centers, intellectual disability research began to grow. Finally, academic medicine became fully involved with other specialties, community organizations, and parent groups to study the etiology of intellectual disability syndromes, establish therapeutic interventions, and develop habilitation and prevention programs.

Legal Rights: Education and Treatment

In the mid-1960s, the Elementary and Secondary Education Act (P.L. 89-10) and its amendments in the following five years initiated funds for the education of children and youths with disabilities and established the Bureau of Education of the Handicapped (BEH) and the National Advisory Council (now the National Council on Disability). The legislative history of special education from 1965 to 2004 is shown in table 2.2.

In the 1970s, additional progress was made in improving the lives of persons with disabilities (Silverstein, 2000). In 1971, the Intermediate Care Facility/ Mental Retardation (ICF/MR) Law was established as part of Title XIX (Medicaid) of the Social Security Act. In 1972, in the Alabama case *Wyatt v. Stickney,* the decision stating that there is a constitutional right to treatment was issued. Discrimination against disabled persons in any program receiving federal financial assistance was prohibited in 1973 in Section 504 of the Rehabilitation Act.

The ICF/MR Law that was passed in 1971 allowed states to receive federal funding for institutional services for persons with intellectual disability as long as the care provided met minimal federal standards for treatment and space. The federal government would reimburse states for 50%–78% of the cost of institutional care. This program resulted in greater efforts toward deinstitutionalization because the minimal space requirements were difficult to meet in overcrowded facilities in most institutions (Rothman and Rothman, 1984). The

Table 2.2 Legislative History of Special Education

Legislation	Title	Provisions
PL. 89-10	The Elementary and Secondary Education Act of 1965 (ESEA)	Provided a comprehensive plan for readdressing the inequality of educational opportunity for economically underprivileged children. It became the statutory basis upon which early special education legislation was drafted.
PL. 89-313	The Elementary and Secondary Education Act Amendments of 1965	Authorized grants to state institutions and state operated schools devoted to the education of children with disabilities. It was the first federal grant program specifically targeted for children and youth with disabilities.
PL. 89-750	The Elementary and Secondary Education Act Amendments of 1966	Established the first federal grant program for the education of children and youth with disabilities at local school level, rather than at state-operated schools or institutions. It also established the Bureau of Education of the Handicapped (BEH) and the National Advisory Council (now called the National Council on Disability).
PL. 90-247	The Elementary and Secondary Education Act Amendments of 1968	Final federal special education legislation of the 1960s, established a set of programs that supplemented and supported the expansion and improvement of special education services. These programs later became known as discretionary.
PL. 91-230	The Elementary and Secondary Education Act Amendments of 1970, which included Title VI of the Civil Rights Act of 1964 and the Education of the Handicapped Act	Established a core grant program for local education agencies, now known as Part B, and it authorized a number of discretionary programs.
PL. 93-280	The Education Amendments of 1974	Established two laws. One was the Education of the Handicapped Act Amendments of 1974, which was the first to mention an appropriate education for all children with disabilities. It also reauthorized the discretionary programs. The second law, the Family Education Rights and Privacy Act, gave parents and students over the age of 18 the right to examine records kept in the student's personal file.
PL. 94-142	The Education for All Handicapped Children Act of 1975	Mandated free appropriate public education for all children with disabilities, ensured due process rights, and mandated IEPs (Individualized Education Plan) and LRE (Least Restrictive Environment). As such, it is the core of federal funding for special education. This law was passed in 1975 and went into effect in October of 1977 when the regulations were finalized.
PL. 98-199	The Education of the Handicapped Act Amendments of 1983	Reauthorized the discretionary programs, established services to facilitate school-to-work transition through research and demonstration projects; established parent training and information centers; and provided funding for demonstration projects and research in early intervention and early childhood special education.

26

Legislation	Title	Provisions
PL. 99-457	The Education of the Handicapped Act Amendments of 1986	Mandated services for preschoolers and established the Part H program to assist states in the development of a comprehensive, multidisciplinary, and statewide system of early intervention services for infants.
PL. 101-476	The Education of the Handicapped Act Amendments of 1990	Renamed the law The Individuals with Disabilities Education Act (IDEA). It reauthorized and expanded the discretionary programs, mandated transition services, defined assistive technology devices and services, and added autism and traumatic brain injury to the list of categories of children and youth eligible for special education and related services.
PL. 102-119	The Individuals with Disabilities Education Act Amendments of 1992	Primarily addressed the Part H (Infants and Toddlers with Disabilities) Program.
PL. 105-17	The Individuals with Disabilities Education Act (IDEA) Amendments of 1997	The reauthorization of IDEA was viewed as an opportunity to review, strengthen, and improve IDEA to better educate children with disabilities and enable them to achieve a quality education. Congress sought to achieve this by accomplishing the following: • Strengthening the role of parents • Ensuring access to the general curriculum and reforms • Focusing on teaching and learning while reducing unnecessary paper work requirements • Assisting educational agencies in addressing the costs of improving special education and related services to children with disabilities • Giving increased attention to racial, ethnic, and linguistic diversity to prevent inappropriate identification and mislabeling • Ensuring schools are safe and conducive to learning • Encouraging parents and educators to work out their differences by using nonadversarial means.
HR.1	The No Child Left Behind Act of 2001, an updated version of the 1965 Elementary and Secondary Education Act (ESEA)	The bill, which passed by large margins in both the House and the Senate, primarily addresses the issue of accountability in schools and help for needy students. Elements of the bill and discussion also touch on issues related to autism and the disability community.
PL. 108-446	Individuals with Disabilities Improvement Act of 2004 (IDEA, 2004; amendments to IDEA, 1997)	In IDEA 2004 Congress added new language to ensure that children with disabilities are taught by teachers who have intensive preservice preparation and ongoing professional development. Scientifically based instructional practice is required to improve academic achievement and functional performance. Early reading programs, positive behavioral interventions and supports, are to be provided to address learning and behavioral needs. Part A (General Provisions), Part B (Assistance for Education of All Children with Disabilities), Part C (Infants and Toddlers with Disabilities).

greatest number of individuals with intellectual disability and developmental disabilities resided in institutional settings in 1967, when there were approximately 195,000 residents. In 1998, the population of public institutions for those with intellectual disability and developmental disabilities had declined to 52,801 persons (Braddock et al., 2002). With the reduction in residents of institutions, community programs that emphasized communication, employment, social integration, and appropriate monitoring of treatment in the community were established (Koegel, Koegel, and Dunlap, 1996). Table 2.3 lists landmark legal decisions regarding care in state and community facilities.

The *Wyatt v. Stickney* (1971, 1972) court decision, one of the most influential cases not decided by the U.S. Supreme Court, focused on the right to treatment for persons with intellectual disability and built on an earlier right to treatment for those with mental illness. The judge wrote that these individuals have "a right to receive such individual treatment as will give each of them a realistic opportunity to be cured or to improve his or her mental condition." Following this case, federal class action suits related to conditions in institutions for those with intellectual disability increased, resulting in more than 70 class action suits in 41 states (Braddock et al., 1998; Braddock et al., 2000). By defining a right to treatment by specifying specific staff ratios and other objective criteria, the court paved the way for massive deinstitutionalization. Subsequently, the Wyatt standards emerged from such legislation. These standards rest on four principles: (1) humane psychological and physical environments; (2) qualified staff in numbers sufficient to administer adequate treatment; (3) individualized treatment plans; and (4) services in the least restrictive environment. Legislation on the right to education was also initiated (Martin, Martin, and Terman, 1996; *Pennsylvania Association of Retarded Children v. Commonwealth of PA*, 1971). Although the U.S. Congress enacted Section 504 of the Rehabilitation Act in 1973, which prohibited discrimination against people with disabilities by any entity receiving public funds, the regulations regarding the operation of Section 504 were delayed. Because of the continuing delay, disabled advocates organized and sued the Secretary of Health, Education, and Welfare (HEW) and began sit-ins and demonstrations (Fleischer and Zames, 1998). People with disabilities occupying federal buildings to secure their rights were seen on television broadcasts. Influenced by such demonstrations, four years after the law was signed, regulations were issued. The coalitions that were built and the advocacy that was shown by disability groups related to the political activity around Section 504 brought together groups that represented various disabilities to work for a unified disability rights agenda. This cross-disability advocacy played an important role in establishing the Americans with Disabilities Act in 1990 (Fleischer and Zames, 1998).

In 1975, the Education for All Handicapped Children Act (P.L. 94-142) was enacted (Braddock, 1986b). In 1986, it was amended to mandate services for preschool children (P.L. 99-457). Such legislation was refined and strengthened over the years and, with the provision of the Education of the Handicapped Act Amendments of 1990 (P.L. 101-476), became known as the Individuals with

Table 2.3 Landmark Legal Decisions Regarding Care in State and Community Facilities

Case	Decision
Pennsylvania Association for Retarded Citizens v. Commonwealth of Pennsylvania, 1971	Determined that every child can be educated; a requirement for appropriate medical and psychological evaluations was instituted.
Wyatt v. Stickney, 1972 and follow-up cases	An Alabama case that established the constitutional right of persons with intellectual disability to appropriate habilitation and treatment. Minimal standards were set for staffing, medical care, and privacy. The indiscriminate use of psychotropic medications, the use of aversive punishment procedures, and institutionalization of persons with mild intellectual disability were prohibited. (The case came to an end on December 5, 2003, when the State had complied with the latest settlement agreement.)
New York Association for Retarded Children v. Rockefeller, 1972	A New York case that established minimal standards of care.
Massachusetts Chapter 766, 1972	Guaranteed public education and all necessary services to all children 3 to 22 years of age; placement is according to service needs rather than diagnostic labeling, interdisciplinary core assessment with parents' participation, and educational plan specifying goals to be achieved. The parents have the right to reject the plan and appeal it.
Souter v. Brennan, 1973	Prohibited involuntary unpaid labor by residents of institutions.
Donaldson v. O'Connor, 1974, 1975	Established the right to treat persons committed to mental hospitals, as well as their right to remain in community settings if they could do so safely, by themselves or with community support.
Halderman v. Pennhurst State Hospital and School, 1979, and follow-up case	Determined that persons in institutions have a right to minimal habilitation and the least restrictive environment; it ordered closing of institutions and placement of their residents in the community. The follow-up case focused on provisions of appropriate care in the community, including psychiatric care and avoidance of unnecessary use of psychotropic agents.
Civil Rights of Institutionalized Persons Act (CRIPA), 1980	Gave authority to the U.S. Department of Justice to sue states to enforce constitutional rights of residents of state institutions.
Wyatt v. Aderholt, 1982	Imposed strict restrictions on sterilization.
Youngberg v. Romeo, 1982	This Pennsylvania case recognized that persons civilly confined in state institutions have specific constitutional rights that include basic necessities, habilitation, reasonable safety, freedom from undue restraints, and appropriate training to enable them to exercise their rights.
Americans with Disabilities Act (ADA), 1992	Prohibits discrimination in employment against persons with disabilities and requires reasonable accommodation for their special needs.
Olmstead v. L.C., and E.W., 1999	The U.S. Supreme Court decided that under ADA the states should provide persons with disabilities with community-based services, and that placement in residential institutions prevented them from participation in the life of the community, social contacts, family, work and educational opportunities. This suit was brought on behalf of *two persons* with mental illness and intellectual disability who were residents of a state hospital. The professionals who treated them felt that they should be discharged to the community, but no place was available to them.

Disabilities Education Act (IDEA). This legislation guarantees children and youths with disabilities, age 3 to 21, a free, appropriate public education. P.L. 94-142 was the first legislation that required compulsory education in the United States for children with disabilities and provided for federal enforcement. This legislation also informed parents that their children were entitled to community services. It was the first legislation regulating the process of evaluation and treatment planning that assured parents the right to examine all relevant records and to approve an individualized education plan. This has resulted in parents becoming advocates for community services and inclusive education in the schools.

The term "developmental disability" as defined in the legislation refers to a severe, chronic disability in an individual five years of age or older (see table 2.4). Inclusion is defined as full participation by persons with disabilities in activities, school, and community settings with persons who do not have disabilities. Such inclusion utilizes the principles of normalization shown in table 2.1 and includes the provision of services and supports necessary to achieve full participation. Inclusion applies to all disabilities: intellectual, cognitive, learning (e.g., reading), psychiatric, and behavioral. Another designation, mainstreaming, refers to purposeful and planned efforts to integrate persons with disabilities into the "mainstream" of society. This term usually is applied to a school setting and

Table 2.4 Federal Definition of Developmental Disability (PL. 95-602)

A. The term "developmental disability" means a severe, chronic disability in an individual five years of age or older that

1. Is attributable to a mental or physical impairment or a combination of mental and physical impairments
2. Is manifested before the person attains age 22
3. Is likely to continue indefinitely
4. Results in substantial functional limitations in three or more of the following areas of major life activity:

   - self-care
   - receptive and expressive language
   - learning
   - mobility
   - self-direction
   - capacity for independent living
   - economic self-sufficiency

5. Reflects the individual's need for a combination and sequence of special, interdisciplinary, or generic services, individualized supports, or other forms of assistance that are of life-long or extended duration and are individually planned and coordinated.

B. INFANTS AND YOUNG CHILDREN: An individual from birth to age 9, inclusive, who has a substantial developmental delay or specific congenital or acquired condition, may be considered to have a developmental disability without meeting three or more of the criteria described in 1–5 above if the individual, without services and supports, has a high probability of meeting those criteria later in life.

refers to the integration of students with disabilities into classrooms with students without disabilities. However, inclusion is the more comprehensive term.

By the 1995–1996 school year, 46% of children with disabilities in the United States were being educated in regular classroom settings, while the others were educated in a combination of other types of settings. These other settings included resource rooms, separate classrooms, and separate schools (U.S. Department of Education, 1998).

Dual Diagnosis

Persons with both intellectual disability and emotional and behavioral problems may not fully benefit from available programs, and their dual diagnosis may prevent participation in school programs. The early child guidance clinics lacked the psychiatric and psychosocial expertise to work with intellectually disabled persons because of their focus on verbal, psychodynamically oriented treatment. At that time it was believed that because of their cognitive deficiencies, intellectually disabled persons were unable to benefit from verbal, conceptually based, and insight-oriented therapy. Yet this is not necessarily true. With greater recognition of the dual diagnosis of intellectual disability and behavioral and psychiatric disorders, recognition of the need for better diagnosis and special programs directed toward treatment of dual diagnosis is greater and interventions (including psychotherapies) are more refined.

COMMUNITY AND FAMILY ORGANIZATIONS

In the 1950s, parents and friends of individuals with disabilities organized and sought better services in many parts of the world for their friends and relatives with impairments. Schools and activity centers were initiated, and international associations that were made up of national organizations that focused on the prevention of disabilities were founded. In Washington State, parents of individuals with intellectual disability organized services for their children as early as in the 1930s (Jones, 1987). Large-scale organization in groups became the focus of the 1950s. Local groups of parents worked together to form the group that became the National Association for Retarded Children, now The Arc of the United States, an organization that seeks to serve children and adults with cognitive, intellectual, and developmental disabilities in every community. Such organizations advocate for better services, better conditions in institutions, better school programs and workshops, and enhanced community services (Goode, 1999). In 1953, the Council of World Organizations Interested in the Handicapped, now the International Council on Disability, was established (Driedger, 1989). Although this international organization initially did not have people with disabilities as its leaders, the United States organizations are increasingly directed by individuals with disabilities.

DEINSTITUTIONALIZATION/RIGHT TO TREATMENT

Public facilities for people with intellectual disability peeked at 194,650 residents in 1967 (U.S. Department of HEW, 1972). An additional 20,000 persons with intellectual disability lived in state and county psychiatric hospitals at that time. Single facilities, such as Willowbrook in New York and Lincoln in Illinois, had 4,000–8,000 residents. In the 1960s, American society continued to treat persons with intellectual disability as a group, and segregation, sterilization, and isolation still occurred (Braddock and Parish, 2002). In the 1970s, institutions for people with intellectual disability began to close, with funds reallocated to community services.

Because of the poor conditions in many institutions for persons with mental illness, the legal right to treatment emerged as a concern for those who lived in these facilities (Birnbaum, 1965). A landmark right-to-treatment case was *Rouse v. Cameron* (1966), which established that if an individual was involuntarily committed to a facility, that person had the right to receive treatment because confinement was based on the need for treatment and not punishment. This right was subsequently upheld and extended in the 1970s to include individuals with intellectual disability (Levy and Rubinstein, 1996). As described earlier, this right was initially extended to persons with intellectual disability in 1972 in *Wyatt v. Stickney.*

The Civil Rights of Institutionalized Persons Act (CRIPA) was created to enforce the rights of institutionalized persons to receive adequate habilitation and active treatment and to be served in the most integrated setting appropriate to their needs. CRIPA authorizes the U.S. Attorney General to conduct investigations and carry out litigation regarding conditions of confinement in locally or state-operated institutions (the statute does not cover private facilities). Under the statute, the Special Litigation Section investigates facilities to determine whether there is a pattern or practice of violating residents' federal rights. The act applies to locally or state-run Developmental Disability and Mental Retardation facilities, mental health facilities, and nursing homes, as well as jails, prisons, and juvenile correctional facilities.

For example, the case of Thomas S. (*Thomas S. by Brooks v. Flaherty* [1990]) highlighted the obligation of states to provide supportive services necessary to enable individuals to transition into the community. The Thomas S. case refers to a court-ordered program of services for persons with intellectual disability and a co-occurring mental illness or substance abuse disorder, which was created in response to a class-action lawsuit that originated in North Carolina. The court specified a constitutional right to the following: safety; protection from harm; treatment under safe conditions; freedom from undue restraint; minimally adequate habilitation or treatment; and any treatment necessary to remedy any injuries caused to individuals for constitutionally inappropriate treatment in the past.

In another case involving the *United States of America v. the State of Wisconsin* (1998), the court ordered adequate care, treatment, and services. This included a comprehensive medical evaluation, an integrated medical plan and emergency services, adequate training of medical staff, neurology consultations and seizure management, psychiatric care and treatment, proper management of psychotropic medication, psychological services, proper management of restraints when indicated, effective record keeping, and involvement in community programs.

SELF-ADVOCACY AND INDEPENDENCE

During the 1970s, independent living for persons with various disabilities increased (Stewart, Harris, and Sapey, 1999). This movement grew out of the Vocational Rehabilitation Act of 1973 (Section 504: Rules), which stated that individuals with disabilities were required to have the supports necessary to live independently in the community. The focus on independent living emphasized that barriers in the community were not only those related to the disability or impairment itself but also those related to social attitudes and architectural, legal, and educational barriers (Braddock and Parish, 2002).

The first independent living center in the United States was established in the 1970s in Berkeley, California. This center and others that followed provided a continuum of services that included advocacy, transportation, training in independent living skills, housing referral, and many others (Roberts, 1989). Those who lived independently could be involved in establishing research and political agendas regarding disability. Four core principles for those in independent living were: self-determination, self-image, public education, and individual and systems advocacy (individual access and removal of community barriers to independent living) (Roberts, 1989). By 2000, centers for independent living served 212,000 individuals and approximately 61% of the nation's counties (Innes et al., 2000). An independent living center serves as a coordinating organization through which disabled persons may be involved in advocacy and educational activities.

Concurrently, by 2000, 125 state institutions for people with intellectual disability had been closed in 37 states (Braddock et al., 2002). With the closure of institutions, the emphasis has been placed on independent community living for persons with intellectual disability. Between 1977 and 1998, there was a tenfold increase in community-based settings for one to six persons. This expansion has been supported by a federal-state partnership in the Medicaid Home and Community-based Services (HCBS) Waiver Program. Similar reductions in residential institutions have occurred in many countries, particularly in Europe. Along with independent living, self-advocacy is critical to establishing autonomy and self-determination (Dybwad and Bersani, 1996). In 1995, a national organization, Self-Advocates Becoming Empowered (SABE), was established. Organized self-advocacy can play a major role in the emergence of autonomy and self-determination, but can be most effective when working closely with national organizations and professional associations.

NATIONAL/INTERNATIONAL DISABILITY PROGRAMS

The Americans with Disabilities Act passed in 1990 has led to improvement in disability rights in the United States and internationally. This law acknowledges discrimination against people with disabilities, recognizing historical patterns of segregation, isolation, and unequal treatment. Segregation and isolation are major problems that confront people with disabilities in addition to their individual impairments (National Council on Disability, 1997). The Americans with Disabilities Act states that there should be no discrimination against people with disabilities in employment, public services, public accommodations, and telecommunications (Parry, 1995). In 1994, the United Nations General Assembly unanimously approved the *Standard Rules on the Equalization of Opportunities for Persons with Disabilities* (United Nations, 1994). These provide an international standard for programs, policy, and laws related to disability. The rules emphasize greater participation and draw on the Declaration on the Rights of Mentally Retarded Persons approved by the United Nations in 1971 (United Nations, 1971). Subsequently, in 1975 the United Nations issued the *Declaration on the Rights of Disabled Persons* (United Nations, 1975) and in 1982, the *World Programme of Action Concerning Disabled Persons* (United Nations, 1982).

The goal of the World Programme of Action (WPA) is to "promote effective measures for prevention of disability, rehabilitation, and the realization of the goals of full participation of disabled persons in social life and development of equality" (Metts, 2000, p. 20). The program proposes opportunities for the disabled that are equal to those of the whole population and applies to each country regardless of its level of development. The program calls for organizing and financing services through legislation and developing the legal basis to carry out these objectives. All barriers to full participation must be removed and the provision of rehabilitation services that link persons with intellectual disability to social, nutritional, medical, educational, vocational assistance, and technical aids must be made available (Metts, 2000).

With the recognition of these needs, by the end of the twentieth century, the public sector in the United States had increased spending for disability services to 293.3 billion dollars and provided income support for more than 41.5 million persons. The spending level was 12.2% of total spending from combined state and federal sources in 1997. Approximately half of these funds supported placement in nursing homes, sheltered workshops, and institutions. In 1996, 61% of students with intellectual disability were in separate facilities. A fine balance is needed in programming to guarantee effective choice, adequate family support, and community participation so that funds are used to facilitate self-determination.

Community-Based Alternatives: Implementing the Olmstead Decision

Community placement in the United States may be facilitated by the Olmstead Decision. In June of 1999, the U.S. Supreme Court ruled in *Olmstead v. L.C.*

& E.W. that it is a violation of the Americans with Disabilities Act for states to discriminate against people with disabilities by providing services in institutions when the individual could be served more appropriately in a community-based setting. States are required to provide community-based services for people with disabilities if treatment professionals determine that it is appropriate, the affected individuals do not object to such placement, and the state has the available resources to provide community-based services. The Court suggests that a state can establish compliance with the Americans with Disabilities Act if it has (1) a comprehensive, effective working plan for placing qualified people in less restrictive settings, and (2) a waiting list for community-based services that ensures people can receive services and be moved off the list at a reasonable pace. In 2001, the New Freedom Initiative expressed a federal commitment to remove barriers to community living for people with disabilities.

On June 18, 2001, Executive Order 13217, "Community-Based Alternatives for Individuals with Disabilities," part of the New Freedom Initiative, called upon the federal government to assist states and localities to swiftly implement the Olmstead decision. It states: "The United States is committed to community-based alternatives for individuals with disabilities and recognizes that such services advance the best interests of the United States."

Executive Order 13217 directed six federal agencies, including the departments of Justice, Health and Human Services, Education, Labor, and Housing and Urban Development, as well as the Social Security Administration, to "evaluate the policies, programs, statutes and regulations of their respective agencies to determine whether any should be revised or modified to improve the availability of community-based services for qualified individuals with disabilities" and to report to the President with their findings. The departments of Transportation and Veterans Affairs, the Small Business Administration, and the Office of Personnel Management, though not named in the Executive Order, have also joined in the implementation effort. Together, these agencies form the Interagency Council on Community Living. Because any plans to improve community integration of people with disabilities must include the ideas and advice of the people who are most affected, the acts ensure that public input is a central component of the federal review.

The short-term effects of the Olmstead decision have not dramatically affected the care settings for people with disabilities. The most important effect thus far is that it has caused providers, consumers, and state officials from various departments to jointly discuss long-term care reforms. It also has caused the federal government to revise its policies in this area and to offer states flexibility and funding to develop innovative solutions. Finally, it has forced states to look at reforms not only in the health arena but also in the areas of transportation, housing, education, and other social supports to fully integrate people with disabilities into the least restrictive settings.

Olmstead implementation (ensuring that individuals receive care in the most integrated setting possible) may take many years, given the array of service delivery systems that require alteration, and the challenge of complying with requirements of complex lawsuits related to the Olmstead Act. State plans will evolve in response to funding, stakeholder input, agency-related initiatives, and continued growth of and demand for community services and supports for people with disabilities.

FUTURE DIRECTIONS

It is essential that the history of past successes and past failures be appreciated in order for effective programs of care to be expanded in the twenty-first century. In the twentieth century, advances in the neurosciences, developmental psychology, developmental psychopathology, phenomenology and classification, family, behavior, and drug treatments have led to a new perspective and a renewed commitment to intellectually disabled persons and persons with both intellectual disability and behavioral and mental disorders (dual diagnosis). Recognition of the brain/behavior/person/community interface, the role of experience on facilitating brain development, and a better understanding of the natural history of specific intellectual disability syndromes have led to the participation of professionals in the habilitation of intellectually disabled individuals. The struggle for rights for persons with impairment in the twenty-first century must emphasize the complex relationship between poverty and cognitive, emotional, and behavioral disability. Unemployment rates for disabled persons frequently approach 80% and personal income is low. Advocacy for persons with disabilities, continuous monitoring of public sector resources, and service commitments are needed in the United States and around the world. This ongoing monitoring is important in continued program planning. The number of disabled people has been estimated at 235 to 549 million in 175 countries; among them are many persons with intellectual disability. Persons who are disabled who are underemployed or unemployed may contribute to society and must have a guaranteed opportunity to participate in society as fully as they can.

KEY POINTS

1. Comprehensive care begins with an empathetic understanding of the long history of stigmatization.
2. Terminology matters. "Mental retardation" should be replaced by "intellectual disability" in discussions with families, other professionals, and schools.
3. Impairment and disability are not the same thing. Interventions for impairment can modify or prevent disability.
4. Understanding early-intervention strategies can prevent later deficits.
5. Familiarity with normalization, inclusion, and the legal rights and remedies available to the family are critical in providing psychological support.
6. Recognizing co-occurring psychiatric and medical conditions is the first step to intervention.
7. Professionals who assist those with intellectual disability must be familiar with the Olmstead decision and legislation that emphasizes a right to treatment.

8. Schools, state, and federal programs must be monitored to assure that they are meeting their responsibilities.

References

American Psychiatric Association. (2000). *Diagnostic and statistical manual of mental disorders,* 4th ed. Text Revision, Author, Washington, DC.

American Psychiatric Association, Committee on Nomenclature and Statistics. (1994). *Diagnostic and statistical manual of mental disorders,* 4th ed. Author, Washington, DC.

ASPIRE/ILIAD IDEA Partnership Projects. (2003). *Discover IDEA–supporting achievement for children with disabilities: An IDEA practices resource guide (Pathway Guide).* Council for Exceptional Children, Arlington, VA.

Bacon, F. [1605] (1900). *The advancement of learning, divine and humane.* Reprint, Clarendon, Oxford, UK.

Barr, M.W. (1904). *Mental defectives.* Blakiston's Sons & Co., Philadelphia, PA.

Binet, A., and Simon, T. (1905). Méthodes nouvelles pour le diagnostic du niveau intellectuel des anormaux. *L'Année Psychologique,* 11:191–244.

Birnbaum, M. (1965). Some comments on the "Right to Treatment." *Archives of General Psychiatry,* 13:33–45.

Bourneville, D.M. (1880). Sclereuse tubereuse des convulsions cérébrales: Idiotie et epilepsie hémiplégique. *Archives of Neurology (Paris),* 1:81–91.

Braddock, D. (1986a). Federal assistance for mental retardation and developmental disabilities: Part I. A review through 1961. *Mental Retardation,* 24:175–182.

Braddock, D. (1986b). Federal assistance for mental retardation and developmental disabilities: Part II. The modern era. *Mental Retardation,* 24:209–218.

Braddock, D., Hemp, R., Parish, S., and Rizzolo, M.C. (2000). *The state of the states in developmental abilities: 2000 study summary.* Department of Disability and Human Development, University of Illinois at Chicago.

Braddock, D., Hemp, R., Parish, S., and Westrich, J. (1998). *The state of the states in developmental disabilities,* 5th ed. American Association on Mental Retardation, Washington, DC.

Braddock, D., Hemp, R., Rizzolo, M.C., Parish, S., and Pomeranz, A. (2002). *The state of the states in developmental disabilities: 2002 study summary.* Coleman Institute for Cognitive Disabilities. University of Colorado, Boulder.

Braddock, D., and Parish, S.L. (2002). An institutional history of disability. In D. Braddock (ed.), *Disability at the dawn of the 21st century and the state of the states.* American Association on Mental Retardation, Washington, DC.

Bromberg, W. (1975). *From Shaman to psychotherapist: A history of the treatment of mental illness.* Henry Regnery, Chicago, IL.

Bryan, C. (1930). *The papyrus Ebers.* D. Appleton, New York.

Carrey, N.J. (1995). Itard's 1828 memoire on mutism caused by a lesion of the intellectual functions: A historical analysis. *Journal of the American Academy of Child and Adolescent Psychiatry,* 34:1655–1661.

Civil Rights for Institutionalized Persons Act, 42 U.S.C. 1997 (CRIPA).

Clarke, A.M., Clarke, D.B., and Berg, J.M. (1985). *Mental deficiency: The changing outlook,* 4th ed. Free Press, New York.

Davis, L. (2000). Dr. Johnson, Amelia, and the discourse of disability in the eighteenth century. In H. Deutsch and F. Nussbaum (eds.), *"Defects": Engendering the modern body,* pp. 54–74. University of Michigan Press, Ann Arbor, MI.

de Condillac, E.B. [1754] (1930). *Treatise on the senses.* Translated by G. Carr. Reprint, University of Southern California, Los Angeles, CA.

Down, J.L.H. (1866). Ethnic classification of idiots. *Clinical Lecture Reports, London Hospital 3,* p. 259.

Driedger, D. (1989). *The last civil rights movement: Disabled peoples' international.* Hurst & Company, London.

Dybwad, G., and Bersani, J. Jr. (eds.). (1996). *New voices: Self-advocacy by people with disabilities.* Brookline, Cambridge, MA.

Edwards, M.L. (1996). The cultural context of deformity in the Ancient Greek World. *Ancient History Bulletin,* 10:79–92.

Esquirol, J.E. (1965). *Mental maladies: a treatise on insanity.* Facsimile of the English edition of 1845. Hafner, New York.

Farmer, S. (1998). Down and out and female in thirteenth-century Paris. *American Historical Review,* 103:344–372.

Fernald, W. (1912). The burden of feeblemindedness. *Journal of Psychoasthenics,* 17: 87–111.

Fernald, W.E. (1915). State care of the insane, feebleminded, and epileptic. *Proceedings of the National Conference of Charities and Correction,* 42:289–297.

Fernald, W.E. (1917). The growth of provision for the feebleminded in the United States. *Mental Hygiene,* 1:34–59

Fernald, W.E. (1919). A state program for the care of the mentally defective. *Mental Hygiene,* 3:566–574.

Fleischer, D.Z. and Zames, F. (1998). Disability rights. *Social Policy,* 28:52–55.

Folling, A. (1934). Uber ausscheidung von Phenylbrenztraubensaure in den Hrn als Stoffwechselanomalie in Verbindung mit imbezillitat. *Hoppe-Seyler's Zeitschrift filer physiologische chemie,* 227:169.

Galton, F. (1883). *Inquiry into human faculty and its development.* Macmillan, London.

Garland, R. (1995). *The eye of the beholder: Deformity and disability in the Graeco-Roman world.* Cornell University Press, Ithaca, NY.

Goddard, H. (1912). *The Kallikak family: A study in the heredity of feeblemindedness.* Macmillan, New York.

Goode, D. (1999). *History of the Association for the Help of Retarded Children of New York City.* Association for the Help of Retarded Children, New York.

Griesinger, W. (1876). *Die pathologie und therapie der psychischen krankheiten,* 4th ed. Braunschweight Vieweg. (Quoted by Kanner, 1964)

Hodgson, K.W. (1953). *The deaf and their problems.* Philosophical Library, New York.

Howe, S.G. (1848). *Report made to the legislature of Massachusetts upon idiocy.* Coolidge and Wiley, Boston, MA.

Innes, B., Enders, A., Seekins, T., Merritt, D.J., Kirshenbaum, A., and Arnold, N. (2000). Assessing the geographical distribution of Centers for Independent Living across urban and rural areas: Toward a policy of universal access. *Journal of Disability Policy Studies,* 10:207–224.

Itard, J.M. (1802). *The wild boy of Aveyron.* Richard Phillips, Paris.

Jones, L.A. (1987). *Doing justice: A history of the Association of Retarded Citizens of Washington.* The Arc of Washington, Olympia, WA.

Kanner, L. (1960). Itard, Seguin, Howe: Three pioneers in the education of retarded children. *American Journal of Mental Deficiency,* 65:2–10.

Kanner, L. (1964). *A history of the care and study of the mentally retarded.* Charles C. Thomas, Springfield, IL.

Kanner, L. (1967). Medicine in the history of mental retardation. *American Journal of Mental Deficiency,* 72:165–170.

Kennedy, J.F. (1961). Statement by the President regarding the need for a national plan in mental retardation. In The President's Panel on Mental Retardation (ed.), *National action to combat mental retardation.* Government Printing Office, Washington, DC.

Koegel, L.K., Koegel, R.L., and Dunlap, G. (1996). *Positive behavioral support: Including people with difficult behavior in the community.* Brookes, Baltimore.

Kroll, J. (1973). A reappraisal of psychiatry in the Middle Ages. *Archives of General Psychiatry,* 29:276–283.

Lane, H. (1976). *The wild boy of Aveyron.* Harvard University Press, Cambridge, MA.

Levy, R.M. and Rubenstein, L.S. (1996). *The rights of people with mental disabilities: The authoritative ACLU guide to the rights of people with mental illness and mental retardation.* Southern Illinois University, Carbondale.

Locke, J. (1690). *An essay concerning human understanding.* Basset, London.

Martin, E.W., Martin, R.T., and Terman, D.L. (1996). The legislative and litigation history of special education. *Special Education for Students with Disabilities,* 6:25–38.

Metts, R.L. (2000). *Disability, issues, trends and recommendations for the World Bank.* World Bank, Washington, DC.

National Council on Disability. (1997). *Equality of opportunity: The making of the Americans with Disabilities Act.* Author, Washington, DC.

Neugebauer, R. (1987). Exploitation of the insane in the New World: Benoni Buck, the first reported case of mental retardation in the American colonies. *Archives of General Psychiatry,* 44:481–483.

Neugebauer, R. (1996). Mental handicap in medieval and early modern England: Criteria, measurement and care. In D. Wright and A. Digby (eds.), *From idiocy to mental deficiency: Historical perspectives on people with learning disabilities,* pp. 22–43. Routledge Kegan Paul, London.

Nirje, B. (1969). The normalization principle and its human management implications. In W. Wolfensberger and R. Kugel (eds.), *Changing patterns in residential services for the mentally retarded,* pp. 181–195. President's Committee on Mental Retardation, Washington, DC.

Nirje, B. (1985). The basis and logic of the normalization principle. *Australia and New Zealand Journal of Developmental Disabilities,* 11:65–68.

Noll, S. (1996). *The feeble-minded in our midst: Institutions for the mentally retarded in the South, 1900–1940.* University of North Carolina Press, Chapel Hill.

Olmstead v. L.C. and E.W. (98–536) 527 U.S. 581 (1999) F. 3d893. Web site: (http://supct.law.cornell.edu/supct/html/98–536.ZS.html).

Parry, J. (1995). *Mental disability law: A primer,* 5th ed. American Bar Association, Washington, DC.

Pennsylvania Association of Retarded Children v. Commonwealth of PA, 334 F. Supp. 1257 (1971).

Pernick, M.S. (1996). *The black stork: Eugenics and the death of "defective" babies in American medicine and motion pictures since 1915.* Oxford University Press, New York.

Pinel, P. [1801] (1977). *Treatise on insanity.* Translated by H. Maudsley. Reprint, University Publications of America, Washington, DC.

Reilly, P.R. (1991). *The surgical solution: A history of involuntary sterilization in the United States.* Johns Hopkins University Press, Baltimore.

Roberts, E.V. (1989). A history of the Independent Living Movement: A founder's perspective. In B.W. Heller, L.M. Flohr, and L.S. Zegans (eds.), *Psychosocial interventions with physically disabled persons,* pp. 231–244. Rutgers University Press, New Brunswick, NJ.

Roberts, J.A.F. (1952). The genetics of mental deficiency. *Eugenics Review,* 44:71–83

Roosens, E. (1979). *Mental patients in town life: Gheel-Europe's first therapeutic community.* Sage, Beverly Hills, CA.

Rosen, G. (1968). *Madness in society: Chapters in the historical sociology of mental illness.* University of Chicago Press, Chicago, IL.

Rothman, D.J. (1990). *The discovery of the asylum: Social order and disorder in the New Republic,* rev. ed. Little, Brown, Boston, MA.

Rothman, D.J., and Rothman, S.M. (1984). *The Willowbrook wars.* Harper & Row, New York.

Rouse v. Cameron, 373 F.2d 451, 452 (D.C. Cir. 1966).

Rushton, P. (1988). Lunatics and idiots: Mental disability, the community, and the Poor Law in North-East England, 1600–1800. *Medical History,* 32:34–50.

Rushton, P. (1996). Idiocy, the family and the community in early modern Northeast England. In D. Wright and A. Digby (eds.), *From idiocy to mental deficiency: Historical perspectives on people with learning disabilities,* pp. 44–64. Routledge Kegan Paul, London.

Scheerenberger, R.C. (1983) *A history of mental retardation.* Paul H. Brookes Publishing, Baltimore, MD.

Séguin, E. (1846). *Traitement moral, hygiène, et éducation des idiots et des autres enfants erroires.* J.B. Baillière, Paris.

Séguin, E. (1866). *Idiocy and its treatment by the physiological method.* William Wood, New York.

Séguin, E. (1870). *New facts and remarks concerning idiocy, being a lecture before The New York Medical Journal Association, October 15, 1869.* William Wood, New York.

Silverstein, R. (2000). *Disability policy framework: A guidepost for analyzing public policy.* Center for the Study and Advancement of Disability Policy and the Arc of the United States, Washington, DC.

Simpson, M.K. (1999). The moral government of idiots: Moral treatment in the work of Seguin. *History of Psychiatry,* 10:227–243.

Skeels, H.M. and Harms, I. (1948). Children with inferior social histories: Their mental development in adoptive homes. *Journal of Genetic Psychology,* 72:283–294.

Social Security Board. (1946). *Recommendations of the Children's Bureau Advisory Committee on Services to Crippled Children: December 1935 to April 1946.* Department of Health and Human Services Archives, Washington, DC.

Stewart, J., Harris, J., and Sapey, B. (1999). Disability and dependency: Origins and futures of "Special Needs" housing for disabled people. *Disability and Society,* 14:5–20.

Thomas S. by Brooks v. Flaherty, 902 F. 2d 250 (4th Cir. 1990).

Trent, J.W. (1995). *Inventing the feeble mind: A history of mental retardation in the United States.* University of California Press, Berkeley, CA.

United Nations. (1971). *Declaration on the rights of mentally retarded persons.* Author, New York.

United Nations. (1975). *Declaration on the rights of disabled persons.* Author, New York.

United Nations. (1982). *World programme of action concerning disabled persons.* Author, New York.

United Nations. (1994). *Standard rules on the equalization of opportunities for persons with disabilities.* Author, New York.

U.S. Department of Education. (1998). *Twentieth annual report to Congress on the implementation of the Individuals with Disabilities Education Act.* Author, Washington, DC.

U.S. Department of Health, Education, and Welfare. (1972). *Mental retardation sourcebook of the DHEW.* U.S. Department of Health, Education, and Welfare, Office of the Secretary, Office of Mental Retardation Coordination, Washington, DC.

Wallace, G.L. (1929). Are the feebleminded criminals? *Mental Hygiene,* 13:93–98.

Wilbur, C.T. (1888). Institutions for the feebleminded. *Proceedings of the Fifteenth National Conference of Charities and Correction,* 17:106–113.

Winzer, M.A. (1993). *The history of special education: From isolation to integration.* Gallaudet University Press, Washington, DC.

Wolfensberger, W. (1972). *The principle of normalization in human services.* National Institute on Mental Retardation, Toronto, Ontario, Canada.

Wolfensberger, W. (1976). On the origin of our institutional models. In R. Kugel and A. Shearer (eds.), *Changing patterns in residential services for the mentally retarded,* rev. ed., pp. 35–82. President's Committee on Mental Retardation, Washington, DC.

Woodside, M. (1950). *Sterilization in North Carolina: A sociological and psychological study.* University of North Carolina Press, Chapel Hill, NC.

World Health Organization. (1992). *The lCD-10 classification of mental and behavioral disorders: Clinical descriptions and diagnostic guidelines.* Author, Geneva, Switzerland.

Wyatt v. Stickney, 325 F. Supp. 781 (M.D. Ala. 1971), enforced in 334 F. Supp. 1341 (1971); 344 F. Supp. 387 (1972); *Wyatt v. Aderholt,* 503 F 2d. 1305 (5th Cir. 1974).

3

The Classification of Intellectual Disability

Although intellectual disability has been recognized since antiquity, interest in its classification did not develop until the nineteenth century, when it became apparent that intellectual disability is not one homogeneous category, as was previously thought, but has many causes. Moreover, it became apparent that intervention could be beneficial and that interventions might be tailored for specific disorders.

EVOLUTION OF CLASSIFICATION

Early authors prepared the way for modern efforts to differentiate specific conditions that differ in both etiology and pathology, yet all result in intellectual disability. Some attempts were misguided. J. Langdon Hayden Down, in his ethnic classification (1866; Jordan, 2000), sought to classify based on the physical appearance of the individuals he examined. His goal was to absolve parents of self-blame for the handicap by emphasizing a constitutional basis for their child's disorder. He proposed an "ethnic classification," suggesting that the various forms of intellectual disability represented regressions to stereotypical racial forms (e.g., mongoloid, Aztec). Although he later abandoned this unfortunate idea, he continues to be known for it. Still, he is credited with drawing scientific attention to the syndrome bearing his name (Jordan, 2000) and for suggesting that the best classification is one based on etiology. Subsequently, he anticipated current efforts at classification by describing three major groups: (1) congenital, which included microcephalic, macrocephalic, hydrocephalic, epileptic, and paralytic types; (2) developmental, with a vulnerability to mental breakdown with stress during a developmental crisis; and (3) accidental (caused by injury or illness). Later, William Weatherspoon Ireland (1877), in his textbook on intellectual disability, suggested 10 subdivisions. Among these are genetous (congential), microcephalic, epileptic, eclamptic, hydrocephalic, paralytic, traumatic, inflammatory, cretinism, and idiocy by social and physical deprivation.

In 1880, tuberous sclerosis complex was identified by Désiré-Maglione Bourneville (1880), who established that intellectual disability might result from brain pathology. Subsequently, many other intellectual disability syndromes were recognized. Thus began a new era, with investigators searching for clearly defined disorders associated with intellectual disability; these were commonly named after their discoverers. It was an era when intellectual disability syndromes were beginning to be recognized, but medicine had little to offer therapeutically. Although some ameliorization was provided by educators, the recognition that brain pathology was linked to specific causes raised questions about the possibility for prevention and medical habilitation as new causes were specified.

In addition to the realization that there are multiple causes for intellectual disability, it was recognized, in the nineteenth century, that there were various degrees of intellectual ability. This led to a classification that focused on levels of severity of intellectual disability. In 1877, new terms were introduced to describe these different levels of intellectual functioning based on language and speech abilities and the extent of cognitive impairment (Field and Sanchez, 1999).

Based on the belief that human intelligence is a single entity that is measurable, tests that quantified levels of intelligence were introduced in the 1900s. Thus, mental age scores replaced earlier measurements used to estimate ability. The Simon-Binet Intelligence Scale appeared at the beginning of the twentieth century (chapter 2). It was later revised for use in the United States as the Stanford-Binet Scale. This test standardized testing, resulting in classification systems based on numerical scores with subcategories. Early classification of levels of functioning emphasized mental age but did not specify adaptive behavioral performance.

In 1910, the Committee on Classification of the Feebleminded, the precursor organization to the current American Association on Mental Retardation (AAMR), established four categories for individuals with intellectual disability. These were feebleminded (mental age of 12 or less), moron, imbecile, and idiot (Field and Sanchez, 1999). However, it soon became apparent that mental age is not on a continuum and does not develop in a linear fashion; instead, during development there are successive reorganizations of specific brain systems as new cognitive abilities emerge. Thus, Intelligence Quotient (IQ) scores, based on standard deviations from the mean score (average range 90–110), replaced mental age scores to classify people by intelligence levels. By the early 1950s, the Diagnostic and Statistical Manual of Mental Disorders (DSM-I) listed different categories of mental retardation (intellectual disability) based on IQ level.

Emergence of the AAMR Definition

In 1961, the AAMR introduced a manual that replaced the older terms, such as "feeblemindedness" and "idiocy" and "mental subnormality," with the term "mental retardation," which was universally adopted (Greenspan and Switzky,

2003). Its goal was to increase uniformity in medical and behavioral classification. For the first time, both intelligence and adaptive behavior were included and objective criteria (test scores) were required to make the diagnosis. The 1961 definition is as follows: "Mental retardation refers to subaverage general intellectual functioning that originates during the developmental period (age 16) and is associated with impairment in adaptive behavior."

Subaverage was defined as an IQ of 85 or less. Moreover, a supplementary classification measured impairments in personal-social (interpersonal) skills and sensorimotor skills (motor, auditory, visual, and speech) that may accompany intellectual disability and influence behavioral and social adaptation. With some modifications, this definition was used in subsequent AAMR definitions until 1983.

The 1961 definition included the category "borderline mental retardation" for those scoring one standard deviation below the mean on a standardized IQ test, theoretically labeling 16% of the population as intellectually disabled. In 1973, the cut-off limit for intellectual disability was adjusted; intellectual disability was defined as scoring two standard deviations below the mean on a standardized IQ test, and the developmental period extended from 16 years of age to 18 years of age. This greatly reduced the number of people with intellectual disability who were eligible for services. By reducing the IQ cut-off to two standard deviations, theoretically 3% of the population would be identified. The 1973 definition stated that intellectual limitations must be *significant* and that adaptive limitations were *concurrent* with intellectual ones.

Subsequently, the 1983 AAMR Manual (1) incorporated an IQ level into the definition. "Significantly subaverage general intelligence" was defined as an IQ of 70 or below on standardized measures of intelligence and (2) suggested that IQ scores for mild-to-profound intellectual disability include the test error of measurement instead of simply listing the single IQ score cut-offs. Consequently, the range was from 50–55 to 70–75 for mild intellectual disability and from 35–40 to 50–55 for moderate intellectual disability. This definition emphasized that biopsychosocial factors and social experiences can impede or facilitate intelligence, and it added a multiaxial coding of social-environmental factors that affect cognition and developmental processes.

Both the 1973 and the 1983 manuals maintained the basic framework laid down in 1961, pairing low IQ with global impairment in adaptive functioning in the definition. For the next revision in 1992 and its refinement in 2002, fundamental changes were made based on changes in service models. With de-institutionalization, more individuals were living in the community and were in need of "supports." The AAMR proposed in 1992 that classifying levels of support is preferable to classifying the severity of intellectual disability. The World Health Organization (WHO) took a different approach. In 1996, WHO introduced ICD-10-MR, which is multiaxial and measures severity of intellectual disability, placing it on Axis I of five axes. In 2001, WHO published the International Classification of Functioning to address supports needed for healthy functioning, similar to the AAMR 1992 proposal. The emergence of the self-advocacy movement is in keeping with this focus on supports and has resulted in greater emphasis on the dignity of persons with intellectual disability. These changes in classification and attitudes toward intellectually disabled persons by others and by themselves are reflected in the sections to follow on the classification systems in current use.

THE DIAGNOSTIC PROCESS

Intelligence has been defined by emphasizing cognitive abilities, measured on standardized testing, or by emphasizing practical "real world" problem solving. Current definitions combine these approaches by including both psychometric measures of intelligence and measures of adaptive (practical) ability. The intellectual disability category chosen should be based on global assessment and not on a single area or specific impairment. IQ levels are provided as a guide, but should not be applied rigidly because they are divisions of a complex developmental process that cannot be defined with absolute preciseness. The intelligence quotient should be determined utilizing standardized, individually administered tests, taking into account local cultural norms. The appropriate test must be selected based on the individual's level of functioning and any associated disabling conditions, such as expressive language difficulties, physical disabilities, and hearing or visual problems. In addition to cognitive tests, scales of adaptive function need to be completed by interviewing parents or care providers who are familiar with the individual's performance of daily activities required for personal and social sufficiency. If both intellectual level and social adaptation are not considered, then the assessment is considered to be a provisional estimate.

Tests of adaptive behavior that are used together with intelligence tests include the AAMR Adaptive Behavior Scales (Lambert, Nihiri, and Leland, 1993; Nihiri, Leland, and Lambert, 1993) and the Vineland Adaptive Behavior Scales (Sparrow, Balla, and Cicchetti, 1984). With the development of these adaptive behavioral instruments, guidelines are provided to determine what constitutes a significant impairment in adaptive functioning. Performance that falls below the third percentile (i.e., standard score below 70 to 75) in two of the following domains is commonly used: communication, daily living skills/self-help, socialization/social functioning/interpersonal, and motor function. Mental disorder co-occurring with intellectual disability (dual diagnosis) is listed on a separate axis in the Diagnostic and Statistical Manual of Mental Disorders (DSM-IVTR) and in the ICD-10-MR Guide.

DIAGNOSIS AND CLASSIFICATION: PURPOSES AND APPLICATIONS

Classification systems may be used for a variety of purposes and based on a number of different factors to meet the varied needs of individuals and their families, researchers, clinicians, and practitioners. Aspects of an individual's intellectual disability might be classified, for example, based on levels of measured intelligence, etiology, levels of assessed adaptive behavior, or functional capacities or on the basis of intensities of needed supports.

The reasons for applying a definition of intellectual disability to a person may include diagnosis, classification, and planning supports. Diagnosis and classification serve many purposes. For example, the diagnosis is used for medical care, to determine eligibility for services, to designate educational programs, for research, and for legal purposes. Likewise, there are different purposes for classification, such as to organize information, to evaluate an individual, to plan research, to plan intervention, and for determination of eligibility for services.

FOUR SYSTEMS OF CLASSIFICATION

Currently, four systems of classification of intellectual disability are commonly used. These systems provide different emphases by classifying intellectual disability medically, functionally, or according to the intensity of supports needed. They are: (1) The International Classification of Diseases (ICD-10) (WHO, 1992); (2) the DSM-IVTR (American Psychiatric Association [APA], 2000); (3) the AAMR Definition, Classification, and Systems of Supports (Luckasson et al., 2002); and (4) the International Classification of Functioning, Disability, and Health (ICF) (WHO, 2001). The World Health Organization provides a specific guide for ICD-10 use with persons with intellectual disability (WHO, 1996), and the Royal College of Psychiatry (2001) offers supplemental Diagnostic Criteria for Psychiatric Disorders for Use with Adults with Intellectual Disability (DC-LD). In the United States the National Association for the Dually Diagnosed (NADD), in association with the American Psychiatric Association, has prepared a manual that provides detailed instruction on how to apply DSM-IV criteria to persons with intellectual disability and has provided modified criteria where applicable. Knowledge of each of these classification systems is important because of differences in emphasis among them.

The classifications of diseases and disorders (ICD-10 and DSM-IVTR) focus on agreed-upon descriptions to recognize the condition and its severity. The application of all these classifications reaches beyond a simple one-dimensional definition of intellectual disability to include multiple axes. The ICD-10 is a classification of diseases with a special supplement that addresses its use in intellectual disability; this guide is *multiaxial*. The DSM-IVTR is a classification of mental disorders. In DSM-IVTR, the diagnosis of intellectual disability is one step in the classification; the full classification uses several axes that in this *multiaxial system* allow classification of intellectual disability and its severity, medical conditions resulting in intellectual disability, associated mental and physical disorders, stressors, and overall global functioning. In contrast, The AAMR system is a *multidimensional* system that includes the measurement of intelligence but places greater emphasis on adaptive functioning and systems of support; its focus is a developmental one that highlights the kinds of positive supports needed for each individual to reach his or her potential. Finally, the ICF/ICIDH (WHO, 2001) is intended to complement the ICD-10. Accepted by 191 countries, it is an international approach to measure health and disability; its emphasis is on how people live and the healthy years of life lost when services are not provided.

A thorough understanding of each of these approaches provides a means to advocate for comprehensive medical and mental disorder diagnoses (the ICD-10, DSM-IVTR, and AAMR), effective supports and treatment planning (the AAMR), and an appreciation of health years lost when positive medical, educational, and community supports are lacking (the ICF). In applying these definitions, specific adaptive abilities often coexist with strengths in other adaptive skills or personal capabilities; therefore, adaptive strengths must be carefully considered. For consistency, the term "intellectual disability" will be used instead of "mental retardation" in the following descriptions of the classification systems even though the classifications themselves use the term "mental retardation."

CLASSIFICATIONS OF INTELLECTUAL DISABILITY

ICD-10 Definition

The Tenth Revision of the International Classification of Diseases (ICD-10) and health-related problems is the latest in a series of classifications initiated in 1893. The ICD-10, Chapter V (Mental Disorders), lists intellectual disability as a disorder of psychological development and takes a somewhat different approach than the DSM-IVTR, placing a greater emphasis on the developmental aspects and discussing the complexity of diagnosis. The ICD-10 definition is as follows:

> Mental retardation [intellectual disability] is a condition of arrested or incomplete development of the mind, which is especially characterized by impairment of skills manifested during the developmental period, contributing to the overall level of intelligence, i.e., cognitive, language, motor, and social abilities.

This definition proposes that intelligence is not a unitary characteristic but is assessed on the basis of a large number of different but more or less specific skills. These skills generally develop to a similar degree in an unaffected individual; however, because intellectual disability is a heterogeneous disorder, one may see large discrepancies in such skills among affected individuals. There may be severe impairments for some in one area, for example, language; in other instances, there may be an area of higher skill level that is maintained (often referred to as a "splinter skill"); for example, disproportionately better visuospatial abilities may be present in a person with severe intellectual disability. This "scatter" in abilities may result in a variable profile, making it difficult to determine which subgroup of intellectual disability is an appropriate diagnosis.

The ICD-10 defines mild (F70), moderate (F71), severe (F72), profound (F73), and unspecified mental retardation [intellectual disability] (F79). Provision is made for a fourth character to be added to the standard diagnostic code to specify the degree of behavioral impairment if another ICD-10 mental disorder diagnosis is not appropriate. For example, intellectual disability with a fourth character "0" indicates no or minimal behavioral impairment. The digit "1" indicates behavioral impairment requiring attention or treatment. The ICD-10 incorporates this definition into a multiaxial system.

ICD-10 Guide for Mental Retardation (Intellectual Disability): Multiaxial Classification

The ICD-10 Guide multiaxial system provides a means to record pertinent information from throughout the ICD-10 classification. Moreover, the ICD-10 Guide (WHO, 1996) takes into account the difficulty in applying diagnostic criteria for mental and behavioral disorders to persons with intellectual disability and provides advice on classifying certain mental and behavioral disorders, placing them on a separate axis.

  Axis I: Severity of retardation and problem behaviors
  Axis II: Associated medical conditions
  Axis III: Associated psychiatric disorders
  Axis IV: Global assessment of psychosocial disability
  Axis V: Associated abnormal psychosocial conditions

The case vignette that follows will be diagnosed using the ICD-10 system first and subsequently each of the other classifications.

CASE VIGNETTE: TINA, AGE 22

Tina is a young woman with Down syndrome who was referred for evaluation by her parents and workshop staff because she was socially withdrawn, refused to eat (lost 20 pounds), exhibited slowing of movements, and lost interest in her usual activities. She also did not respond to loud noises in her environment. Early onset Alzheimer's disease was suspected. Psychometric testing showed a full-scale IQ of 40 during her final year in school before leaving for placement in a workshop program. The diagnosis of Down syndrome was made at birth, leading to enrollment in special education preschool and school programs in small classroom settings. Other than separation anxiety on elementary school entry, which resolved after several weeks, she had done well in school in a small classroom setting with other students of her own age and intellectual ability; she had been socially engaged with peers before the onset of her current disorder.

    When she reached age 21, she left her protective school environment and made the transition into a community workshop program where she was exposed for the first time to people of all ages with many different types of developmental disorders; many of these residents had behavioral difficulties. It was in that setting that she became symptomatic. Alzheimer's disease was ruled out, and she was diagnosed with a depressive disorder that was successfully treated with positive behavioral supports and an antidepressant medication. After treatment, her functioning returned to her baseline level of abilities.

    In the ICD-10 multiaxial system, Tina would be classified as follows:

  Axis I: F11.1 moderate mental retardation
  Axis II: Q90.0 trisomy 21, meiotic nondisjunction
              H80 otosclerosis
  Axis III: F32.1 moderate depressive episode with somatic features

Axis IV: Psychosocial disability: Personal care: 4 (severe)
Occupation: 4 (severe)
Family and household: 4 (severe)
Broad social context: 4 (severe)
Duration: Less than 1 year
Strength: Interpersonal skills before illness onset
Axis V: Z86.5 History of depression
Z73 Problems in lifestyle (workshop stressors)
Z74.1 Need for assistance in personal care
Z74.3 Need for continuous supervision

The diagnostic criteria used to diagnose Tina with major depression are best based on the diagnosis of depression outlined in the Diagnostic Criteria for Psychiatric Disorders for Use with Adults with Learning Disability/Mental Retardation (DC-LD), as described in the section that follows.

Diagnostic Criteria for Psychiatric Disorders for Use with Adults with Learning Disability/Mental Retardation (DC-LD)
Hierarchical Approach to Diagnosis

Persons with intellectual disability, especially those with moderate-to-profound intellectual disability, may be difficult to classify using the criteria for mental disorder. Intellectual disability specialists in the United Kingdom and Ireland have prepared DC-LD to provide an approach to classification that is more appropriate for these individuals whose cognitive and communication difficulties make classification problematic. The criteria were developed for use with adults in the more severe ranges of intellectual disability, but they are used to complement the ICD-10 for persons who are mildly intellectually disabled. Therefore, the classifications can be used side by side, depending on case presentation. The DC-LD is a classification system that provides operationalized diagnostic criteria. A hierarchical approach is taken to diagnosis through and within the axes shown in table 3.1.

The first axis emphasizes the severity of intellectual disability, the second the etiology, and the third the psychiatric disorders. Five levels are listed under psychiatric disorders. Level A, Developmental Disorders, is a separate level in

Table 3.1 DC-LD Hierarchical Approach to Diagnosis

Axis I: Severity of [intellectual disability]
Axis II: Cause of [intellectual disability]
Axis III: Psychiatric disorders
Level A: Developmental disorders
Level B: Psychiatric disorders
Level C: Pesonality disorders
Level D: Problem behaviors
Level E: Other disorders

From Royal College of Psychiatry (2001).

recognition of the fact that a developmental disorder, for example, pervasive developmental disorder, may co-occur with a syndrome such as fragile X syndrome, and is not always associated with intellectual disability. Moreover, developmental disorders are distinct from psychiatric disorders even though they may co-occur. The other levels (Psychiatric disorders, Personality disorders, Problem behaviors, and Other disorders) clarify the nature of the problem.

In the DC-LD, Tina would be classified as follows:

Axis I: F11.1 Moderate mental retardation (intellectual disability)
Axis II: Q90.0 trisomy 21, meiotic nondisjunction
Axis III: A. No additional developmental disorder
           B. III B4.1 Depressive episode
           C. None
           D. III D1.7 Oppositional behavior
           E. None

Although depression is diagnosed in both ICD-10 and the DC-LD, the criteria in the DC-LD are more descriptive of the presentation in a person with moderate intellectual disability, focusing as they do on depressed mood and loss of interest in pleasure activities and not on cognitive symptoms of depression. Also, oppositional behavior can be more specifically identified as a focus for treatment, since the DC-LD allows for classification of specific problem behaviors.

DSM-IVTR Definition

The DSM-IVTR is the standard classification for mental disorders in the United States. The definition of mental retardation (intellectual disability) is as follows: significantly subaverage intellectual functioning: an IQ of approximately 70 or below on an individually administered IQ test (for infants, a clinical judgment of significantly subaverage intellectual functioning). There are concurrent deficits or impairments in present adaptive functioning.

Table 3.2 shows the DSM-IVTR (APA, 2000) diagnostic criteria.

DSM-IVTR Multiaxial Assessment

One of the major advances in DSM-III (APA, 1980) and subsequent editions of the DSM system was the establishment of the multiaxial classification system (Part V) to address complex cases. A multiaxial system differs from a multiple category system in that it provides specific axes and rules for their use. This system was derived from an earlier triaxial classification (Rutter et al., 1969). It provides a means to categorize both the intellectual and adaptive disability of intellectual disability, associated psychiatric conditions, associated brain disorder, and global functioning. Although, in general, the multiaxial classification system has been viewed from the perspective of the Axis I diagnosis, when dealing with developmental disorders its benefits become particularly clear because the major areas involved in treatment planning and predicting outcome can be designated on different axes. It provides a convenient format for organizing and communicating clinical information, and if all five axes are used, offers

Table 3.2. DSM-IVTR Diagnostic Criteria for Mental Retardation

A. Significantly subaverage intellectual functioning: an IQ of approximately 70 or below on an individually administered IQ test (for infants, a clinical judgment of significantly subaverage intellectual functioning).

B. Concurrent deficits or impairments in present adaptive functioning (i.e., the person's effectiveness in meeting the standards expected for his or her age by his or her cultural group) in at least two of the following areas: communication, self-care, home living, social/interpersonal skills, use of community resources, self-direction, functional academic skills, work, leisure, health, and safety.

C. The onset is before age 18 years.

Code based on degree of severity reflecting level of intellectual impairment:

317	**Mild Mental Retardation:**	IQ level 50–55 to approximately 70
318.0	**Moderate Mental Retardation:**	IQ level 35–40 to 50–55
318.1	**Severe Mental Retardation:**	IQ level 20–25 to 35–40
318.2	**Profound Mental Retardation:**	IQ level below 20 or 25
319	**Mental Retardation, Severity Unspecified:** when there is strong presumption of Mental Retardation but the person's intelligence is untestable by standard tests	

From APA (2000). Reprinted with permission of author from the *Diagnostic and Statistical Manual of Mental Disorders, Fourth Edition, Text Revision.* American Psychiatric Association. Copyright © 2000.

a far more comprehensive description than does a single diagnostic axis. For intellectual disability, it highlights the need to plan for features associated with cognitive impairments.

In DSM-IVTR, the multiaxial system is maintained. The diagnosis of intellectual disability is on Axis II in DSM-IVTR, as was the case with earlier editions. Psychiatric diagnoses are placed on Axis I to emphasize the importance of making specific diagnoses for intellectually disabled persons, rather than simply focusing on associated behaviors. If known, a particular intellectual disability syndrome is coded on Axis III, general medical disorders. The Axis IV and V categories are domains that should be included for all intellectually disabled persons. Axis IV refers to specific stressors, psychosocial, and environmental problems, and Axis V to global assessment of functioning (GAF) scale, which provides an additional means to measure adaptive abilities. By using the multiaxial classification, factors that influence functioning can be better specified in the diagnostic system. Moreover, the complexity of a clinical situation can be demonstrated by describing co-occurring conditions and comorbidity to highlight the heterogeneity of persons with a similar or the same diagnosis. The multiaxial system is of particular value in evaluating long-term prognosis because the axes contribute to evaluating outcome risks.

The DSM-IVTR axes are as follows:

Axis I: Clinical disorders
          Other conditions that may be a focus of clinical attention
Axis II: Personality disorders
          Mental retardation [intellectual disability]
Axis III: General medical conditions

Axis IV: Psychosocial and environmental problems
Axis V: Global assessment of functioning (GAF)

Axis I is used for all disorders and conditions in the classification except personality disorders and intellectual disability, which are placed on Axis II. If there is more than one Axis I diagnosis, all are listed with the principal reason for the visit listed first. While the ICD-10 provides a specific guide to its use for intellectual disability, the DSM-IVTR does not. In DSM-IVTR the psychiatric disorder is listed on Axis I and other conditions that may be a focus of treatment are listed as "V codes" and also coded on this axis. V codes include relational problems that may be secondary to a mental disorder and interpersonal problems between parent and child, marital problems, and sibling problems. Problems of neglect or abuse that may be an issue for intellectually disabled persons also are coded as V codes.

The listing of intellectual disability on the second axis ensures that intellectual disability is always considered when making a diagnostic assessment. If there is more than one Axis II diagnosis, all should be listed. If intellectual disability is the primary diagnosis, it should be listed with the qualifying phrase (principal diagnosis).

Axis III is used for current general medical conditions that are pertinent to understanding and managing the individual's condition. Syndrome diagnosis, such as Down syndrome or fragile X syndrome, would be placed on this axis.

Axis IV is for reporting psychosocial and environmental problems that may impact the diagnosis, treatment, and prognosis of mental disorders on Axis I and Axis II. These include personal stressors, lack of social support or personal resources, or other problems that relate to the context in which a person's difficulties have occurred. Moreover, a psychosocial problem may be the result of intellectual disability or behavior and emotional problems associated with it. All psychosocial and environmental problems present during the year preceding the current evaluation are listed. When a psychosocial or environmental problem is the primary focus of clinical attention, it is recorded on Axis I as a V code diagnosis.

The following categories are used in DSM-IVTR on Axis IV:

1. Problems with primary support group (e.g., neglect, parental over-protection, sexual or physical abuse, death of a family member).
2. Problems related to the social environment (e.g., inadequate social support, problems with social environment, discrimination, adjustment to life transition).
3. Educational problems (e.g., discord with teacher or classmates, academic problems).
4. Occupational problems (e.g., threat of job loss, dissatisfaction with job or workshop).
5. Housing problems (e.g., inadequate housing, discord with neighbors).
6. Economic problems (e.g., poverty).
7. Problems with access to health care services (e.g., inadequate health care, inadequate health insurance, lack of transportation).

8. Problems related to interaction with the legal system/crime (e.g., arrest, victim of crime).
9. Other psychosocial or environmental problem (e.g., discord with non-family caregivers, lack of social services).

Axis V is used to report the clinical judgment of the individual's overall level of functioning. This information is used to plan treatment and measure its impact over time to assess and predict outcome. The DSM-IVTR provides a Global Assessment of Functioning (GAF) scale. This scale is rated in regard to psychological, social, and occupational functioning but not impairment due to physical or environmental limitations (e.g., having no friends or being disruptive in class). If there are discrepancies between an individual's symptom severity and level of function, the final GAF always indicates the worse of the two.

Severity of Intellectual Disability

Intellectual disability is divided into four levels of severity in DSM-IVTR (APA, 2000). The DSM-IVTR reflects the extent of intellectual impairment: mild, moderate, severe, or profound. The levels of severity are the same as in ICD-10.

Mild Intellectual Disability. Utilizing properly standardized intelligence tests, an IQ range for mild intellectual disability is 50 to 69. For mild intellectual disability, DSM-IVTR lists the IQ range from 50–55 to approximately 70. For mildly intellectually disabled persons, previously referred to as educable, problems with the use of language and speech difficulties may limit independence in adult life. This group makes up approximately 85% of those who are classified as intellectually disabled. In the early months of life, these individuals may not be distinguishable from normal children; they may only be recognized at school entry or in the preschool years (0 to 5) when social and communication skills develop.

Persons with mild intellectual disability may acquire academic skills up to the fifth- or sixth-grade level by their late teenage years. During their adult years, mildly intellectually disabled persons may develop sufficient social and vocational abilities to work and live independently or in supervised apartments and group homes and need a minimum of external support. Still, ongoing guidance is needed under stressful social conditions or during economic hardship. Their developmental achievements allow them to engage others in conversation and participate in clinical interviews. Their learning difficulties may become evident in academic work. Socioculturally, when academic achievement is not required, their problems may be minimal. Yet there may be a noticeable degree of social and emotional immaturity, leading to difficulties in coping in a community setting. There may be difficulty in coping with the demands of marriage or child rearing or to meet specific cultural expectations. Still, for the most part, behavioral, emotional, and social problems of persons with mild intellectual disability and their need for psychosocial and behavior treatment and support are similar to those of persons with normal intelligence. Brain abnormalities are identifiable in a minority of this group. Associated conditions include autistic disorder, other developmental disorders, epilepsy, conduct disorders, or physical disability.

Moderate Intellectual Disability. The IQ range for moderate intellectual disability is from 35 to 49. The DSM-IVTR indicates an IQ range spanning from 35–40 to 50–55. However, the full-scale IQ score can be deceptive because variable cognitive profiles of abilities are common for this group, e.g., some individuals may have better visuospatial skills than language skills. Moreover, some the functioning of some moderately intellectually disabled persons may be underestimated due to motor incoordination. Those with this degree of cognitive impairment may be socially interactive and communicative with appropriate assistance. Language development is variable across this IQ range, spanning from the capacity to carry on simple conversations to language limited to communication of basic needs. Those who never learn language may understand simple instructions or learn to use sign language or language devices to compensate for communication difficulties. There are also limitations in their achievement of self-care and motor skills. School progress is limited, but the higher functioning individual may learn basic skills in reading, writing, and counting. As adults, moderately intellectually disabled individuals may participate in simple, practical work that is carefully structured, but they generally need consistent supervision by others. Completely independent living is rarely achieved in adulthood. Moderately intellectually disabled individuals make up approximately 10% of the intellectually disabled population.

In regard to etiology, brain abnormality can be identified in the majority of affected individuals. Seizure disorder and other neurological and physical disabilities also commonly occur. Autistic disorder and other pervasive developmental disorders may be associated with moderate intellectual disability, leading to further problems in social adaptation. Psychiatric diagnosis may be difficult because of their limited language development, which often requires the use of other informants. In the past, the term "trainable" was used for moderately intellectually disabled persons, but it should be avoided because many individuals in this group can benefit from educational programs. Efforts should be made to identify appropriate sheltered workshops, group homes, and supportive employment programs.

Severe Intellectual Disability. The IQ range for severe intellectual disability is 20 to 35. In DSM-IVTR, this is listed as IQ 20–25 to 35–40. This group is similar to that of persons in the moderately intellectually disabled group in regard to their clinical picture and presence of brain abnormality. A significant number of severely intellectually disabled persons has marked motor impairment and other associated deficits.

During the preschool years, poor motor development and lack of communicative speech are readily recognized. During the school-age years, verbal language may emerge and elementary self-care skills may be taught. Depending on their cognitive ability, basic survival skills, including sight-reading of essential words, such as *stop, man,* and *woman*, may be learned. In adulthood, supervision is needed to aid in task performance. Community programs and group homes are frequently needed, or in some cases, specific in-home assistance to families is required. Associated disabilities may require specialized nursing care.

The severely intellectually disabled group makes up 3% to 4% of persons with intellectual disability.

Profound Intellectual Disability. The IQ range for profound intellectual disability is below 20. DSM-IVTR lists an IQ below 20–25. Language comprehension and use is generally limited to understanding simple commands and making simple requests. Adaptive function is variable, although certain visuospatial skills, such as matching and sorting, may be acquired. With supervision and guidance, the child, and later the adult, may take part in practical tasks and domestic routines. As a result of their various disabilities, a highly structured environment with continual aid and supervision is necessary. Individualized relationships with caregivers are emphasized to facilitate optimal development. Self-care, communication skills, and motor abilities may require training in a structured setting. Living arrangements include small group homes in the community, intermediate care facilities, or living with their families along with day-program support.

Brain abnormality can be identified in the majority of profoundly intellectually disabled persons. Neurological and physical disabilities that affect mobility are common, as are associated seizure disorder and visual and hearing impairment. Pervasive developmental disorders, especially autistic-like behavior, are frequent. This group constitutes 1%–2% of those diagnosed as intellectually disabled.

Unspecified Intellectual Disability. Overall, the younger the person, the more difficult it is to make a diagnosis of intellectual disability, except for the most severe cases. The unspecified category is used when there is a presumption of intellectual disability, but the person cannot be tested on standardized instruments. This may occur when children, adolescents, or adults are uncooperative or too impaired to participate in testing. This category may also be used for infants when available tests, such as the Catell or Bayley, that do not provide IQ values are used. If the individual's IQ is thought to be over 70, unspecified intellectual disability should not be utilized. This category is most commonly used when an assessment of the degree of intellectual disability, using the standard procedures, is difficult or impossible because of age and associated physical and sensory disabilities; for example, in blind, deaf, mute, severely behaviorally disturbed, or physically disabled individuals.

In the DSM-IVTR system, Tina (case vignette, page 48) would be classified as follows:

Axis I: 296.2x Major depressive disorder, single episode, moderate without psychotic features
          V61.9 Relational problem related to mental disorder
Axis II: 318.0 Moderate mental retardation (intellectual disability)
Axis III: Otosclerosis
Axis IV: Problems related to social environment
          Educational problems
Axis V: GAF: 40

It should be noted that persons under 18 who meet diagnostic criteria for dementia and whose IQ is below 70 are given both the diagnosis of dementia and intellectual disability. However, an individual over 18 who develops multiple cognitive impairments, with a drop in IQ to below 70, receives only the diagnosis of dementia. The diagnosis of dementia can be made any time after the IQ is fairly stable (usually by age 3 or 4). Clarification of a diagnosis of dementia is important because intellectual disability is a developmental disability. Although referred for a diagnosis of Alzheimer's disease (dementia), Tina does not have this diagnosis; instead, her primary diagnosis is depression.

2002 AAMR Definition

The DSM-IVTR and ICD-10 use comparable diagnostic codes but vary in their definitions of intellectual disability. The approach of the AAMR differs from both of these in providing an extended definition of intellectual disability that focuses on the individual's needs, as shown in table 3.3, and what can be done to improve functioning. The 2002 revision (Luckasson et al., 2002) replaces their 1992 definition (Luckasson et al., 1992). The 1992 AAMR definition (1) emphasized that intellectual disability is a state of functioning; (2) classified intensity of supports and described the supports that intellectually disabled people require; (3) focused on intellectual disability as an expression of the interaction between the affected person and the environment; and (4) emphasized particular adaptive skills that may be impaired.

The 2002 AAMR 2002 definition in *Mental Retardation: Definition, Classification, and Systems of Support, 10th edition* (Luckasson et al., 2002), retains the term "mental retardation." Although the AAMR Board of Directors proposed that a name change be considered, the membership voted to keep this terminology for the 2002 classification in keeping with the current international classification. The functional orientation introduced in their 1992 definition the three diagnostic criteria describing intellectual functioning, adaptive behavior, and age of onset, and continued emphasis on the intensities of required supports were

Table 3.3 AAMR Multidimensional Classification System

Dimension		Classification
Dimension I:	Intellectual Abilities	Cognitive Tests
Dimension II:	Adaptive Behavior (conceptual, social and practical skills)	Adaptive Behavior Scales
Dimension III:	Participation, Interactions, and Social Roles	Ecological Analysis
Dimension IV:	Health (physical health, mental health, and etiology)	ICD-10, DSM-IVTR
Dimension V:	Context (environments and culture)	ICF

refined. Persons with intellectual disability were included in discussions on the 1992 definition where they emphasized their desire for community inclusion, access to services, independence, and needed supports (Reiss, 1994). This focus on inclusion was continued in developing the 2002 definition. Families and consumer organizations are particularly interested in the AAMR emphasis on community-based supports as it may result in better services.

The 2002 AAMR definition is as follows:

> Mental retardation is an intellectual disability characterized by significant limitations, both in intellectual function and adaptive behavior expressed in conceptual, social, and practical adaptive skills. The disability originates before age 18.

The 2002 system includes standard deviation criteria for intellectual and adaptive behavior components and a fifth dimension of participation, interactions, and social roles, and it describes adaptive behavior in greater detail. It proposes that adaptive behavior includes conceptual, social, and practical skills. It provides a framework of assessment and describes how to assess supports and intensity of supports. There is an expanded discussion of mild intellectual disability. The 2002 definition reviews the use of clinical judgment in assessment and discusses the interface of the AAMR definition with other definitions of intellectual disability. The 2002 system includes commentary that has developed over the past 10 years on the 1992 system and more clearly operationalizes the multidimensional views of intellectual disability. Best practice guidelines are provided in regard to diagnosis, classification, and planning supports. However, the 2002 system is still a work in progress as research continues to define the nature of intelligence, how intelligence relates to adaptive behavior, how supports are best implemented, how we should conceptualize disabling conditions, how participation of families and caregivers impacts functioning, and how diagnostic labels become stigmatizing.

The definition emphasizes the risks of a unidimensional approach that focuses only on disability. In contrast to the ICD-10 and DSM-IVTR approaches that maintain the levels of intellectual disability as "mild, moderate, severe, and profound," its emphasis is on function and support systems. Yet, from a developmental perspective, the inclusion of levels of impairment is helpful, so a complete diagnostic assessment should draw on either ICD-10 or DSM-IVTR multiaxial classifications and the AAMR multidimensional classification and include both levels of impairment and systems of support.

Table 3.4 compares DSM-IVTR criteria with the 2002 AAMR criteria, pointing out differences between them. The change from global concepts of adaptive behavior toward adaptive skill areas from the AAMR definition was incorporated into the DSM-IVTR definition of intellectual disability. Having a specific list of psychosocial and environmental problems (as noted in the DSM-IVTR description in the previous section) encourages evaluators to assess psychosocial skills in addition to academic abilities.

Table 3.4 Diagnostic Criteria for Mental Retardation (Intellectual Disability)

	DSM-IVTR	AAMR
Adaptive Function	Concurrent impairment in *present* adaptive functioning in at least 2 of 11 areas listed in table 3.2.	Significant limitations in adaptive behavior as expressed in conceptual, social, and practical skills.
Intelligence Quotient		
Child/Adolescent	IQ of *approximately* 70 or below on individually administered tests.	Significant limitations in intellectual functioning demonstrated by scoring approximately two standard deviations below the mean on standardized tests, considering the standard error of measurement of the instrument.
Infants	Clinical judgment of sub-average function.	Level estimated as below the 3rd percentile by clinical judgment.
Levels of Mental Retardation	Mild, moderate, severe, profound.	Rather than levels, categories of intensity of needed supports are designated.

Key Elements and Assumptions of the AAMR Approach

The AAMR approach addresses the following: (1) instrumental competence (cognition and learning) and social competence (practical and social intelligence) that make up adaptive skills; (2) environments where an individual lives, works, and learns; and (3) overall functioning, which refers to the ability to cope with ordinary challenges of everyday living in the community. It is essential to remember that intellectual disability is not a static condition; the developmental goal is to establish a "best fit match" of the person with environmental supports to maximize adaptive ability.

The 2002 AAMR definition is based on five assumptions that take into account community setting, cultural issues, and the expectation of improvement with appropriate supports because each person has unique strengths, as well as limitations. These assumptions also apply to the DSM-IVTR definition. The assumptions are as follows:

1. Limitations in present functioning must be considered within the context of community environments typical of the individual's age, peers, and culture.
2. Valid assessment considers cultural and linguistic diversity, as well as differences in communication, sensory, motor, and behavioral factors.
3. Within an individual, limitations coexist with strengths.
4. An important purpose of describing limitations is to develop a profile of needed supports.
5. With appropriate personalized supports over a sustained period, the life functioning of the person with intellectual disability will generally improve.

Appropriate supports are matched to an individual's needs and include supportive individuals and services. Although intellectual disability may not be lifelong,
these supports may be needed for an extended period, and in some instances,
throughout life. Improvement in function is expected for the majority but, for
some, supports are needed to maintain a basic level of function or primarily to
slow the regression process.

The 2002 AAMR definition (Luckasson et al., 2002) suggests that supports
planning should relate to an individual's strengths and needs in each of five
dimensions: (1) intellectual abilities, (2) adaptive behavior (conceptual, social,
and practical skills), (3) participation, interactions, and social roles, (4) health
(physical health, mental health, and disease etiology), and (5) context (environments and culture). The definition indicates that supports planning should be
focused on desired person-referenced outcomes. Clinical judgment plays a key
role in diagnosis, classification, and planning supports.

ISSUES REGARDING CLASSIFICATION OF LEVELS OF INTELLECTUAL
DISABILITY AND/OR LEVELS OF SUPPORT

Professionals working with intellectually disabled persons have criticized the
removal of the mild, moderate, severe, and profound levels of severity in the
AAMR definition (McMillan, Gresham, and Siperstein, 1993; 1995). The 2002
AAMR definition maintains the elimination of levels of intellectual disability
severity based on IQ scores, a proposal first introduced by the AAMR in 1992.
The AAMR proposes that the definition of intellectual disability relies on limitations in IQ and adaptive skills, while an individual's level of severity is based
on IQ alone. Opposing this viewpoint, it should be noted that the levels of
severity are subclassifications of the category "intellectual disability," and that
adaptive functioning is included in the larger category of intellectual disability
from which they are derived. Thus, severity level infers limitations in both IQ
and adaptative functioning. Moreover, the AAMR suggests that IQ scores at the
extremes of measurement are less accurate than those measures that are closer
to the mean.

Although the AAMR indicates that levels of support are not meant to be
substituted for levels of severity (Luckasson et al., 1996; Luckasson and Spitalnik, 1994), levels of support have been misinterpreted as a replacement for
such levels of impairment. Overall, the AAMR suggests that too much emphasis
has been placed on subclassification by levels of impairment in special education
placement and in determining the types of services provided for both children
and adults. Therefore, the 2002 AAMR manual proposes that the IQ score be
used to make the diagnosis of intellectual disability and that adaptive ability be
clearly described and linked to supports in special education. An individual's
adaptive skills should be determined by an interdisciplinary team, using observation, interviews, and reports of those who know the individual well.

In 1992, the AAMR initially proposed that the identification of strengths and
the need for supports across the life dimensions should be included in the assessment. Intellectual functioning and adaptive skills, psychological and emo-

tional considerations, health and physical considerations, and environmental considerations, were used to create a profile of the person's needed supports for optimal functioning. This approach is further refined in the 2002 definition. The AAMR considers the 1992 AAMR definition to be a "paradigm shift" in how intellectual disability and adaptive behavior are described. Previously, a global concept of adaptive behavior was utilized, but in the 1992 definition, "adaptive behavior" was replaced by the term "adaptive behavioral skill." Several competencies were defined to indicate how an individual functions in a particular social context. The capacity of the individual to change their behavior to meet environmental and situational demands was emphasized. Ten broad adaptive behavioral skill areas were included with the requirement of significant limitations in at least two of these developmentally appropriate areas. Moreover, the term "maladaptive behavior" was eliminated. Rather than emphasizing IQ-based subgroups (mild, moderate, severe, and profound), professionals were encouraged to describe needed supports for individuals with intellectual disability. The 1992 definition assumed valid assessment, that adaptive skills were assessed in a context typical of age peers, that limitations coexist with strengths, and that appropriate supports over time would result in improved adaptive functioning. After establishing the diagnosis, the support profile was prepared to include strengths and needs not only in regard to intellectual functioning and general adaptive skills but also with respect to psychological, emotional, physical, and environmental skills. Comprehensive classification of an individual entails multiple assessments and clinical judgment; this is preferable to reliance only on standardized measures on a single test with a single evaluator.

The 1992 and 2002 AAMR diagnostic system proposals for elimination of IQ levels in their classification and increased emphasis on clinical judgment have been controversial. Still, a greater emphasis on needed supports rather than the the extent of impairment has been seen as a positive feature, especially by families. The elimination of IQ levels was proposed to reduce the error of IQ-based classification practices that segregate by levels, and the potential stigma from the utilization of levels. However, others argue strongly that to provide appropriate services, it is critical to emphasize what the person's capacity level is, both intellectually and adaptively.

In regard to adoption of the 1992 AAMR definition, a survey of directors of special education in the 50 states showed that 44 states have continued to use the 1983 AAMR definition and four use the 1992 AAMR definition. None used the levels-of-support model proposed by the AAMR. Three states did not base their diagnosis of intellectual disability during the school age years on either of these models (Denning, Chamberlain, and Polloway, 2000). Moreover, less than 1% of investigators carrying out research on those with intellectual disability applied the 1992 AAMR classification (Polloway et al., 1999).

What are the reasons for the limited adoption of the 1992 definition? The 2002 AAMR manual suggests that the change in the definition required new assessment devices to measure adaptive skills. Yet no standardized or accepted ways to assess strengths and limitations in these skill areas are generally available, and as a result only nonspecific existing measures, informal observation, and clinical judgment could be used for assessment. In addition, eliminating the IQ-based levels of functioning suggested a change in commonly used terminology, with no clear substitute. Others found that the existing legally required education programs for children in schools and individualized habilitation plans for adults seemed sufficient in identifying support profiles for persons with intellectual disability.

Finally, severity levels have been the fundamental way that educators, psychologists, adult service providers, and those conducting research classify individuals with intellectual disability. Substitution of levels of support for levels of severity has been faulted because support levels lack psychometric qualities needed for measurement and because of their lack of precision (McMillan, Gresham, and Siperstein, 1993). The American Psychiatric Association in DSM-IVTR (APA, 2000) adopted the 1992 AAMR definition and its proposals for adaptive behavior but maintained the levels of severity (Jacobson and Mulick, 1996).

Another issue relates to the continued use of the term "mild mental retardation" (intellectual disability). McMillan and others (McMillan et al., 1998; McMillan, Gresham, and Siperstein, 1993) question the use of the term "mild mental retardation," just as the use of the term "borderline mental retardation" was questioned in the past. The mildly intellectually disabled group represents at least 75% of those with a diagnosis of intellectual disability (Field and Sanchez, 1999). These individuals are increasingly classified by schools as having learning disabilities rather than intellectual disability because of concerns about stigma. McMillan, Siperstein, and Gresham (1996) suggested schools are hesitant to use the term "mental retardation" for those in the mild intellectually disabled range. The term "mental retardation," for the general public, applies to individuals who function in lower, more severe ranges of intellectual disability. Such questions of terminology have been dealt with differently in other countries, such as the United Kingdom, by substituting the term "learning disability" generically to describe all individuals with intellectual disability. However, the term "learning disability" in the United States is applied primarily to individuals who test in the normal range of intelligence but have learning disabilities in academic skills, such as reading and mathematics.

In keeping with such questions raised by schools about classification, the U.S. Department of Education found that the percentage of school aged children classified as having intellectual disability decreased 40% between the 1976–1977 school year and the 1994–1995 school year (Beirne-Smith, Ittenbach, and Patton, 1998). During the same period, the percentage of students with learning disabilities increased as much as 200% (McMillan, Siperstein, and Gresham, 1996). The 1992 AAMR definition, if applied, by abandoning levels and focusing on needs, may have resulted in fewer diagnoses of "mild mental retardation." Those with mild intellectual disability or mild cognitive limitations do experience different problems in daily life than those with moderate-to-profound intellectual disability and might well be seen as sufficiently distinct by school programs to be placed in other school categories.

Mild intellectual disability has been diagnosed in a disproportionate number of children who belong to minority groups. Changes in the IQ cut-off point of the definition may affect minorities disproportionately if IQ scores alone are inappropriately used for diagnosis. Using an IQ cut-off of 75, McMillan, Gresham, and Siperstein (1993) proposed that 18.4% of African-American children and 2.6% of Caucasian children would be diagnosed with intellectual disability.

Because intellectual disability has many causes, ability profiles and behavior vary considerably among the various etiologies. Using etiology and levels of intellectual disability, it is estimated that those with mild intellectual disability constitute 75%–89% of those diagnosed, whereas those with moderate-to-profound intellectual disability make up 11%–25% of those diagnosed. An identifiable cause is found in 25%–40% of those with mild intellectual disability. In contrast, specific causes are recognized for 60%–75% of those with moderate-to-profound intellectual disability. Whether the AAMR can fully represent the interests of all persons with intellectual disability by eliminating the differentiation between those groups has been questioned (McMillan, Gresham, and Siperstein, 1993). Without specifying levels, the specific needs of individuals with different degrees of cognitive handicap may not be fully appreciated, particularly when the levels of support are not designated by IQ level along with level of adaptive functioning. Maintaining levels but emphasizing supports for an individual is the most comprehensive approach.

McMillan, Siperstein, and Gresham (1996) suggest that a new terminology is needed to include heterogeneous groups (those with multiple etiologies), particularly for mildly intellectually disabled persons. Among the terminologies suggested for mild intellectual disability are "cognitive impairment" and "general learning disability." Others have suggested that those with mild intellectual disability be excluded from the category of intellectual disability entirely. Concerned about these questions of terminology, the AAMR continues to seek agreement on the most inclusive and least stigmatizing designation.

Regarding cognitive levels, the AAMR suggests that mild intellectual disability has been a misleading term in many individuals who have mild cognitive impairment (Tymchuk, Lakin, and Luckasson, 2001) and better adaptive functioning. They suggest further study of the diagnostic classification regarding this category, particularly in regard to use of adaptive abilities, and not basing the diagnosis on IQ alone; for example, an individual with good adaptive behavior and IQ of 70 might not receive an intellectual disability diagnosis. For such individuals with good adaptive skills, the term "mild cognitive disability" may be less confusing to the general population than the term "mild mental retardation."

Taking into account all these issues regarding classification, perhaps the best solution is to maintain levels of intellectual disability from a developmental point of view along with the AAMR's categories that emphasize means to enhance individual functioning by providing supports. This is the approach taken by the World Health Organization by introducing the ICF categories to be used in conjunction with ICD-10, as described in the next section.

ICF/ICIDH

In 2001, the World Health Organization introduced its ICF/ICIDH. Its approach to the issue of levels is to provide two classifications: one of diseases that includes levels of intellectual disability and another separate classification of functioning. The 2002 AAMR classification is consistent with the WHO classification, now simply referred to as the International Classification of Functioning (ICF). Thus, the most comprehensive approach may be to follow the WHO model and use the ICD-10 or DSM-IVTR to classify levels of intellectual disability and the AAMR approach that emphasizes intensity of supports for treatment planning.

The ICF is accepted by 191 countries as an international standard to describe and measure health and disability. Using this framework, the World Health Organization estimated that the healthy years of life lost each year due to disability is double the years lost due to premature death. The ICF places its emphasis on how people actually live. The classification describes mental and physical functioning, activities and participation (e.g., communication, self-care, domestic life, interpersonal interactions, and relationships), and environmental factors (e.g., attitudes, services, systems, and policies). Environmental factors are included because functioning and disability occur in the context of an individual's life. The ICD-10 classifies disease, while the ICF classifies health. Together, the two systems provide a way to assess the health of individuals and how they relate to their environment. A focus on functioning places the emphasis on the effectiveness of interventions. The ICF is aimed at linking medical models and social models to a psychobiological or biopsychosocial approach that offers a coherent view of various dimensions of health at biological, individual, and social levels. The goal is to describe the dimensions that affect how an individual lives with a health condition and how these can be improved to lead a healthy life. In the ICF classification, mental retardation (b117) (intellectual disability) is listed under intellectual functions that include "general mental functions required to understand and constructively integrate the various mental functions, including all cognitive functions and their development over the life span."

Impairment and Disability

Intellectual disability has been conceptualized as impairment and disability. The impairment involves the central nervous system and results from genetic, chromosomal, or environmental reasons that have affected the acquisition of skills and learning ability. The impairment has implications for treatment and prognosis and, in many instances, genetic counseling. An impairment may be psychological, physiological, or functional. It represents a deviation from the norm.

The term "disability" refers to the limitations that an individual shows in functioning within a social context or setting. Disability occurs at the interface between the demands of a specific impairment, society's interpretation of that impairment, and the larger political and the economic context of disability (Braddock and Parish, 2001), while impairment refers to a known biological condition. Disability was not a social category prior to the eighteenth century, although impairments were well recognized. A disability is the consequence of the impairment of the person's ability to learn and acquire new skills. It is the way functional limitation expresses itself in everyday life. The extent to which an impairment results in a loss of function (disability) is influenced by the nature and extent of available interventions that enhance functioning. The extent of the disability can be ameliorated by others who help the individual or by environmental modifications, such as wheelchair ramps, that diminish the impact of physical disabilities. Interventions and environmental modifications maximize independence and enhance qualify of life.

When considering a person with intellectual disability, the immediate social setting that involves the person and family, the neighborhood school and community, and social systems and influences in the larger society are assessed. When establishing the context for behavior, one must take into account the degree of intellectual ability, specific syndrome, and adaptive functioning. The context is assessed through clinical judgment and an understanding of the individual and his or her capacity to function in a designated setting.

The ICF suggests that a medical model focuses on disabilities caused by a health condition that requires medical care, while a social model considers disability as a socially created problem and is concerned with integrating individuals into society. Moreover, disability can become a political issue involving human rights, as well as health care (Baxter, 2004).

A disability is conceptualized as a significant problem in functioning and is characterized in the ICF model by marked and severe problems in the capacity to perform (impairment), the ability to perform (activity limitations compared to people without the health condition), and the opportunity to perform (participation restrictions). Social and environmental influences on a person's health and well-being are indicated in the model's four sections: body functions, body structures, activities, and participation and environmental factors. The latter include health and other professionals. Adaptive behavior encompasses the application of conceptual, social, and practical skills to daily life. Its assessment should relate to an individual's typical performance during daily routines and changing circumstances, not to maximum performance. Intellectual functioning is still best represented by IQ scores when obtained from appropriate standardized assessment instruments. The criterion for diagnosis of intellectual disability is approximately two standard deviations below the mean of a corresponding group of people (for example, matched in age, culture, and context) considering the standard error of measurement for the specific assessment instruments used and the instruments' strengths and weaknesses.

ICF–Functioning and the Environment

The ICF considers environmental factors that influence a person on an individual level and in the context of "services and systems." Individually, the focus is on the immediate environment where the person lives—his or her home, school, or work place as well as on supports, relationships with others, values, and attitudes toward disability. The services and systems level refers to both formal and informal services and social systems. There are several levels of organization: (1) the immediate social setting (e.g., family and advocates); (2) the neighborhood, the local community, and rehabilitation organizations; and (3) the larger society, with its sociopolitical influences. These systems may facilitate communication, provide transportation, and offer education, health, and religious opportunities. Critically, they include national programs that establish services that must be provided through law, regulations, and national health and educational programs. Finally, personal factors refer not to an individual's medical diagnosis or adaptive functioning per se but to lifestyle, educational achievement, coping style, and social background.

Past and current life experiences are considered in the context of age, race, gender, individual fitness, and capacity. How can this person make the best use of positive supports? What positive environmental supports (e.g., adaptive equipment) and personal supports (e.g., encouragement) are needed for this particular person? In summary, the emphasis is on appreciating what personal qualities an individual brings to his or her engagement with the outside world and how these interactions can be facilitated to enhance independence, interpersonal relationships, success in school and community life, and personal well-being. When assessing contextual supports, both the strengths and limitations of the individual must be evaluated. The purpose of assessing limitations is to determine which supports are needed.

COMPARISON OF THE AAMR MULTIDIMENSIONAL MODEL AND ICF MODEL

The 2002 AAMR definition is consistent with the ICF model. In fact, the fifth dimension, contextual factors, in the AAMR Multidimensional model was added for consistency with the WHO's ICF model of disability. The AAMR definition emphasizes the person's functional ability and, in so doing, considers the congruence of intellectual and adaptive abilities and stressors that impact the capacity to function. The assessment of adaptive functioning is essential because IQ tests alone are not an accurate measure of an intellectually disabled person's adaptive ability, although adaptive skills are closely related to intellectual limitations. Adaptive ability has been defined as "the effectiveness or degree with which an individual meets the standards of personal independence and social responsibility expected of his age and cultural group" (Grossman, 1983). This includes the areas of social/interpersonal skills and responsibility, communication, self-care, home living, use of community resources, self-direction, functional academic skills, work, leisure, health, and safety. As in DSM-IVTR, these areas must be considered to diagnose a generalized limitation in adaptation. Because skills in these areas vary with chronological age, the assessment also must take age into account. The low intelligence score and limited adaptive ability must have their onset before 18 years of age, the age when adult roles are typically assumed.

Both the 2002 AAMR definition and ICF classifications emphasize human

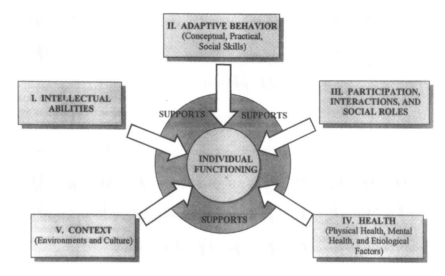

Figure 3.1 Theoretical Model. Source: Luckasson et al. (2001). Reprinted by permission of Ad Hoc Committee on Terminology and Classification, *Proposed New Edition of Mental Retardation: Definition, Classification, and Systems of Support,* AAMR News & Notes, Vol. 14, No. 5. American Association on Mental Retardation, 2001, Washington, DC.

functioning as a person interacts with, and experiences, his or her physical and psychosocial environment. Both systems emphasize an ecological approach to functioning and disability. Both systems offer a dynamic concept of disability that recognizes strengths and limitations. Similar concepts are used in both systems to understand and assess disability as a problem in human functioning, and both systems emphasize an integrated biopsychosocial model. Thus, the 2002 AAMR system does fit in the same frame of reference in classifying functioning and disability as the ICF.

The theoretical model used in the 2002 AAMR definition (figure 3.1) describes the relationship among individual functions, supports, and the five dimensions that are used in a multidimensional approach to intellectual disability. These five dimensions are similar to the four dimensions in the 1992 AAMR classification, where the four dimensions were: intellectual functioning and adaptive skills, psychological and emotional considerations, health and physical considerations, and environmental considerations.

Context and Behavioral Phenotype

The 2002 AAMR system has five dimensions: intellectual abilities; adaptive behavior; participation, interactions, and social roles; health; and contextual factors. This final dimension puts each individual life in context (Luckasson et al., 2002). Its focus is on how current adaptation and functioning can be understood based on (a) environmental or external influences that have affected development and (b) personal qualities or internal influences, both of which make them the person that they are. There are many external influences that affect a person's development. Among these are the physical environment (e.g., coping with getting around in a wheelchair), the social environment made up of family and community members, and the "attitudinal environment" that may or may not be supportive of individual endeavors. Positive factors in the environment facilitate personal growth and negative factors are obstacles to that growth.

In the AAMR definition, "context" refers to social settings (e.g., family, neighborhood, sociopolitical); however, it is also critical that the specific syndrome and its natural history be understood in these settings. When individual rights and responsibilities are considered in a social context, an understanding of the behavioral phenotypes characteristic of specific disorders is essential. For example, the National Prader-Willi Association has expressed concern about therapeutic food restriction protocols not being enforced to prevent complications from compulsive overeating. Hyperphagia, compulsive eating without apparent satiation, is a behavioral phenotype in Prader-Willi syndrome that has a physiological basis. In Lesch-Nyhan disease, where self-biting is a behavioral phenotype, life-threatening self-mutilation may occur if physical restraints are not utilized properly. For this syndrome, standard procedures for use of physical constraints must be modified to allow appropriate restraints to be used. It is the affected child or adult who must be consulted about when it is safe to remove restraints. In these examples, context requires consideration of both the social setting and the characteristic features of the disorder.

FRAMEWORK FOR ASSESSMENT—2002 AAMR

In the 2002 AAMR system, each of the multidimensional influences on an individual's functioning is mediated through the support system provided for that person. Thus, this is an interactive model that focuses on the emergence of the person in adapting to tasks in the real world.

The framework for assessment that is used in the 2002 AAMR system involves three elements: diagnosis, classification, and planning supports, as shown in table 3.5.

A diagnosis of intellectual disability is essential to establish eligibility for services, benefits, and needed legal protections. The classification is utilized to communicate among professionals working with intellectually disabled individuals to carry out research and to establish funding for services. For classification purposes, IQ levels, special education categories, environmental assessments, levels of adaptive behavior, mental health measures, and intensity of support skills are important. To plan supports, one must consider the best personal outcome for an individual leading to independence, enhanced relationships, participation in school and community activities, and a sense of well-being. Measures for planning supports include self-appraisals, support-intensity scales, and individualized education programs. The AAMR provides operational definitions for intelligence, adaptive behaviors, supports, disability, and contexts.

In the AAMR definition, intelligence is described as a general mental capac-

Table 3.5 Framework for Diagnosis, Classification, and Planning Supports

Function	Purposes	Assessment	
		Matching Measures to Purposes	*Guidelines and Considerations That May Be Important*
Diagnosis	Establishing eligibility: • Services • Benefits • Legal protections	IQ Test[a] Adaptive behavior scales[a] Documented age of onset[a]	Match between measures and purpose Psychometric characteristics of measures selected Appropriateness for person (age group, cultural group, primary language, means of communication, gender, sensori-motor limitations) Qualifications of examiner Examiner characteristics and potential for bias Consistency with professional standards and practices Selection of informants Relevant context and environments Social roles, participation, interactions Opportunities/experiences
Classification	Grouping for: • Service reimbursement or funding • Research • Services • Communication about selected characteristics	Support intensity scales IQ ranges or levels Special education categories Environmental assessments Etiology–risk factor systems Levels of adaptive behavior Mental health measures Funding levels Benefits categories	Clinical and social history Physical and mental factors Behavior in assessment situation Personal goals Team input
Planning Supports	Enhancing personal outcomes: • Independence • Relationships • Contributions • School and community participation • Personal well-being	Person-centered planning tools Self-appraisal Assessment of objective life conditions measures Support intensity scales Required individual plan elements (IFSP, IEP, ITP, IPP, IHP)	

Source: Modified from Luckasson et al. (2002). Reprinted by permission of author from *Mental Retardation: Definition, Classification, and Systems of Support, 10th edition*. American Association on Mental Retardation, Washington, DC. Copyright © 2002.
Note: IFSP = individualized family service plan; IEP = individualized education program; ITP = individualized transition plan; IPP = individualized program plan; and IHP = individualized habilitation plan.
[a] Required assessments to establish diagnosis of intellectual disability.

ity that includes reasoning, planning, problem solving, abstract thinking, comprehension, and learning from experience. Limitations in intelligence affect participation and interaction in social activities, as well as adaptive behavior. Intellectual functioning is best represented by intelligence test scores, using appropriate test instruments.

Adaptive behavior involves conceptual, social, and practical skills that must be learned to carry out everyday activities. Limited adaptive behavior in persons with intellectual disability affects their daily lives as they respond to environmental demands and demonstrate their capacity to adapt to challenges, both physical and psychosocial. Adaptive behavior is related to intellectual ability and affects participation in social activities. Adaptive abilities are measured on standardized scales, such as the Vineland Social Maturity Scale and the AAMR Adaptive Behavioral Scale. On these scales, limitations are operationally defined through performance that is at least two standard deviations below the mean in conceptual, social, or practical adaptive behavior, or in the overall score on the standardized tests.

Support systems should include resources and strategies that promote personal development, education, and well-being. To participate in social life at home, in school, and in the community, supports must be keyed to intellectual ability, adaptive capacity, and an aggregate of characteristic features of a syndrome.

There is continuing effort to refine the measurement of adaptive behavioral skills. The 10 adaptive skills listed by the AAMR were not determined empirically and require clinical judgment with input from professionals working with the person with intellectual disability and their family members.

Assessment is needed in each of the 10 skill areas. The requirement that there be significant weakness in two or more skill areas has been criticized as it does not uniformly deal with younger children, school-aged children, and adult individuals (McMillan, Siperstein, and Leffert, 2002).

INCORPORATING SYSTEMS OF SUPPORT RATINGS WITHIN THE AAMR DIAGNOSTIC SYSTEM

In the AAMR system, Tina (case vignette, page 48) would be classified as follows:

Function I: **Diagnosis of Mental Retardation (Intellectual Disability)**
Moderate mental retardation: IQ score 40
Adaptive Behavior Scales of Independent Behaviors-Revised: SS 35
> Limitations in conceptual adaptive skills, social adaptive skills, and overall adaptive behavior. These limitations occur in the context of community settings for typically developing peers in the same cultural setting.

Function II: **Classification and Description**
Dimension I: Intellectual Abilities

Strengths: Performance subscales on WISC-IIIR
Limitations: Verbal subscales

A full classification for Tina would also require a description of the following areas:

Dimension II: Adaptive Behavior
Conceptual Adaptive Behavior Skills (cognitive and communication/academic skills)
1. Receptive Language
   Strengths
   Limitations
2. Expressive Language
   Strengths
   Limitations
3. Reading
4. Writing
5. Money concepts
6. Self-Direction
7. Other
Social Adaptive Behavior Skills
Interpersonal
Responsibility
Self-esteem
Gullibility (likely to be tricked or manipulated)
Naïveté (limited logic, understanding of cause and effect, foresight, strategic planning)
Follows rules
Obeys laws
Avoids victimization
Other
Practical Adaptive Behavior Skills
Activities of Daily Living
1. Eating
2. Transfer/mobility
3. Toileting
4. Dressing
Instrumental Activities of Daily Living (behaviors related to independent and/or community living)
1. Meal preparation
2. Housekeeping
3. Transportation
4. Taking medication
5. Money management
6. Telephone use
7. Occupational skills

8. Maintain safe environments (includes fire, poisons, home maintenance, home security)

Dimension III: Participation, Interactions, Social Roles Participation (e.g., activities, events, organizations) Interactions (e.g., friends, family, peers, neighbors) Social Roles:

1. Personal roles
2. School roles
3. Community roles
4. Work roles
5. Leisure and recreation
6. Spiritual life
7. Other

Dimension IV: Health (Physical Health, Mental Health, and Etiology) (list health-related diagnoses, mental health diagnoses, risk factors leading to diagnosis)

1. Physical Health–Down syndrome, otosclerosis
2. Mental Health–Major depressive disorder, first episode
3. Etiology
   Biomedical
   Behavioral
   Educational
4. Interactions Among Risk Factors

Dimension V: Context (strengths and limitations of individual's environment)
   Immediate surroundings
   Community, Neighborhood
   Society

Function III: Support Needs Profile (Support areas, activities, intensities of support)

Support Areas:
1. Human Development
2. Teaching and Education
3. Home Living
4. Community Living
5. Employment
6. Health and Safety
7. Behavioral
8. Social
9. Protection and Advocacy

Implications of the 2002 AAMR System

The AAMR suggests that there are nine implications that relate to their 2002 classification system. These include (1) focusing the approach to intellectual disability on a multidimensional perspective; (2) employing an ecological approach to understand and investigate the impact of the living environment on the individual functioning of the person, and the individual supports; (3) recognizing differences and relevance for assessment of three diagnostic features (diagnosis, classification, and planning supports); (4) integrating further support systems into special education and habilitation; (5) modifying research designs to reflect an emphasis on inclusion and appropriate supports; (6) establishing a needs-based approach to eligibility; (7) funding services on the basis of individual support needs; (8) incorporating current thinking about intellectual disability into legal procedures and the justice system; and (9) addressing the needs of those individuals with higher IQ levels who avoid the label of intellectual disability but still require services for their cognitive limitations.

Issues in Applying the Multidimensional Approach

In utilizing the AAMR multidimensional approach, there are several issues that must be considered:

1. Appreciation of the parallel aspects of intelligence and adaptive behavior is essential.
2. Etiology is a critical factor in carrying out diagnosis, classification, and planning individual supports.
3. Environments must be analyzed for the individual person with intellectual disability.
4. An individual's desired outcomes must be included in the provision of environmental supports.

When considering intelligence, the tripartite model of intelligence (Sternberg, 1988) may be helpful. The three elements are conceptual intelligence, social intelligence, and practical intelligence. Moreover, there is a tripartite model of adaptive behavior that includes personal independence (practical), responsibility in the community (social), and academic (conceptual) achievement (Luckasson et al., 2002). Thus, models of intelligence and adaptive behavior may be linked, especially in regard to conceptual similarities between practical intelligence and the element of adaptive behavior involving independent living skills. Conceptual intelligence is linked to cognitive and communication ability and academic skills, and social intelligence is linked to social competence. Intelligence and adaptive behavior may be considered as aspects of personal competence. In testing intelligence, an intelligence profile that shows strengths and limitations in the various subscale scores of tests such as the WISC-R and WAIS-III is commonly used. These tests emphasize how a person learns and processes information. Such intellectual and cognitive profiles are used in planning to facilitate learning and personal outcomes. The same is true for adaptive behavior profiles. Merging intelligence and adaptive behavior helps to facilitate program planning.

Etiology and Health Factors

It is essential to consider the impact of a specific etiology and to review the biomedical, social, behavioral, and educational consequences of that etiology. For example, Down syndrome, fragile X syndrome, and Prader-Willi syndrome may have different outcomes and effects on family functioning. An understanding of both health and behavioral characteristics over the life span is essential for parents, caregivers, and community programs.

Individual competence is affected by the person's physical health. Health management requires consideration of the person's living environment, his or her coping abilities, his or her communication style, and problems engaging the health care system. Appreciating the health care needs of persons with various etiologies may lead to preventing complications and removing aversive factors that impact health.

Environmental Analysis

The individual's environment must be fully characterized to facilitate personal growth, meaningful participation, and meaningful social interactions. The specific setting where individual services are provided, whether it is school, the home environment, the work place or the recreation setting, must be considered. The diagnostic assessment process characterizes how these environments facilitate or restrict an individual's growth, development, and well-being. An optimal environment provides opportunities to facilitate independence, relationships, community and school participation, and personal well-being.

Personal Outcomes

Individualized supports are best based on an individual's personal wishes. This includes the desire for independence, for relationships, for school and community participation, and for personal well-being. A focus on personal choice may be a challenge to both those providing services and to professionals. However, organizing supports is critical to helping each individual make choices and master important challenges.

Providing Supports: Support Needs

The AAMR has provided a Supports Intensity Scale (SIS) (Thompson et al., 2004) to implement supports needed in each of the categories previously described in Function III of the multidimensional classifications. In each of the activity domains (home living activities, community living activities, lifelong learning activities, employment activities, health and safety activities, and social activities), frequency, daily support time, and type of support necessary for the person to be successful are listed. Frequency is rated on a scale of 0–4, ranging from more than monthly to hourly or more frequently. The amount of daily support time is rated on a scale of 0–4, ranging from none to 4 hours or more on a typical day. Finally, the type of support is indicated, ranging from none to monitoring, verbal/gesture prompting, and partial physical assistance to full physical assistance.

For example, home living activities include dressing, toileting, eating, and grooming. Community living activities include transportation, visiting friends, access to public buildings, and recreation. Lifelong learning activities address actions involved, such as interacting with others, participating in decision-making, learning to count or to read signs, and using self-management strategies. Employment activities include learning and using specific job skills, interacting with coworkers/supervisors, completing work-related tasks with acceptable speed and quality, and seeking information and assistance from an employer.

Health and safety activities are frequently situational. Technology and reminders or individualized cueing are needed. Taking medication, avoiding health hazards, accessing emergency services, and maintaining physical and emotional well-being are included. Social activities focus on making friends, using appropriate skills, and communicating with others about personal needs in various settings (at home, in the community).

In addition to the Support Needs Scale, there is a Supplemental Protection and Advocacy Scale. This subscale includes self-advocacy, managing money, protecting oneself from exploitation, making one's own choices and decisions, obtaining legal services, and advocating for others.

Finally, there are support scales for exceptional medical support needs, such as specialized respiratory care (oxygen therapy or suctioning), feeding assistance (jaw positioning or tube feeding), dialysis, and seizure management. Categories are provided for exceptional behavioral support needs, such as assault toward others, property destruction, prevention of self-injury, sexual aggression, and emotional outbursts.

Upon completion of this detailed Support Needs interview, a Supports Intensity Scale Scoring Form and Profile is completed; this consists of (a) Support Needs Ratings, (b) Support Needs Profile, (c) Support Considerations Based on Protection and Advocacy Scores, and (d) Support Considerations Based on Exceptional Medical and Behavioral Support Needs. Final recommendations are made based on each of these ratings.

SUMMARY

In summary, both medical and functional classifications of persons with intellectual disability are needed. The medical classification is needed for defining the disorder, indicating levels of severity, designating medical conditions, designating associated syndromes, communication among professionals, obtaining comprehensive services, and conducting research. Specifically, the medical classifications, ICD-10 and DSM-IVTR, provide a means to indicate associated medical problems, behavioral problems (ICD-10) or associated mental disorders, and stressors and global functioning (DSM-IVTR). The functional classifications are important for highlighting needed supports and for better specification of service needs. The ICF classification emphasizes individual functioning, and, in addition, the AAMR multidimensional classification emphasizes supports to help the individual reach his or her potential. Each of the systems of classification should be understood by professionals and parents. For a person with intellectual disability, both proper diagnostic classification and functional classification are important in establishing a network of supports. As we look to the future of new knowledge in gene-brain-behavior-environment relationships, we can expect to have a better understanding of the brain mechanisms that result in intellectual disability. Such new knowledge may result in a classification system that is not only descriptive but also based on the etiology of the intellectual disability.

KEY POINTS

1. The classification of intellectual disability began in earnest in the nineteenth century with the identification of discrete etiologies.
2. Recognition that intelligence is measurable resulted in the identification of levels of severity and allowed standardized testing into categories based on numerical scores.
3. Mental age is not a continuum but is linked to successive reorganizations of brain regions during development.
4. Individuals with the same IQ score may differ in a range of cognitive and language abilities.
5. It was not until 1961 that objective test scores and the dual criteria of intelligence and adaptive behavior were introduced into the AAMR classification. The term "mental retardation" was introduced in the 1961 classification.
6. In 1983, multiaxial coding of social-environmental factors that affect cognitive and developmental processes was added to the AAMR Diagnostic Manual.
7. By 1992, the emphasis in the definition had shifted to substantial limitations in present functioning and adaptive skills (rather than adaptive behavior), and a multidimensional approach was introduced that highlighted the importance of providing systems of support.
8. The DSM-IVTR and ICD-10 definitions list four levels of severity and provide multiple axes. The DSM-IVTR provides a greater emphasis on co-occurring psychiatric and behavioral problems; the ICD-10 Guide to Mental Retardation provides extensive links to classify both co-occurring medical conditions and psychiatric disorders. When making psychiatric diagnoses in persons with moderate-to-profound intellectual disability, diagnostic criteria must be operationalized to take into account cognitive ability and community skills.
9. The DSM-IVTR is a classification of mental disorders; the ICD-10 is a classification of diseases. The 2002 AAMR definition includes both of these but emphasizes needed supports to enhance functioning.
10. The 2002 AAMR definition continues to emphasize classification based on intensities of needed supports. Its multidimensional system now has five dimensions: (1) intellectual abilities; (2) adaptive behavior (rather than

skills); (3) participation, interactions, and social roles; (4) health; and (5) context (added to be consistent with the ICF classification).

11. The term "intellectual disability" is used to designate the federal advisory committee to the Secretary of HHS and the President of the United States, i.e., The President's Committee for People with Intellectual Disabilities (PCPID). This committee was previously known as The President's Committee on Mental Retardation (PCMR). As noted in chapter 1, the name change is indicative of the growing consensus for the use of the term "intellectual disability."

References

American Psychiatric Association (2000). *Diagnostic and statistical manual of mental disorders,* 4th ed., text revision. Author, Washington, DC.

American Psychiatric Association, Committee on Nomenclature and Statistics. (1980). *Diagnostic and statistical manual of mental disorders,* 3rd ed. Author, Washington, DC.

Baxter, P. (2004). ICF: Health vs. disease. *Developmental Medicine and Child Neurology,* 46:291.

Beirne-Smith, M., Ittenback, R.F., and Patton, J.R. (1998). *Mental retardation,* 5th ed. Merrill/Prentice Hall, Upper Saddle River, NJ.

Bourneville, D.M. (1880). Sclerose tubereuse des circonvolutions cerebrales: Idiotie et epilepsie hemiplegique. *Archives of Neurology (Paris),* 1:81–91.

Braddock, D., and Parish, S. (2001). An institutional history of disability. In G. Albrecht, K. Seelman, and M. Bury (eds.), *Handbook of disability studies,* pp. 11–68. Sage, New York.

Denning, C.B., Chamberlain, J.A., and Polloway, E.A. (2000). An evaluation of state guidelines for mental retardation: Focus on definition and classification practices. *Education and Training in Mental Retardation and Developmental Disabilities,* 35: 226–232.

Down, J.L.H. (1866). Reports observations of the ethnic classification of idiots. *London Hospital,* 3:259–262.

Field, M.A., and Sanchez, V.A. (1999). *Equal treatment for people with mental retardation: Having and raising children.* Harvard University Press, Cambridge, MA.

Greenspan, S. and Switzky, H.N. (2003). Forty years of American Association on Mental Retardation Manuals. In H.N. Switzky and S. Greenspan (eds.), *What is mental retardation: Ideas for an evolving disability.* AAMR, Washington, DC. (Published on the AAMR web site.)

Grossman, H.J. (1983). *Manual on terminology and classification in mental retardation,* revised ed. American Association on Mental Deficiency, Washington, DC.

Ireland, W.W. (1877). *On idiocy and imbecility.* Churchill, London

Jacobson, J.W., and Mulick, J.A. (1996). Psychometrics. In J.W. Jacobson and J.A. Mulick (eds.), *Manual of diagnosis and professional practice in mental retardation,* pp. 75–84. American Psychological Association, Washington, DC.

Jordan, T.E. (2000). Down's (1866) essay and its sociomedical context. *Mental Retardation,* 38:322–329.

Lambert, N., Nihiri, K., and Leland, H. (1993). *AAMR Adaptive Behavior Scales—school.* Pro-Ed, Austin, TX.

Luckasson, R., Borthwick-Duffy, S., Buntinx, W.H.E., Coulter, D.L., Craig, E.M., Reeve, A., Schalock, R.L., Snell, M.E., Spitalnik, D.M., Spreat, S., and Tasse, M.J. (2001). Theoretical Model. Proposed new edition of *Mental retardation: Definition, classification, and systems of support.* Committee on Terminology and Classification, *AAMR News & Notes,* Volume 14, No. 5, American Association on Mental Retardation, Washington, DC.

Luckasson, R., Borthwick-Duffy, S., Buntinx, W.H.E., Coulter, D.L., Craig, E.M., Reeve, A., Schalock, R.L., Snell, M.E., Spitalnik, D.M., Spreat, S. and Tasse, M.J. (2002). *Mental retardation: Definition, classification, and systems of supports,* 10th ed. American Association on Mental Retardation, Washington, DC.

Luckasson, R., Coulter, D.L., Polloway, E.A., Reiss, S., Schalock, R.L., Snell, M.E., Spitalnik, D.M., and Stark, J.A. (1992). *Mental Retardation: Definition, classification, and systems of supports,* 9th ed. American Association on Mental Retardation, Washington, DC.

Luckasson, R., Schalock, R.L., Snell, M.E., and Spitalnik, D. (1996). The 1992 AAMR definition and preschool children: A response from the Committee on Terminology and Classification. *Mental Retardation,* 34:247–253.

Luckasson, R., and Spitalnik, D. (1994). The 1992 definition of mental retardation. In V.J. Bradley, J.W. Ashbaugh, and B.C. Blaney (eds.), *Creating individual supports for people with developmental disabilities,* pp. 81–95. Paul H. Brooks, Baltimore.

McMillan, D.L., Gresham, F.M., Bocain, K.M., and Lambros, K.M. (1998). Current plight of borderline students: Where do they belong? *Education and Training in Mental Retardation and Developmental Disabilities,* 33:83–94.

McMillan, D.L., Gresham, F.M., and Siperstein, G.N. (1993). Conceptual and psychometric concerns about the 1992 AAMR definition of mental retardation. *American Journal of Mental Retardation,* 98:325–335.

McMillan, D.L., Gresham, F.M., and Siperstein, G.N. (1995). Heightened concerns over the 1992 AAMR definition: Advocacy versus precision. *American Journal on Mental Retardation,* 100:87–97.

McMillan, D.L., Siperstein, G.N., and Gresham, F.M. (1996). A challenge to the viability of mild mental retardation as a diagnostic category. *Exceptional Children,* 62:356–371.

McMillan, D.L., Siperstein, G.N., and Leffert, J.S. (2002). Children with mild mental retardation: A challenge for classification practices. In H. Switzky and S. Greenspan (eds.), *What is mental retardation?* American Association on Mental Retardation, Washington, DC.

Nihiri, K., Leland, H., and Lambert, N. (1993). *AAMR Adaptive Behavior Scale—residential and community.* Pro-Ed, Austin, TX.

Polloway, E.A., Smith, J.D., Chamberlain, J., Denning, C.B., and Smith, T.E.C. (1999). Levels of deficits or supports in the classification of mental retardation: Implementation practices. *Education and Training in Mental Retardation and Developmental Disabilities,* 34:200–206.

Reiss, S. (1994). Issues in defining mental retardation. *American Journal on Mental Retardation,* 99:1–7.

Royal College of Psychiatrists. (2001). *DC-LD (diagnostic criteria for psychiatric disorders for use with adults with learning disabilities/mental retardation).* Gaskell Press, London.

Rutter, M., Lebovici, S., Eisenberg, L., Sneznevskij, A.V., Sadoun, R., Brooke, E., and Lin, T-Y. (1969). A triaxial classification of mental disorders in childhood. *Journal of Child Psychology and Psychiatry,* 10:41–61.

Sparrow, S.S., Balla, D.A., and Cicchetti, D.V. (1984). *Interview edition. Expanded form manual. Vineland Adaptive Behavior Scales.* American Guidance Service, Circle Pines, MN. (Available at www.vinelandforum.com)

Sternberg, R.J. (1988). *The triarchic mind: A new theory of human intelligence.* Penguin, New York.

Thompson, J.R., Bryant, B.R., Campbell, E.M., Craig, E.M., Hughes, C.M., Rotholz, D.A., Schalock, R.L., Silverman, W.P., Tasse, M.J., and Wehmeyer, M.L. (2004). *AAMR Supports Intensity Scale.* American Association on Mental Retardation, Washington, DC.

Tymchuk, A.J., Lakin, K.C., and Luckasson, R. (2001). *The forgotten generation: The status and challenges of adults with mild cognitive limitations.* Paul H. Brookes, Baltimore.

World Health Organization. (1992). *The international classification of diseases (ICD-10) classification of mental and behavioral disorders: Clinical descriptions and diagnostic guidelines.* Author, Geneva, Switzerland.

World Health Organization. (1996). *ICD-10 guide for mental retardation.* Division of Mental Health and Prevention of Substance Abuse. Author, Geneva, Switzerland.

World Health Organization. (2001*). International classification of functioning, disability, and health (ICF).* Author, Geneva, Switzerland.

4

Epidemiology: Who Is Affected?

Intellectual disability is the most common developmental disorder and the most handicapping of the disorders beginning in childhood. It ranks as first among chronic conditions that limit full participation in society. Epidemiologic approaches provide a basis for understanding the distribution and dynamics of health, disease, and disorder for persons with intellectual disability; epidemiology is the foundation of public health practice. Because it relies largely on statistical methods, accurate data and clear definitions are essential. The interpretation of epidemiologic information requires background knowledge of demography, social sciences, environmental science, and the clinical sciences.

Although epidemiologic studies are essential in establishing prevalence, and in describing the demography of a disorder, the role of epidemiology is far more extensive than this. Epidemiology can teach us about the nature and scope of intellectual disability and associated general medical, behavioral, emotional, and psychiatric problems. In so doing, epidemiologic approaches may be combined with neurobiologic and psychosocial measures. Moreover, epidemiologic studies can disclose individual developmental trajectories and the influences that shape those trajectories. Some of these influences promote risk; others provide protection and promote resiliency in the individual. Finally, experimental approaches in epidemiology allow the study of causative processes, factors that influence the course of the disorder, and service needs. It is these more extensive uses of epidemiology that are called for in future research.

Chapter 3 outlines the classification of intellectual disability. This chapter will discuss the use of definitions of intellectual disability in establishing its prevalence, factors affecting prevalence, variability in rates in the various states, demographic features including the impact of increasing life expectancy, associated physical, behavioral, and emotional impairments, and new research directions.

PREVALENCE

Accurate estimates of the number of intellectually disabled individuals are required for planning purposes and to gain better knowledge of the impact of interventions. Studies of the prevalence and incidence of intellectual disability date back to at least 1811, when Napoleon ordered a census of "cretins" to be made in one of the Swiss cantons (Kanner, 1964). Although little information is available about how this census was used, many surveys have been carried out since that time. In modern studies, there continues to be wide variability between prevalence estimates. This variability stems from the multiple causes of intellectual disability and variations in screening methods.

The methods used to define intellectual disability to collect prevalence data are critical to interpreting results (Munro, 1986). The population prevalence of intellectual disability in general and of specific intellectual disability syndromes, such as Down syndrome and fragile X syndrome, must be known. Moreover, screening for intellectual disability in children who have very low birth weight or experience early trauma, neonatal screening for metabolic disorders (Holtzman, 2003), and screening for exposure to drugs in utero or for diseases beginning in utero are critical. Gestational substance abuse, especially alcohol abuse, results in the most preventable form of intellectual disability. Population studies must be careful to consider the various terms that are or have been used for intellectual disability, that is, mental retardation, mental deficiency, mental handicap, mental subnormality, developmental delay, cognitive disability, and learning disability. When reviewing published studies, the definition used in case findings to make the diagnosis must be carefully scrutinized.

DEFINING INTELLECTUAL DISABILITY

At least three approaches have been used in research to define cases of intellectual disability: (1) statistical models, (2) pathological models, and (3) social systems models. The most pragmatic definitions of intellectual disability are those provided by the statistical model, which considers psychometric (psychological) test scores, and the pathological model, which emphasizes adaptive functioning and focuses on specific causes of the intellectual disability. A fourth model, the developmental model, has received less emphasis. The developmental model assesses fluid intelligence and the processes involved in problem solving; it is more commonly used in interventions than in case finding.

Currently, the statistical model, which utilizes an IQ score two standard deviations below the mean (an IQ of 70 or lower), along with an assessment of adaptive function to identify intellectual disability, is the accepted system. Yet this statistical model implies a continuum of cognitive abilities that may not exist; the occurrence of intellectual disability does not follow a clear bell curve with an even percentage of people at each level of intellectual disability. Although general categories such as mild, moderate, severe, and profound degrees of intellectual disability are important, variability in cognitive profile and associated conditions complicate assessment and may make categorization difficult.

Thus, additional neuropsychological testing may be needed to designate ability profiles.

The pathological model focuses on specific syndromes, such as Down syndrome, or a particular etiology, such as intraventricular hemorrhage in the postpartum period. It is important in establishing behavioral phenotypes and the natural history of a syndrome. Using a pathological model, Yeargin-Alsopp et al. (1997) sought to identify biomedical causes of intellectual disability among school-aged children and associated medical conditions in children where no cause was reported. These authors studied 715, 10-year-old children, born between 1975 and 1977, who had been diagnosed with intellectual disability (IQ <70). Biomedical causes were investigated based on whether the "event" was prenatal, perinatal, or postnatal. When there was no identifiable biomedical cause, the frequency of associated medical conditions was studied. No associated medical condition was identified in 78% of children with intellectual disability (87% of whom were classified as mild, IQ 50–70; 57% of whom were classified as severe, IQ <50). Prenatal causes were identified in 12%, perinatal causes in 6%, and postnatal causes in 4%. Based on the results, the authors concluded that public health strategies might reduce the number of children identified with intellectual disability. Future studies are expected to diagnose larger numbers of cases based on more sophisticated procedures.

The social systems model designates individuals as intellectually disabled if they are so labeled by a social system, most commonly the school. For these purposes, many children are not regarded as intellectually disabled until they start school and may no longer carry the diagnosis after they leave school if they are functioning adequately in society and have sufficient physical and social skills to work independently; the majority of this group would be classified as mildly intellectually disabled under the social systems model.

The developmental approach to intellectual disability is a dynamic one that focuses on the engagement of the person with intellectual disability with other people and environmental challenges. Unlike the statistical approach (looking backward from the population mean), it looks forward developmentally. This dynamic approach to intelligence emphasizes fluid intelligence, the general inferential and reasoning ability (Demetriou et al., 2002; Gustafson and Undheim, 1996) that underlies thinking and problem solving in novel situations. Fluid intelligence is closely associated with general intelligence (Demetriou et al., 2002; Gustafson and Undheim, 1996), and it is strongly associated with working memory and processing efficiency. It should be contrasted with crystallized intelligence, which refers to knowledge that is already possessed. Intelligence tests measure crystallized intelligence. Considering fluid intelligence as it relates to processing efficiency and working memory in intellectual disability suggests a re-evaluation of the stage model of intellectual disability proposed by Barbel Inhelder.

In her classic text, *The Diagnosis of Reasoning in the Mentally Retarded,* Inhelder (1943, 1968) provided a functional analysis of the dynamics of the development of reasoning by analyzing its failure to progress in persons with intellectual disability, and she discussed cognitive inefficiency as an important feature. She proposed, based on the reasoning tests of conservation that she used, that what are generally termed levels of mental retardation (mild, moderate, severe, and profound) represent a lack of cognitive progression that corresponds to failures on certain tests of reasoning (modes of problem solving). Thus, failure to advance beyond trial-and-error reasoning (sensorimotor operations) is indicative of profound intellectual disability; failure to advance beyond early symbolic operations characterizes severe mental retardation. Attaining symbolic capacity (preoperational thinking) suggests reaching the level of representation with the capacity to decenter, that is, to keep two units of information in mind simultaneously, which is an early form of working memory. Moderate intellectual disability refers to reasoning that results in carrying out reversible operations in the mind (concrete operations). This entails the utilization of working memory, a prefrontal lobe function, with executive functioning and sufficient cognitive efficiency to allow the individual to keep mental objects in mind to solve problems. An example is carrying out the mental processes involved in subtraction or tasks of divided attention (Schretlen, Hobholz, and Brandt, 1996). Mild intellectual disability entails the ability to perform more advanced operations of this kind but the failure to reach levels of abstract reasoning for problem solving. Pasnak, Wilson-Quayle, and Whitten (1998) found correlations of 0.66 with IQ and 0.77 with mental age in a group of mildly intellectually disabled students when they compared measurements obtained using Piagetian tests (categorization, seriation, and conservation of discrete quantities) to those obtained using standardized IQ tests (discussed in chapter 6). The only commonly used standardized test that focuses on this developmental approach is the Uzgiris-Hunt scale (Uzgiris and Hunt, 1975) that is used to evaluate individuals with severe-to-profound intellectual disability. A dynamic developmental approach tests how an individual reasons when faced with a task to solve.

MEASURING THE PREVALENCE OF INTELLECTUAL DISABILITY

Despite the various definitions used in population studies, there is general agreement between international studies of prevalence rates (Baird and Sadovnick, 1985; Koller et al., 1983). The overall population prevalence of intellectual disability is less than 1% (fewer than 10 per 1,000 persons). If the population in the United States is approximately 250 million, a 1% prevalence identifies 2.5 million people with intellectual disability. Yet a 3% prevalence has often been chosen, using the statistical approach and basing the diagnosis on an IQ below 70. The 3% rate assumes the death rate for intellectually disabled individuals is similar to that of the general population, considers that intellectual disability is routinely identified in infancy, and assumes the diagnosis does not change with increasing age. None of these assumptions can be supported. Because there are many etiologies, the survival rate may be similar to that of the general population only for those with milder forms of intellectual disability. Because intellectual disability is not always diagnosed in preschool children, its prevalence may be higher during the school years due to the inclusion of mildly intellectually disabled persons whose adaptive abilities may improve with education. For the mildly intellectually disabled group, the diagnosis may no longer apply after leaving school if adaptive function improves. Thus, the diagnosis of intellectual disability may change over time and, in this example, is age dependent.

VARIABILITY IN RATES AMONG THE STATES

The number of children with intellectual disability in each state may be determined from the U.S. Department of Education listings of children with intellectual disability who are enrolled in special education programs; for adults, the number can be determined from listings by the Social Security Administration. Using the standard definition "significantly subaverage intellectual functioning with deficits in adaptive behavior" (Frankenberger and Harper, 1988), the U.S. Centers for Disease Control (CDC) analyzed reports from the Department of Education that included the number of children aged 6–17 who were enrolled in special education programs during the 1993–1994 school year. For adults aged 18–64, a similar analysis was based on information obtained by the Social Security Administration in 1993 and used the same definition but emphasized onset in the developmental period (before age 22). Included were adults with intellectual disability who received Supplementary Social Security Income (SSI) and/or Social Security Disability Insurance (SSDI). To receive Social Security benefits for intellectual disability, adults must have an IQ of less than or equal to 59, or an IQ of 60–70, along with other physical or mental impairments that lead to additional, and substantial, work-related limitations in function (Committee on Disability for Mental Retardation, 2002).

The number of intellectually disabled children and adults identified in each of the states and the District of Columbia were combined to establish an overall estimate of the number of intellectually disabled persons receiving services in the total population in the United States. The prevalence for children ages 6–17 and for adults ages 18–64 was estimated using the 1990 census. According to this approach, in 1993 in the United States, 1.5 million people ages 6–64 were diagnosed with intellectual disability. The overall rate was 7.6 cases per 1,000 persons. However, the rates varied considerably among the states. For example, there is a fivefold difference between Alaska (3/1,000) and West Virginia (16.9/1,000). The 10 states with the highest rates were located in the eastern, southern, and central parts of the United States; the lowest rates were found in the Pacific and Mountain regions. For children, the overall rate was 11.4/1,000, ranging ninefold from 3.2/1,000 in New Jersey to 31.4/1,000 in Alabama. For adults, the rate was 6.6/1,000, ranging sixfold with a rate of 2.5/1,000 in Alaska and 15.7/1,000 in West Virginia. In 84% of the states, the rates were higher for children than for adults. Seventy percent of the state-specific variation in rate for adults was accounted for by median household income, percentage of total birth to teen-aged mothers, and the percent of the population with less than a ninth grade education. These findings are consistent with a relationship between prevalence and socioeducational factors, especially low maternal education levels (Drews et al., 1995).

Understanding the Basis of Variability

The interpretation of these findings must take the following into account: (1) Although there are national guidelines to determine eligibility for services, they are interpreted locally; (2) the Department of Education information does not include those who drop out of school or never enroll in public education (enrollment in private schools varies in the individual states); (3) eligibility for Social Security Administration funding is based on personal income and the presence of a disability, so some individuals could be excluded if earned income exceeds eligibility requirements; and (4) data limitations may be the result of complicated state and federal cooperative arrangements. Still, the large state-to-state differences most likely do represent some real differences among the states.

METROPOLITAN ATLANTA DEVELOPMENTAL DISABILITIES SURVEILLANCE PROGRAM

To clarify prevalence in a defined population, the CDC developed the Metropolitan Atlanta Developmental Disabilities Surveillance Program, utilizing the statistical method and multiple data sources, to track intellectual disability rates for children aged 3–10 years (Yeargin-Allsopp et al., 1992). Rates were calculated by race, sex, and age. This program focused on establishing how common intellectual disability is by tracking the number of children with intellectual disability in a five-county area in Metropolitan Atlanta, Georgia. Both the overall rate and level of severity of intellectual disability were calculated. Between 1991 and 1994, an average 1% (9.7/1,000) of children ages 3–10 were diagnosed with intellectual disability. Intellectual disability was more common in older children (ages 9–10) (12.3/1,000) than in younger children (ages 3–4) (5.2/1,000), more common in boys than in girls, and more common in African-American than in Caucasian children. Regardless of age, race, or sex, severe intellectual disability (IQ below 50) accounted for one-third of all cases (Boyle et al., 1996). Two-thirds of the cases were in the mild range of intellectual disability. The increase in prevalence with advancing age occurred in children with mild-to-moderate intellectual disability; however, it did not occur for those with severe-to-profound intellectual disability in whom the rate was essentially constant with advancing age. Overall, only 10% of the children with intellectual disability were diagnosed before 2 years of age; among these, 36% were diagnosed with profound intellectual disability, and 7% were diagnosed with mild intellectual disability. By five years of age, 67% of children with intellectual disability had been identified. These findings are consistent with a previous CDC study carried out as part of the Metropolitan Atlanta Developmental Disabilities Surveillance Program that studied disabilities in 10-year-old children; the rate among 10-year-olds was 12/1,000 (Murphy et al., 1995). Similarly, mild intellectual disability was three times more common than severe intellectual disability; the rates were higher in boys and in African Americans. These findings are also consistent with rates in other studies (Kiely, 1987; Reschly and Jipson, 1976; Yeargin-Allsopp et al.,

1995). Ethnic differences on tests of intelligence have been linked to economic deprivation, home environment, and maternal characteristics (Brooks-Gunn, Klebanov, and Duncan, 1996), so these *issues,* not *race,* are the important factors.

FACTORS AFFECTING PREVALENCE

Many factors, such as normalization programs (see chapter 2), mainstreaming, and improved interventions for those who have been educationally and socially deprived, influence the prevalence of intellectual disability. The reduction of poverty, improvement in nutrition, early intervention, and more refined medical diagnoses may also influence prevalence rates. Greater availability of genetic counseling, prenatal diagnosis, and abortion services for high-risk pregnancies also are factors, as are postnatal dietary/hormonal treatments for inborn errors of metabolism such as galactosemia, phenylketonuria, and endocrine disorders like congenital hypothyroidism. Improved obstetrical techniques have lowered the incidence of brain damage at birth, yet improvements in care for extremely premature infants have led, in some instances, to an increased rate of intellectual disability in those with very low birth weights who survive. For some disorders, such as Down syndrome, prenatal diagnosis with pregnancy termination has some impact on incidence; however, improved qualify of life, which increases the life span of affected individuals, also has affected prevalence.

Demographic considerations that influence prevalence include age, sex, socioeconomic level, race, and variations between urban and rural populations (Munro, 1986). In regard to age, most surveys show an increase in prevalence from the preschool years (0 to 4) to middle childhood (5 to 12). Prior to school entry, children with severe intellectual disability are most likely to be identified. Because performance expectations are greater on school entry, milder developmental disabilities may not be recognized until that time. In the midteen years, there may also be an apparent increase in the rate when new and increasing cognitive demands are made by the school system. During the teen years, adaptive difficulties related to social judgment and behavior control may become more apparent. In young adulthood (22 to 34), population prevalence rates generally decrease following the completion of school. Finally, in older persons, rates decrease as a result of reduced demands from vocational programs and early death in some intellectual disability syndromes. Because of all these considerations, population studies must consider age-specific rates of intellectual disability for planning purposes.

The rate of intellectual disability has been reported to be higher in males than in females, perhaps because congenital anomalies are more prevalent in boys, as are prematurity, neonatal death, and stillbirth. Another important factor in males is the presence of X-linked forms of intellectual disability. Moreover, due to aggressive behavior, boys may come to the attention of authorities more often than girls and may be more likely to be diagnosed. Still, not all studies show an increased prevalence among males, possibly because age, as well as extent and type of intellectual disability, must be considered. Higher rates among males have been reported in mildly intellectually disabled persons, but the gender difference is less apparent among persons who are more severely intellectually disabled.

Socioeconomic level is important as it relates to intellectual disability because of possible differences in sensory and psychosocial experiences. In the past, the terms "retarded due to psychosocial disadvantage" (Grossman, 1983) or "cultural familial mental retardation" (Zigler, 1967) were used. Psychosocial factors, such as poor living conditions, overcrowding, and lack of educational opportunity, may correlate with intellectual disability, particularly in the mild range; however, genetic factors must be taken into account for all persons with intellectual disability. For the more severe levels of intellectual disability, clear-cut differences in socioeconomic status are less common than in milder degrees of intellectual disability. Prevalence rates have been reported to be higher among racial minorities, but these are more clearly linked to socioeconomic level and not to race. Similarly, differences between urban and rural populations may be influenced by educational, occupational, and cultural opportunities. In some surveys, reported rates have been higher in rural areas, and in others, in inner-city populations.

LIVING ARRANGEMENTS

Living arrangements may vary, with the higher functioning groups (those with better cognitive functioning) tending to live in community residences or with family members. Individuals with moderate intellectual disability are more often placed in foster and group homes, whereas the most severely and profoundly intellectually disabled individuals may be placed in community settings in foster and group homes as they grow older. Thus, the percentage living with family members and in the communities has been reported to be inversely related to the degree of intellectual deficit.

INCREASING LIFE EXPECTANCY

By the year 2040, approximately 25% of the general population will be over age 60, compared to approximately 12% at the turn of the twenty-first century; a similar trend is expected in intellectual disability. It is expected that the cohort age 60–70 will represent the largest segment of individuals with intellectual disability (Davidson et al, 2003). The life expectancy of intellectually disabled persons is correlated with their level of intellectual functioning and the etiology of the disorder (Eyman et al., 1990). In a 1983 Canadian study, 98% of identified individuals with mild and moderate intellectual disability and 92% in the severe range reached age 20. From ages 1 to 19, the death rate among individuals with mild and moderate intellectual disability was twice that of the general population, whereas the rates for those with severe and profound intellectual disability were 7 and 31 times higher, respectively (Herbst and Baird, 1983). Yet life expectancy among intellectually disabled persons is increasing, particularly for those who survive beyond the first years of life. Janicki et al., (1999) studied

2752 adults with intellectual disability, age 40 and older, who died over a 10-year period in New York State. The average age at death was 66.6 years; this was lower than the general population, but many individuals lived as long as their peers, especially if there were no severe associated features linked to their intellectual disability. For persons with Down syndrome, the average age at death was 55.8 years, reflecting increased longevity. The cause of death for this group was similar to the general population (cardiovascular disease, respiratory illness, and neoplastic disease).

Patja et al. (2000) reported on a 35-year follow-up study (1963–1997) based on a nationwide population study of the life expectancy of people with intellectual disability in Finland. This is the longest population-based follow-up study reported for persons with intellectual disability; it involved a nationwide cohort with a high retention of subjects. The population studied consisted of a total of 60,969 person years. This was a prospective cohort study with mortality follow-up at 35 years of age, and life expectancy was calculated based on different levels of intellectual disability. People with mild intellectual disability did not have shorter life expectancies than the general population. People with profound intellectual disability had a decreased life span in all age groups. This is most likely the result of neurological disorders and more severe associated disorders. Severe and moderately intellectually disabled persons had reduced life span for similar reasons.

A survey in Western Australia (Bittles et al., 2002) calculated the survival possibilities of 8,724 individuals. Stratification by level of IQ showed that 54.7% were categorized as mild, 27.8% as moderate, and 17.5% as severe. A genetic disorder was diagnosed in 16% of mild, 33.8% of moderate, and 27.5% of severe cases. Down syndrome was the most common genetic disorder, accounting for 12.5% of the total number of cases. The 50% survival probability for the population with intellectual disability was 68.8 years, but it was 75.6 years for men and 81.2 years for women in the general Australian population. Male participants with intellectual disability had an average life span of 66.7 years and females of 71.5 years. Fifty percent survival probabilities were related to the extent of intellectual disability (mild, moderate, and severe levels) in persons 74.0, 67.6, and 58.6 years of age, respectively. The median survival was 60.1 years for those with a genetic disorder and 72.2 years for persons with no genetic disorder. The authors note that, by middle age, individuals with intellectual disability had a greater likelihood of being obese and were less physically fit than the general population. Moreover, increased rates of psychiatric problems, osteoporosis, thyroid problems, nonischemic heart disease, and early onset of dementia were reported. With more individuals in community placement, the demand for health services is likely to increase, requiring long-term planning.

In regard to health risk factors other than the increased risk of obesity and reduced physical activity, people with intellectual disability may have less exposure to certain environmental risk factors, such as smoking and alcohol use (although this is a growing problem). Children may have less exposure to domestic accidents as they are often supervised; traffic accident exposure is less common, as are occupational deaths, and suicide is less common.

Finally, studies of aging in intellectually disabled persons may contribute to better understanding of disorders as they occur not only in a particular syndrome but also in the general population. For example, women with Down syndrome and early onset menopause (46 years or younger) had earlier onset and a greater risk of Alzheimer's disease than did women with onset of menopause after 46 years (rate ratio, 2.7; 95% confidence interval [CI], 1.2–5.9) (Scupf et al., 2003). Women with Down syndrome and dementia had higher mean serum sex hormone binding globulin levels than did nondemented women (86.4 nmol/L vs. 56.6 nmol/L, p 0.02) but similar levels of total estradiol, suggesting that bioavailable estradiol, rather than total estradiol, is associated with dementia. These findings in Down syndrome support the hypothesis that reductions in estrogens after menopause might contribute to pathological processes leading to Alzheimer's disease.

FREQUENCY OF ASSOCIATED IMPAIRMENTS

Population surveys of intellectual disability usually consider associated physical disability, such as visual impairment, hearing loss, speech and language problems, seizure disorder, and cerebral palsy. Twenty to twenty-five percent of persons with blindness are also intellectually disabled, with the highest rates of visual impairment occurring in those who are more severely intellectually disabled. Moreover, subtle problems in visual acuity and color blindness may be overlooked in individuals with intellectual disability. The rate of visual disability, depending on the level of intellectual disability, has been reported to be 15 times greater than the general population rate.

Hearing impairment occurs at three to four times the general population rate and is present in approximately 10% of intellectually disabled persons. Hearing problems in older individuals may be more common in certain syndromes, such as Down syndrome, in which there is an increased risk of otosclerosis. Like blindness, hearing impairment is also greatest among severely and profoundly intellectually disabled persons. Rates of hearing impairment are five to eight times greater in severe-to-profoundly intellectually disabled individuals and may require special diagnostic tests, such as evoked response audiometry, because of their unreliability in responding to standard assessment techniques. Speech and language disorders are among the most common disabilities of intellectually disabled persons, with rates of up to 80% in institutionalized severely and profoundly intellectually disabled individuals. Prevalence information on communication skills in nonverbal populations is limited. In noninstitutionalized intellectually disabled persons, rates for speech problems are triple that of the general population prevalence.

Seizure disorders are common in intellectually disabled persons. In institutional settings, approximately one-third (most often, severely intellectually disabled individuals) have seizure disorders. In noninstitutionalized groups, the rate of seizures is approximately 15% vs. 1.5% for a control group. Rates in the mild-to-moderately intellectually disabled group range from 3%–6% to 12%–18%, depending on the population studied. For more severely intellectually disabled individuals, approximately 33% have seizures. Patja et al. (2000) found that seizure disorders and hearing loss increased the relative risk for death at all levels of intellectual disability.

Cerebral palsy frequently co-occurs with intellectual disability. Severely intellectually disabled persons have a rate of cerebral palsy ranging from 30% to 60%. Certain forms of cerebral palsy are more often related to intellectual disability; for example, children with spastic quadriplegia and diplegia have a higher rate than those with the extrapyramidal forms.

PSYCHOPATHOLOGY IN INDIVIDUALS WITH INTELLECTUAL DISABILITY

The prevalence of psychopathology, the presence of both mental and behavioral disorders in children, adolescents, and adults with intellectual disability, is an important consideration. Basic information on the frequency or prevalence and the impact of psychopathology is limited. However, children with intellectual disability have a three- to fourfold greater risk of emotional and behavioral problems than do those who are not affected, using standard rating scales. Overall, the estimates of psychiatric disorders in those with intellectual disability, using the DSM Classification (DSM-IIIR) (American Psychiatric Association, 1987), range from 4% to 18% (Borthwick-Duffy and Eyman, 1990; Eaton and Menolascino, 1982; Jacobson, 1982; Rojahn et al., 1993). Fewer studies address the commonality of more specific disorders. For example, estimates of attention deficit/hyperactivity disorder range from 0.5% to 11%, disorders of conduct and oppositional defiant disorder from 0.5% to 12%, for anxiety disorders from 0.5% to 10%, and for mood disorders from 0.5% to 4% (Myers and Pueschel, 1991; Rojahn et al., 1993). These published estimates are in the same range or lower than studies of typically developing children in the general community. The reason for these differences and the accepted three- to fourfold increased risk may be linked to community-based studies that review clinical records rather than doing standardized assessments as proposed by the American Psychiatric Association and the National Association of Dual Diagnosis. The DSM criteria must be modified for use in intellectual disability, as have the ICD-10 criteria (World Health Organization, 1992).

Prevalence of Psychopathology

Until recently, comprehensive epidemiologic studies of mental disorders in persons with intellectual disability were limited in number and scope. These limitations are being reduced by study designs in prevalence studies that recognize that diagnosis is affected by the issues previously noted (Cooper, Melville, and Einfeld, 2003; Sovner, 1986) and by "diagnostic overshadowing" (Jopp and Keys, 2001; Reiss, Levitan, and Szysko, 1982). This term refers to situations in which the presence of severe intellectual disability is so clear that the significance of an associated mental disorder is minimized; for example, intellectual disability is given greater credence than concurrent emotional and behavior disorders that may be minimized in the context of the severity of intellectual disability. A severely intellectually disabled person who is withdrawn and asocial may be less likely to be diagnosed as depressed than a person with a normal IQ. The application of the DSM-IVTR multiaxial system that includes a separate axis for intellectual disability was designed to address this issue, allowing the diagnostic focus to specify mental or behavior disorder on Axis I and mental retardation (intellectual disability) on Axis II. As described in chapter 3, the DC-LC was designed to better account for the nature of the developmental disability when applying diagnostic criteria. The APA/NADD classification fulfills this purpose for DSM-IVTR.

Systematic studies are providing an appreciation for the true prevalence and complexity of psychopathology in persons with intellectual disability. Epidemiologic studies involving community samples indicate that children, adolescents, and adults with developmental disorders are at significant risk for the development of emotional and behavioral disturbances. Prevalence rates of psychiatric and behavior disorders generally range between approximately 10% and 39% (Borthwick-Duffy, 1994) depending on specific assessment procedures, diagnostic criteria, and the degree of intellectual disability manifested by the person. These rates vary greatly and represent up to a four- or fivefold increase over the prevalence of psychopathology in the general population, as shown in table 4-1. Kerker et al. (2004) carried out a systematic review of peer-reviewed materials on mental health status of people with intellectual disability. The authors point out two problems with published studies. First, evaluators have difficulty in making the diagnoses, and second, there are methodological limitations in published studies. Some studies with representative samples and systematic and reliable assessment procedures are available. An early report by Rutter, Tizard, and Whitmore (1970) reported that 30% to 40% of all 9- to 11-year-old children with intellectual disability living on the Isle of Wight manifested a psychiatric disorder, a prevalence several times higher than that found among children of average intelligence, in whom the rate was 6%.

Lund (1985) identified an epidemiologic sample of 302 adults with intellectual disability living in a region of Denmark. The sample was representative of the country as a whole and included subjects with a wide age and IQ range. Comprehensive neuropsychiatric evaluations were conducted. Twenty-seven percent of the subjects received psychiatric diagnoses using modified DSM-III criteria. A wide range of disorders was diagnosed, including affective, anxiety, schizophrenic, organic, and pervasive developmental disorders. Gostason (1985) applied a similar evaluation procedure to randomly selected groups of adults with and without intellectual disability who were living in Sweden. Psychiatric disorders were identified among three-fourths of the severely intellectually disabled subjects, one-third of the mildly intellectually disabled subjects, and one-fourth of the typically developing subjects. The severity of psychopathology paralleled the degree of intellectual impairment, as was the case in other studies.

With deinstitutionalization, it is critical to evaluate prevalence of mental disorder in community settings. Community surveys of noninstitutionalized persons with psychiatric and behavioral disorders also have found rates of 20% to 35% for behavioral and emotional disturbance in persons with intellectual disability

Table 4.1. Prevalence Studies of Psychiatric Disorder in Intellectual Disability

Study	Number	Sample Characteristics	Prevalence
Rutter, Tizard, & Whitmore (1970)	3,271	Population based; Isle of Wight	30–42% of 9- to 11-year-olds vs. 6–7% of controls
Jacobson (1982)	27,023	New York DD system case records (66% aged 21–64 years)	12.4% of adults (psychological symptoms)
Eaton & Menolascino (1982)	798	Participants in community-based ID programs	21% (referred for psychiatric diagnosis) 14% (psychiatric diagnosis)
Gostason (1985)	51 with severe ID 64 with mild ID 64 control cases	Swedish population-based adult sample	71% with severe ID 33% with mild ID 23% controls (DSM-III) 37% of severe ID 14% of mild ID 8% of control (CPRS)
Lund (1985)	302 (>19 years of age)	Danish population-based sample	28% (modified DSM-III)
Iverson & Fox (1989)	165	Random sample of adults receiving ID services in the midwestern U.S. (PIMRA survey)	36% of total sample 55% with mild ID 32% with moderate ID 26% with severe/profound ID
Reiss (1990)	205	Community-based day program, random selection (96% adults)	39% (using Reiss screen) 40% (psychological evaluation) 12% (using case records)
Borthwick-Duffy & Eyman (1990)	78,603	California DD system case records	10% of total cohort 16% with mild ID 9% with moderate ID 5% with severe ID 6% with profound ID
Cooper and Bailey (2001)	207	Population-based in the UK	49.2% (according to PPS-LD)
Deb, Thomas, & Bright (2001)	90 (Ages 16–64)	Random selection community sample Mini-PAS-ADD for psychiatric disorder	16% ICD-10 diagnosis 4.4% schizophrenia 2.2% depressive disorder 2.2% GAD 4.4% phobic disorder 1.0% delusional disorder
Deb, Thomas, & Bright (2001)	101 (Ages 16–64)	Random selection community sample (Disability Assessment Schedule)	60.4% one behavior 23% aggression 24% self-injury 26% temper tantrum 26% overactivity 29% screaming 38% attention seeking 20% objectionable habits 18% nighttime disturbance 12% destructiveness

Key: (PAS-ADD) Psychiatric Assessment Schedule for Adults with Developmental Disability; (CPRS) Comprehensive Psychopathological Rating Scales; (DSM-III-R) Diagnostic and Statistical Manual, 3rd edition-Revised; (PIMRA) Psychopathology Instrument for Mentally Retarded Adults; (DD) developmental disability; (ID) intellectual disability; (PPS-LD) Present Psychiatric State for Adults with Learning Disabilities; (Mini-PAS-ADD) Mini-Psychiatric Assessment Schedule for Adults with Developmental Disability.

(Parsons, May, and Menolascino, 1984). Symptomatic forms (symptoms linked to brain) of mental disorder related to associated brain dysfunction occur at high rates. Schizophrenia has been reported in 2% to 3% of persons with intellectual disability (Reid, 1989), a prevalence that includes symptomatic forms. Both major depression and bipolar disorder may occur, but prevalence rates have not been systematically determined and vary by syndrome. Anxiety disorders, obsessive compulsive, and repetitive behavior disorders and phobias may be diagnosed at higher rates than in the general population; however, there is no established evidence that, overall, persons with intellectual disability have greater vulnerability to affective or anxiety disorders (Stark et al., 1988). However, there is variability among syndromes in the rates of these disorders.

Case studies from clinical records may underrepresent the true frequency of psychopathology (Reiss, 1990). Dekker and Koot (2003) sought to estimate the one-year prevalence of anxiety disorders, mood disorders, and disruptive behavioral disorders, including AD/HD, using DSM-IV (American Psychiatric Association, 1994) criteria in persons with intellectual disability. They wanted to evaluate differences in frequency in a community-based sample of children with borderline-to-moderate degrees of intellectual disability using the standardized instrument, the DISC-IV-P (Shaffer et al., 2000a and 2000b). Dekker and Koot (2003) further assessed prevalence, comorbidity and impact of DSM-IV disorders in 7–20-year-olds with borderline-to-moderate intellectual disability. A total of 474 individuals were randomly selected among students in Dutch schools for the intellectually disabled. Parents completed anxiety, mood, and disruptive behavior modules of the Diagnostic Interview Schedule for Children. In this study, 21.9% met DSM-IV symptom criteria for anxiety disorder, 4.4% for mood disorder, and 25.1% for disruptive behavior disorder. More than 50% of those meeting criteria for a DSM-IV disorder were severely impaired in their everyday living, and 37% of this group had a comorbid disorder diagnosis. Those with multiple diagnoses were more likely to be impaired. In regard to service delivery, 25% of those diagnosed had received mental health care in the previous year. The authors concluded that most disorders can be observed in children, adolescents, and young adults and that impairment and comorbidity are high. It is of concern that less than one-third of those with identified psychopathology had received mental health attention.

FUTURE RESEARCH

The NIH workshop Emotional and Behavioral Health in Persons with Mental Retardation and Developmental Disabilities: Research Challenges and Opportunities (2001) identified needed areas for future research in epidemiology. The participants emphasized the identification of risk and protective factors and the establishment of the natural history of various etiologies of intellectual disability. They asked that careful attention be paid to the consideration of research designs, research strategies, and approaches. Noting that there are few studies on service utilization, and taking into account the emphasis on supports in the AAMR definition and the International Classification of Functioning, a crucial research question is: Which new data are needed in order to design and conduct research aimed at improving the functioning of persons with mental retardation?

The expert group identified the following critical issues:

1. There is a lack of adequate data on risk and protective factors in people at different developmental stages, including preschool, school entry, school-to-work transition, and aging.
2. Study of the interaction between genes and the environment is needed. It is expected that variations in the heritability of behavioral or cognitive traits will be observed across different social levels and environmental conditions.
3. Issues in sampling and measuring behavior and related characteristics, including adaptative behavior, are critically important.
4. Ensuring adequate sample sizes is paramount. For example, many individuals with mild intellectual disability may be difficult to identify beyond the school years. In addition, recruiting adequate numbers of individuals with more rare neurogenetic syndromes may be difficult.
5. There is a need to examine behavioral features, emotional problems, and psychiatric diagnoses in groups with specific neurodevelopmental syndromes, including Down syndrome, fragile X, and Prader-Willi syndrome.
6. Systems research studies, including investigations focusing on state systems, residential units, group homes, supported living and prison settings, are needed.

To address these critical issues, the group recommended the following:

1. Conduct longitudinal studies to examine key life-stage transitions regarding risk and protective factors. Comparisons of such factors as time of diagnosis of the disorder, residential status, and family functioning should be made. Both concurrent longitudinal designs and case-control designs for behavioral genetics research and nonconcurrent longitudinal designs that make use of record linkages are needed.
2. Use informative samples and innovative research designs for behavioral genetic research, including twin pairs studied from birth and informative family and sibling studies.
3. Develop and refine an array or measures of outcomes and measures of hypothesized risk and protective factors.
4. Ensure that those with mild intellectual disability or rare neurogenetic disorders are sampled adequately. Utilize opportunities to piggyback on existing surveys, such as the CDC health risk behavior surveys and the National Health Interview Survey.
5. Conduct syndrome-specific cohort studies to ascertain specific vulnerabilities to common disorders, inform analysis of interactions between genes, brain, and behavior, and improve understanding of functioning.
6. Target state systems, schools, residential units, group home, supported living, and prison settings using system research studies. Understudied

areas in systems research include factors leading to the success or failure of de-institutionalization and the probable increase in use of medications during the past decade.

SUMMARY

Establishing how common intellectual disability is and who is affected depends on the age group being considered (infant, preschool, school age, adult, or elderly), the person's gender, the method used to define cases (statistical, pathological, social systems, or developmental), the state one lives in, the purpose of the survey (planning services), local environmental risk factors (eg., lead poisoning and alcohol abuse), psychosocial and socioeconomic considerations, the extent of intellectual disability (mild, moderate, severe, or profound), and the availability of preventive services. Although the average rate is approximately 1% of the general population, the use of this percentage for planning purposes is not precise; utilizing prevalence based on age cohort and demographic factors is more appropriate. Because there are many causes, there are many opportunities for prevention. As new causes are determined and new treatments are developed, the overall rate may be reduced in the general population. Additional studies are needed to determine the extent of the dual diagnosis of psychiatric or behavioral disorder and intellectual disability and the impact of the co-occurring diagnosis on the ability to utilize and participate in preventive services. Finally, a developmental model that focuses on early and continuing intervention with positive supports may result in more individuals working at their capacity. If so, it will be important to ask whether a person with intellectual disability who is working at his or her ability level and using his or her full capacity should be referred to as intellectually disabled.

KEY POINTS

1. Epidemiology:
   A. Provides a basis for understanding the distribution and dynamics of health and illness in persons with developmental disability.
   B. Enhances our understanding of the nature and scope of intellectual disability and of associated general medical, behavioral, emotional, and psychiatric disorders.
   C. Establishes prevalence of disorders and determines developmental trajectories of disorders and factors that influence those trajectories.
   D. Emphasizes both risk and protective factors; these may be neurobiologic, environmental, or a combination of both.
   E. Facilitates our understanding of the working and impact of health services on the lives of persons with intellectual disability.
2. Intellectual disability is the most common developmental disorder and ranks first among chronic conditions beginning in childhood that limit full participation in society.

3. There is a wide variability in prevalence estimates due to the multiple causes of intellectual disability and variations in methods used for screening.

4. Prevalence studies require both general population surveys and separate prevalence surveys for specific syndromes, such as Down syndrome and fragile X syndrome.

5. At least three approaches have been used to identify cases: statistical models, pathological models, and social systems models.

6. A developmental approach to intellectual disability is critical; it is a dynamic one and emphasizes personal engagement with other persons and the environment.

7. A developmental approach emphasizes fluid intelligence. It addresses how cognitive inefficiency affects social and environmental adaptation and how an individual reasons when faced with a task that must be understood and solved.

8. Due to differences in case identification, state prevalence estimates vary considerably.

9. Reduction in poverty, improved nutrition, newborn-screening programs, improved obstetrical care, and preschool interventions affect prevalence.

10. Among the psychosocial factors affecting prevalence are normalization programs, mainstreaming, and inclusion programs for persons who have been educationally and socially deprived.

11. Improved quality of life through early interventions that result in a longer life span affects prevalence rates.

12. The prevalence of emotional, behavioral, and psychiatric disorders is three- to fourfold greater in persons with intellectual disability.

References

American Psychiatric Association. (1994). *Diagnostic and statistical manual of mental disorders,* 4th ed. (DSM-IV). Author, Washington, DC.

American Psychiatric Association, Committee on Nomenclature and Statistics. (1987). *Diagnostic and statistical manual of mental disorders,* 3rd ed., revised. Author, Washington, DC.

Baird, P.A., and Sadovnick, A.D. (1985). Mental retardation in over half-a-million consecutive live births: An epidemiologic study. *American Journal of Mental Deficiency,* 89:323.

Bittles, A.H., Petterson B.A., Sullivan, S.G., Hussain, R., Glasson, E.J., Montgomery, P.D. (2002). The Influence of Intellectual Disability on Life Expectancy. *The Journals of Gerontology, Series A Biological Sciences and Medical Sciences,* 57A: M470–M472.

Borthwick-Duffy, S.A. (1994). Epidemiology and prevalence of psychopathology in people with mental retardation. *Journal of Consulting and Clinical Psychology,* 62:17–27.

Borthwick-Duffy, S.A., and Eyman, R.K. (1990). Who are the dually diagnosed? *American Journal on Mental Retardation,* 94:586–595.

Boyle, C.A., Yeargin-Allsopp, M., Doernberg, N.S., Holmgreen, P., Murphy, C.C., and Schendel, D.E. (1996). Prevalence of selected developmental disabilities in children 3–10 years of age: The Metropolitan Atlanta Developmental Disabilities Surveillance Program, 1991. *Morbidity and Mortality Weekly Report CDC Surveillance Summaries,* 45:1–14.

Brooks-Gunn, J., Klebanov, P., and Duncan, G.J. (1996). Ethnic differences in children's intelligence tests: Role of economic deprivation, home environment, and maternal characteristics. *Child Development,* 67:396–408.

Committee on Disability Determination for Mental Retardation (2002). *Mental Retardation: Determining Eligibility for Social Security Benefits,* p. 140. D.J. Reschly, T.G. Myers, and C.R. Hartel (eds.). National Academy Press, Washington, DC.

Cooper, S.A., and Bailey, N.M. (2001). Psychiatric disorders amongst adults with learning disabilities—prevalence and relationship to ability level. *Irish Journal of Psychological Medicine,* 18:45–53.

Cooper, S.A., Melville C.A., and Einfeld S.L. (2003). Psychiatric diagnosis, intellectual disabilities and diagnostic criteria for psychiatric disorders for use with adults with learning disabilities/mental retardation (DC-LD). *Journal of Intellectual Disability Research,* 47:3–15.

Davidson, P.W., Heller, T., Janicki, M.P., and Hyer, K. (2003). The Tampa Scientific Conference on Intellectual Disability, Aging and Health, p.5. Chicago: Rehabilitation and Research Training Center on Aging with Developmental Disabilities, University of Illinois at Chicago.

Deb, S., Thomas, M., and Bright, C. (2001). Mental disorder in adults with intellectual disability. I: Prevalence of psychiatric illness among a community based population aged between 16 and 64 years. *Journal of Intellectual Disability,* 45:495–505.

Dekker, M.C., and Koot, H.M. (2003). DSM-IV disorders in children with borderline to moderate intellectual disability. I: Prevalence and impact. *Journal of the American Academy of Child and Adolescent Psychiatry,* 42:915–922.

Demetriou, A., Christou, C., Spanoudis, G., and Platsidou, M. (2002) The development of mental processing: Efficacy, working memory, and thinking. *Monographs of the Society for Research in Child Development,* 67(1, Serial No. 268):122–133.

Drews, C.D., Yeargin-Alsopp, M., Decoufle, P., and Murphy, C.C. (1995). Variation in the influence of selected socio-demographic risk factors for mental retardation. *American Journal of Public Health,* 85:329–334.

Eaton, L.F., and Menolascino, F.J. (1982). Psychiatric disorders in the mentally retarded: Types, problems, and challenges. *American Journal of Psychiatry,* 139:1297–1303.

Eyman, R.F., Grossman, H.J., Choney, R.H., and Call, T.L. (1990). The life expectancy of profoundly handicapped people with mental retardation. *New England Journal of Medicine,* 323:584–589.

Frankenberger, W., and Harper, J. (1988). States' definitions and procedures for identifying children with mental retardation: Comparison of 1981–1982 and 1985–1986 guidelines. *Mental Retardation,* 26:133–136.

Gostason, R. (1985). Psychiatric illness in the mentally retarded: A Swedish population study. *Acta Psychiatrica Scandinavia,* 71:3–117.

Grossman, H.J. (1983). *Manual on Terminology and Classification in Mental Retardation,* revised ed. American Association on Mental Deficiency, Washington, DC.

Gustafson, J.E., and Undheim, J.O. (1996). Individual differences in cognitive functions. In D.C. Berliner and R.C. Calfee (eds.). *Handbook of Educational Psychology,* pp. 186–242. MacMillan. New York.

Herbst, D.S., and Baird, P.A. (1983). Nonspecific mental retardation in British Columbia as ascertained through a registry. *American Journal of Mental Deficiency,* 87:506–513.

Holtzman, N. (2003). Expanding newborn screening: How good is the evidence? JAMA. 290:2606–2608. (http://genes-r-us.uthscsa.edu/resources/newborn/screenstatus.htm)

Inhelder, B. [1943] (1968). (B. Stephens, trans.) *The diagnosis of reasoning in the mentally retarded.* The John Day Company, New York.

Iverson, J.C., and Fox, R.A. (1989). Prevalence of psychopathology among mentally retarded adults. *Research in Developmental Disabilities*, 10:77–83.

Jacobson, J.W. (1982). Problem behavior and psychiatric impairment within a developmentally disabled population. I: Behavior frequency. *Applied Research in Mental Retardation,* 3:121–139.

Janicki, M.P., Dalton, A.J., Henderson, C.M., and Davidson, P.W. (1999). Mortality and morbidity among older adults with intellectual disability: Health services considerations. *Disability and Rehabilitation,* 21:284–94.

Jopp, D.A., and Keys, C.B. (2001). Diagnostic overshadowing reviewed and reconsidered. *American Journal of Mental Retardation,* 106:416–433.

Kanner, L. (1964). *A history of the care and study of the mentally retarded.* Charles C. Thomas, Springfield, IL.

Kerker, B.D., Owens, P.L., Zigler, E., and Horwitz, S.M. (2004). Mental health disorders among individuals with mental retardation: Challenges to accurate prevalence estimates. *Public Health Report,* 119:409–417.

Kiely, M. (1987). The prevalence of mental retardation. *Epidemiology Review,* 9:194–218.

Koller, H., Richardson, S.W., Katz, M., and McLaren, J. (1983). Behavioral disturbance since childhood among a 5-year birth cohort of all mentally young adults in a city. *American Journal of Mental Deficiency,* 87:386.

Lund, J. (1985). The prevalence of psychiatric morbidity in mentally retarded adults. *Acta Psychiatrica Scandinavia,* 72:563–570.

Myers, B.A., and Pueschel, S.M. (1991). Psychiatric disorders in persons with Down syndrome. *Journal of Nervous and Mental Disease,* 179:609–613.

Munro, J.D. (1986). Epidemiology and the extent of mental retardation. In C. Stavrakaki (ed.), Psychiatric perspectives on mental retardation. *Psychiatric Clinics of North America,* 9:591–624.

Murphy, C.C., Yeargin-Allsopp, M., Decoufle, P., and Drews, C.D. (1995). Administrative prevalence of mental retardation in 10-year-old children, metropolitan Atlanta, 1985 through 1987. *American Journal of Public Health,* 85:319–23.

NIH Workshop. (2001). *Emotional and behavioral health in persons with mental retardation and developmental disabilities: Research challenges and opportunities.* Nov. 29–Dec. 1, 2001, Rockville, MD. http://ord.aspensys.com/asp/workshops/search.asp

Parsons, J.A., May J.G., and Menolascino, F.J. (1984). The nature and incidence of mental illness in mentally retarded individuals. In F.J. Menolascino and J.A. Stark (eds.), *Handbook of mental illness in mentally retarded individuals,* pp. 3–44. Plenum Press, New York.

Pasnak, R., Wilson-Quayle, A. and Whitten, J. (1998) Mild retardation, academic achievement, and Piagetian or psychometric tests of reasoning. *Journal of Developmental and Physical Disabilities.* 10:23–33.

Patja, K., Ivanainen, M., Vesala, H., Oksanen, H. and Ruoppila, I. (2000). Life expectancy of people with intellectual disability: a 35-year follow-up study. *Journal of Intellectual Disability Research,* 44:591–599.

Reid, A. (1989). Schizophrenia in mental retardation: Clinical features. *Research in Developmental Disabilities,* 10:241–249.

Reiss, S., (1990). Prevalence of dual diagnosis in community-based day programs in the Chicago metropolitan area. *American Journal on Mental Retardation,* 94:578–585.

Reiss, S., Levitan, G.W., and Szysko, I. (1982). Emotional disturbance and mental retardation: Diagnostic overshadowing. *American Journal of Mental Deficiency,* 86: 567–574.

Reschly, D.J., and Jipson, F.J. (1976). Ethnicity, geographic locale, age, sex, and urban-rural residence as variables in the prevalence of mild retardation. *American Journal of Mental Deficiency,* 81:154–161.

Rojahn, J., Borthwick-Duffy, S.A., and Jacobson, J.W. (1993). The association between psychiatric diagnoses and severe behavior problems in mental retardation. *Annals of Clinical Psychiatry,* 5:163–170.

Rutter, M, Tizard, J., and Whitmore, K. (eds.). (1970). *Education, health and behaviour.* Longman, London.

Schupf, N., Pang, D., Patel, B.N., Silverman, W., Schuber, R., La, F., Kline, J.K., Stern, Y., Ferin, M., Tycko, B., and Mayeux, R. (2003). Onset of dementia is associated with age at menopause in women with Down's syndrome. *Annals of Neurology,* 54: 433–438.

Schretlen, D., Hobholz, J.H., and Brandt, J. (1996). Development and psychometric properties of the Brief Test of Attention. *The Clinical Neuropsychologist,* 10:80–89.

Shaffer, D., Fisher, P., Lucas, C., and Comer, J. (2000a). *Scoring Manual Diagnostic Interview Schedule for Children (DISC-IV).* Columbia University, New York.

Shaffer, D., Fisher, P., Lucas, C., Dulcan, M.K., and Schwab-Stone, M.E. (2000b). NIMH Diagnostic Interview Schedule for Children Version IV (NIMHDISC-IV): description, differences from previous versions, and reliability of some common diagnoses. *Journal of the American Academy of Child and Adolescent Psychiatry,* 39:28–38.

Sovner, R. (1986). Limiting factors in the use of DSM-III criteria with mentally ill/mentally retarded persons. *Psychopharmacology Bulletin,* 22:1055–1059.

Stark, J.A., Menolascino, F.J., Albarelli, M.H., and Gray, V.C. (1988). *Mental retardation and mental health: Classification, diagnosis, treatment, services.* Springer-Verlag, New York.

Uzgiris, I.C., and Hunt, J.M. (1975). *Assessment in infancy: Ordinal scale of psychological development.* University of Illinois Press, Urbana.

World Health Organization. (1992). *The ICD-10 classification of mental and behavioral disorders: clinical descriptions and diagnostic guidelines.* Author, Geneva, Switzerland.

Yeargin-Allsopp, M., Drews, C.D., Decoufle, P., and Murphy, C.C. (1995). Mild mental retardation in black and white children in metropolitan Atlanta: A case-control study. *American Journal of Public Health,* 85:324–328.

Yeargin-Allsopp, M., Murphy, C.C., Codero, J.F. Decoufle, P., and Hollowell, J.G. (1997). Reported biomedical causes and associated medical conditions for mental retardation among 10-year-old children, Metropolitan Atlanta, 1985–1987. *Developmental Medicine and Child Neurology,* 39:142–149.

Yeargin-Allsopp, M., Murphy, C.C., Murphy, C.C., Oakley, G.P., and Sikes, R.K. (1992). A multiple source method for studying the prevalence of developmental disabilities in children: The Metropolitan Atlanta Developmental Disabilities Study. *Pediatrics,* 89:624–630.

Zigler, E. (1967). Familial mental retardation: A continuing dilemma. *Science,* 155:292–298.

5

Etiology and Assessment

Intellectual disability is a general term that describes intellectual capacity and adaptive functioning. There are many causes and many co-occurring conditions. To appreciate and respect the uniqueness of each individual and to choose appropriate interventions, it is critical that, if possible, the cause for intellectual disability be identified or the conditions that led to or sustain it be recognized. This chapter begins with an overview followed by an approach to understanding causation, a description of how etiology is determined, consideration of the neurobiological/environmental interface, a discussion of the evaluation process to determine causes and conditions related to diagnoses, and a discussion of risk factors.

OVERVIEW

Intellectual disability is an intellectual, cognitive, and developmental disability that profoundly affects an individual's functioning and adaptation to everyday life. Intellect refers to mental ability or capacity, the power of thought, and the ability to reason and solve problems. Mental capacity is distinguished from perception, emotions, and feelings. Intelligence refers to facility and quickness in understanding and problem solving. In intellectual disability, there is reduced mental capacity. Cognition refers to the use or handling of knowledge through mental activities associated with thinking, learning, and memory, which are necessary processes to acquire knowledge. In intellectual disability, there are cognitive disabilities that vary depending on the individual syndrome. The extent of intellectual disability varies among syndromes, and there may be variations within a syndrome. Both cognition and intellect are linked to cortical brain function. Intellectual disability is a developmental disability with onset during the developmental period. Thus, there are delays in meeting developmental milestones in motor, fine motor, language, and psychosocial areas. Finally, there are difficulties in adaptive function and in the mastery of developmental tasks as a result of intellectual, cognitive, and developmental disabilities. A focus on the etiology of intellectual disability is needed for research, clinical, and administrative purposes.

This chapter will review the multiple causes of intellectual disability, considering the interface between genetic, neurobiologic, and environmental factors and causation. It emphasizes the importance of a comprehensive evaluation and provides guidelines for conducting an evaluation. Associated mental, emotional, and behavioral disorders are discussed in chapter 6.

MULTIPLICITY OF CAUSES

Multiple causes of intellectual disability reflect a complex interaction involving genetic predisposition, environmental insults, developmental vulnerability, heredity, and environment. The AAMR considers biomedical, social, behavioral, and educational risk factors (Luckasson et al., 2002). Genetic predisposition must take into account individual susceptibilities to the influence of environmental agents. Genetic damage is particularly likely when exposure occurs during periods of gene (DNA) replication or of gene expression. Genetic influences may be based on the failure of expression of specific genes in neurogenetic syndromes involving single genes, such as phenylketonuria (PKU), or contiguous genes, as in Williams syndrome, or they may involve multiple genes or gene-environmental interactions.

Genetics and Epigenesis

Genes play a major role in the transmission of intelligence, as documented in studies of twin pairs and adoption studies. General intelligence, Spearman's g, is a better predictor and is implicated in a wider range of behaviors than any other psychological construct. General intelligence is made up of basic cognitive processes that are integrated into a complex system in the brain. The general intelligence factor accounts for up to 50% of the variance between individuals on intelligence tests. General cognitive ability is a key factor in learning and memory and is among the most heritable behavioral traits. It is thought that much of the association between intelligence and speed of information processing is due to a common gene or set of genes. Genetic effects on various cognitive abilities are general rather than involving specific modules (Plomin and Craig, 2001).

From an evolutionary perspective, there may be sufficient continuity in development that animal studies may contribute to the understanding of human intelligence. Indeed, in mice studies, Matzel et al. (2003) found that a single factor accounted for 38% of the total variance among mice on tests of associative fear conditioning, operant avoidance, path integration, discrimination, and spatial navigation. Moreover, two genes, *ASPM* and *microcephalin*, have been implicated in the evolution of brain size. Both are associated with genetic forms of microcephaly in humans (Evans et al., 2004)

Research on the molecular basis of intellectual disability has focused on differences in gene sequences that may occur with chromosomal aberrations (e.g., Down syndrome), deletions (e.g., Cri du Chat syndrome), or microdeletions (e.g., Williams syndrome); however, it is non–sequence-based or "epigenetic" mechanisms that regulate gene transcription, resulting, for example, in instances of discordance in monozygotic twins and non-Mendelian forms of heredity. Epigenetic mechanisms, including methylation (important in fragile X syndrome), acetylation, and phosphorylation of protein-DNA complexes, may be involved in the environmental regulation of gene expression. Such changes are time-dependent and may be localized to a particular cell type or gene region. Therefore, it is important not only to find gene sequence variations but also to understand how both environmental and developmental factors alter gene expression.

Understanding epigenesis is especially important. The term "epigenetic" was introduced in 1939 by Conrad Waddington when he contrasted genetics with epigenetics. Epigenetics is the study of processes by which genotypes give rise to phenotypes as the developmental program unfolds. It refers to the processes in which more complex structures emerge during development.

Epigenetic changes, in comparison with genetic changes, are more gradual. For example, fragile X syndrome is the result when a CGG repeat in the *FMR1* 5' untranslated region expands and is methylated de novo, causing the gene to be silenced and producing a "fragile" site on the X chromosome. The fact that a chromosomal anomaly is produced indicates that epigenetic factors may affect chromosomal architecture.

Epigenetic may refer to developmental modulation of cell phenotype that is always nuclear but not sequence-related (Holliday, 2002); Lederberg (2001) proposes the term "epinucleic" as a more specific descriptor for this developmental process. In this sense, it refers to changes in nuclear inheritance that are not coded in the DNA sequence itself. In the sense that Waddington initially used the term "epigenetic," there are also developmental processes that do depend on sequence-related changes, such as cellular senescence following telomere shortening. Overall, three systems interact and stabilize each other to regulate genes (Egger et al., 2004). These include DNA methylation, RNA-associated silencing of genes, and histone modification. Histones are important parts of the DNA control system and associate with DNA, enabling the packaging of DNA into chromosomes.

Endogenous and Exogenous Toxins

Nutritional status, exposure to endogenous and exogenous toxins, microorganisms, radiation, and other psychosocial stressors impact the developing brain. The developmental timing of exposure to potentially hazardous environmental agents is a crucial consideration. The severity of resulting intellectual disability may be related to the timing of the insult to the central nervous system. Prenatal factors that affect the developing fetal brain are responsible for 55%–75% of persons with severe intellectual disability and for 25%–40% of persons with mild intellectual disability. The time during the developmental period when exposure to a risk factor occurs can be critical. Exposure of the fetus to the rubella virus during the first trimester of pregnancy can lead to major congenital anomaly and intellectual disability, and exposure to the same virus later in gestation or during the postnatal period leads to a mild infectious disease. Thalidomide embryopathy affecting the fetus at approximately day 20–24 after conception has been associated with autistic disorder (Stromland et al., 1994).

Identifying Neurobiological Etiologies

Advances in biomedical technology now allow identification of a neurobiological etiology for an increasing number of intellectual disability syndromes. A specific cause for intellectual disability can be identified in approximately two-thirds of cases. The more severe the degree of intellectual disability, the greater the likelihood a specific cause will be uncovered. For example, a cause can be confirmed for approximately 80% of those with severe intellectual disability. Neurobiological factors also play a significant etiological role in mild intellectual disability and in borderline intellectual functioning. A variety of biomedical abnormalities, including chromosomal abnormalities, perinatal trauma, and exposure to toxic substances, may be responsible for 30%–45% of cases of mild intellectual disability (Hagberg et al., 1981; Lamont and Dennis, 1988), and in 25%–30% of those with borderline intellectual functioning. These results have led to a reexamination of the causative role of psychosocial disadvantage and polygenic inheritance in mild intellectual disability and borderline functioning.

Intellectual disability is associated with immature morphology of synaptic spines, structures involved in neurotransmission and memory processes, suggesting that intellectual disability is linked to a deficiency in neuronal network formation. Dendritic abnormalities are proposed as anatomical correlates of intellectual disability in several syndromes. Although dendritic spine dysgenesis initially was associated with unclassified intellectual disability, it is found in specific genetic syndromes associated with intellectual disability (Kauffman and Moser, 2000). Well-defined dendritic anomalies that involve dendritic branches and/or spines include Down syndrome, Rett's disorder, and fragile-X syndrome. Dendritic pathology is suggested in Williams and Rubinstein-Taybi syndromes based on cytoarchitectonic analyses. Such dendritic abnormalities in syndromes seem to have syndrome-specific evolution and pathogenesis that might correlate with their cognitive deficit profile. Animal models of specific syndromes are being used to document abnormalities in dendritic architecture.

The recent cloning of eight genes which cause nonspecific intellectual disability, when mutated, may provide a window into the cellular mechanisms that result in dendritic abnormalities that may underlie intellectual disability. Investigation of the roles of these genes in neuronal development and function may lead to a better understanding of the cellular mechanisms underlying intellectual disability. Three of the encoded proteins, oligophrenin1, PAK3 and alphaPix, interact directly with Rho GTPases. Rho GTPases are key signaling proteins which integrate extracellular and intracellular signals to orchestrate coordinated changes in the actin cytoskeleton, essential for directed neurite outgrowth and the generation/rearrangement of synaptic connectivity. It is becoming more clear how mutations that cause abnormal Rho signaling result in abnormal neuronal connectivity which may result in deficient cognitive functioning.

These Rho proteins act as molecular switches which integrate extracellular and intracellular signals to regulate rearrangement of the actin cytoskeleton. Since the actin cytoskeleton mediates neuronal motility and morphogenesis, one can envision how mutations in proteins involved in Rho-dependent signaling result in intellectual disability by altering neuronal network formation (van Galen and Ramakers, 2005; Ramakers, 2002).

CLASSIFICATION OF ETIOLOGIES

The classification of causes of intellectual disability has generally focused on the timing of the damage to the central nervous system. It has been estimated that between 30% and 50% of developmental disorders involve some temporal risk factors. The AAMR (Luckasson et al., 1992; Luckasson et al., 2002) includes prenatal causes (chromosomal disorders, single-gene disorders, syndrome disorders, inborn errors of metabolism, developmental disorders of brain formation, gestational substance abuse, and environmental influences); perinatal causes (intrauterine disorders, prematurity, birth injury, and neonatal disorders); and postnatal causes (traumatic brain injury, infections, demyelinating disorders, degenerative disorders, seizure disorders, toxic metabolic disorders, malnutrition, environmental deprivation, and hypoconnection syndrome). Some disease categories involve abnormalities that, although prenatal in origin, may not be evident until postnatal life. The best known of these include single-gene metabolic disorders (e.g., PKU) whose manifestations are not seen at birth. Some chromosomal syndromes may increase susceptibility to perinatal trauma; for example, inadequate central respiratory control in a syndrome may increase the risk of brain damage due to lack of oxygen (hypoxic, ischemic damage).

More than 750 genetic disorders are associated with intellectual disability. Approximately 25% of known genetic conditions exert their primary clinical effects on the brain, and others may lead to secondary effects to the central nervous system (table 5.1). Table 5.1 lists four clusters of prenatal causes for intellectual disability, which are primarily genetic disorders. Among these are chromosomal disorders, syndromic disorders whose genetics are increasingly being identified, inborn errors of metabolism, developmental disorders of brain formation, and disorders caused by environmental influences.

The section that follows provides background information on classic Mendelian and non-Mendelian forms of inheritance that is needed to understand genetic disorders. Examples of these mechanisms in particular syndromes are provided in table 5.2.

Table 5.1 Disorders Associated with Intellectual Disability with Selected Examples

I. PRENATAL CAUSES

A. Chromosomal Disorders
 1. Autosomes
   a. 4p-
   b. Ring 13
   c. Trisomy 18 (Edwards)
   d. Trisomy 21 (Down)
   e. Translocation 21 (Down)
 2. X-Linked Mental Retardation
   a. Fragile X syndrome
   b. Glycerol kinase deficiency
   c. Juberg syndrome
   d. Renpenning syndrome
 3. Other X Chromosome Disorders
   a. XO syndrome (Turner)
   b. XYY syndrome
   c. XXY syndrome (Klinefelter)
   d. XXXXX syndrome (penta-X)
 4. Uniparental Dysomy
   a. Prader-Willi syndrome
   b. Angelman's syndrome

B. Syndrome Disorders
 1. Neurocutaneous Disorders
   a. Klippel-Trenaunay syndrome
   b. Neurofibromatosis (Type 1)
   c. Sturge-Weber syndrome
   d. Tuberous sclerosis
   e. Xeroderma pigmentosum
 2. Muscular Disorders
   a. Congenital muscular dystrophy
   b. Duchenne muscular dystrophy
   c. Myotonic muscular dystrophy
 3. Ocular Disorders
   a. Aniridia-Wilms' tumor syndrome
   b. Anophthalmia syndrome (X-linked)
   c. Lowe syndrome
 4. Craniofacial Disorders
   a. Acrocephalosyndactyly (e.g., Apert type)
   b. Craniofacial dysostosis (Crouzon)
   c. Multiple synostosis syndrome
 5. Skeletal Disorders
   a. Hereditary osteodystrophy (Albright)
   b. Klippel-Feil syndrome
   c. Osteopetrosis (Albers-Schonberg)
   d. Radial hypoplasia-pancytopenia syndrome (Fanconi)

C. Inborn Errors of Metabolism
 1. Amino Acid Disorders
   a. Phenylketonuria
   b. Histidinemia

   c. Branched-chain amino acid disorders
    1. Hyperleucine-isoleucinemia
    2. Maple-syrup urine disease
   d. Biotin-dependent disorder
   e. Propionic acidemia
   f. Methylmalonic acidemia
   g. Folate-dependent disorders
   h. Homocystinurian
   i. Hartnup disease
 2. Carbohydrate Disorders
   a. Glycogen storage disorders
   b. Galactosemia
   c. Pyruvic acid disorders
 3. Mucopolysaccharide Disorders
   a. Alpha-L-iduronidase deficiency (e.g., Hurler type)
   b. Iduronate sulfatase deficiency (Hunter type)
   c. Heparan N-sulfatase deficiency (Sanfilippo 3A type)
 4. Mucolipid Disorders
 5. Urea Cycle Disorders
   a. Ornithine transcarbamylase deficiency
   b. Arginase deficiency (argininemia)
 6. Nucleic Acid Disorders
   a. Lesch-Nyhan syndrome (HGPRTase deficiency)
   b. Orotic aciduria
 7. Copper Metabolism Disorders
   a. Wilson disease
   b. Menkes disease
 8. Mitochondrial Disorders
   a. Kearns-Sayre syndrome
 9. Peroxisomal Disorders
   a. Zellweger syndrome
   b. Adrenoleukodystrophy

D. Developmental Disorders of Brain Formation
 1. Neural Tube Closure Defects
   a. Anencephaly
   b. Spina bifida
 2. Brain Formation Defects
   a. Hydrocephalus
   b. Lissencephaly
   c. Polymicrogyria
 3. Cellular Migration Defects
   a. Abnormal layering of cortex
   b. Cortical microdysgenesis
 4. Intraneuronal Defects
   a. Dendritic spine abnormalities
   b. Microtubule abnormalities

5. Acquired Brain Defects
   a. Hydranencephaly
   b. Porencephaly
6. Primary (Idiopathic) Microcephaly

E. Environmental Influences
1. Intrauterine Malnutrition
   a. Maternal malnutrition
   b. Placental insufficiency (see Perinatal Causes)
2. Drugs, Toxins, and Teratogens
   a. Thalidomide
   b. Phenytoin (fetal hydantoin syndrome)
   c. Alcohol (fetal alcohol syndrome)
   d. Cocaine
   e. Methylmercury
3. Maternal Diseases
   a. Varicella
   b. Diabetes mellitus
   c. Hypothyroidism (fetal iodine deficiency)
   d. Maternal phenylketonuria
4. Irradiation During Pregnancy

II. PERINATAL CAUSES

A. Intrauterine Disorders
1. Acute Placental Insufficiency
   a. Placenta previa/hemorrhage
   b. Toxemia/eclampsia
2. Chronic Placental Insufficiency (marginal reserve)
   a. Postmaturity (involution)
   b. Erythroblastosis (edema)
   c. Maternal diabetes
3. Abnormal Labor and Delivery
   a. Premature labor (prematurity)
   b. Premature rupture of membranes
   c. Abnormal presentation (especially breech)
   d. Obstetrical trauma
4. Multiple Gestation (smaller, later, or male infant)

B. Neonatal Disorders
1. Hypoxic-Ischemic Encephalopathy
2. Intracrancial Hemorrhage
3. Posthemorrhagic Hydrocephalus
4. Periventricular Leukomalacia
5. Neonatal Seizures
6. Respiratory Disorders
   a. Hyaline membrane disease
7. Infections
   a. Septicemia
   b. Meningitis
   c. Encephalitis

8. Head Trauma at Birth
9. Metabolic Disorders
   a. Hyperbilirubinemia (kernicterus)
   b. Hypoglycemia
   c. Hypothyroidism
10. Nutritional Disorders
   a. Intestinal disorders
   b. Protein-calorie malnutrition

III. POSTNATAL CAUSES

A. Head Injuries
1. Cerebral concussion (diffuse axonal injury)
2. Cerebral contusion or laceration
3. Intracranial hemorrhage
4. Subarachnoid (with diffuse injury)

B. Infections
1. Encephalitis
   a. Herpes simplex
   b. Measles
   c. Human immunodeficiency virus
2. Meningitis
   a. Streptococcus pneumoniae
   b. Haemophilus influenzae, type B
   c. Mycobacterium tuberculosis
3. Parasitic Infestations
   a. Malaria
4. Slow or Persistent Virus Infections
   a. Measles (subacute sclerosing panencephalitis)
   b. Rubella (progressive rubella panencephalitis)

C. Demyelinating Disorders
1. Postinfectious Disorders
2. Postimmunization Disorders
   a. Postpertussis encephalopathy

D. Degenerative Disorders
1. Syndromic Disorders
   a. Rett syndrome
   b. Disintegrative psychosis (Heller)
2. Poliodystrophies
   a. Friedreich ataxia
3. Basal Ganglia Disorders
   a. Hallervorden-Spatz disease
   b. Huntington disease (juvenile type)
   c. Parkinson disease (juvenile type)
   d. Dystonia musculorum deformans
4. Leukodystrophies
   a. Pelizaeus-Merzbacher disease
   b. Adrenoleukodystrophy
   c. Galactosylceramidase deficiency (Krabbe)

(continued)

Table 5.1 (*continued*)

5. Sphingolipid Disorders
   a. Beta-galactosidase deficiency (GM1 gangliosidosis)
   b. Hexosaminidase A deficiency (Tay-Sachs)
6. Other Lipid Disorders
   a. Abetalipoproteinemia (Bassen-Kornzweig)

E. Seizure Disorders
1. Infantile Spasms
2. Myoclonic Epilepsy
3. Lennox-Gastaut Syndrome
4. Progressive Focal Epilepsy (Rasmussen)
5. Status epilepticus–induced brain injury

F. Toxic-Metabolic Disorders
1. Reye Syndrome
2. Intoxications
   a. Lead
   b. Mercury
3. Metabolic Disorders

G. Malnutrition
1. Protein-Calorie (PCM)
   a. Kwashiorkor
   b. Marasmus

H. Environmental Deprivation
1. Psychosocial Disadvantage
2. Child Abuse and Neglect
3. Chronic Social/Sensory Deprivation

I. Hypoconnection Syndrome

Adapted from Luckasson et al., 1992. Reprinted by permission of author from *Mental Retardation: Definition, Classification, and Systems of Support, 9th edition*. American Association on Mental Retardation, Washington, DC. Copyright © 1992.

Table 5.2 Mode of Inheritance of Selected Intellectual Disability Syndromes

Syndrome	Mode of Inheritance
Down	
95%	Trisomy 21
1.0%	Mosaic
4.0%	Robertsonian
	Translocation 21q/21q
Tay-Sachs Disease	Autosomal recessive
Hurler	Autosomal recessive
Hunter	X-Linked recessive
PKU	Autosomal recessive
Rett	Transcriptional derepression
Lesch-Nyhan	X-linked recessive
Prader-Willi	Cytogenetic
	Deletion/genomic imprinting (maternal)
Fragile X	Trinucleotide repeat expansion (heritable unstable DNA sequences)

PRENATAL CAUSES–GENETIC DISORDERS

There are three main types of genetic disorders.

Single-Gene Disorders (Abnormal Gene and Gene Product)

These are caused by mutant genes. The mutation may be on one of a pair of chromosomes, matched with a normal allele on the homologous chromosome, or on both of the chromosomes of a pair. In both instances, the result is an error in genetic information. Family studies show abnormal pedigree patterns. These conditions are rare, although for some disorders, their occurrence may be as frequent as 1/500 births. Over 3,000 of the more than 4,000 single-gene phenotypes are genetic disorders (McKusick, 1998). In many of these conditions, the gene has been isolated and cloned, that is, segments have been purified so that large amounts of the purified segment can be produced for study. In addition to nuclear genes, mitochondrial genes have been recognized as abnormal. These mitochondrially transmuted genes lead to another type of single-gene disorder.

Single-gene traits are often referred to as Mendelian because these traits segregate within families and on average are found in specific and fixed proportions when offspring whose parents have the trait are studied. Many single-gene diseases result in abnormalities at the protein or DNA levels. Contiguous gene disorders (microdeletion syndromes) may show a pedigree pattern that simulates a single-gene disorder even though the disorder does not have a single-gene basis. This type of disorder involves multiple gene loci that are adjacent to one another. Inherited single-gene disorders can usually be identified from other types of familial disorders by their typical Mendelian segregation ratios. Confirmation that it is a single-gene disorder may require demonstration of defects at the level of the gene product or gene.

The patterns of single-gene transmission depend on the location of the chromosomal locus, either autosomal or X-linked, and whether the phenotype is dominant or recessive. Dominant inheritance is expressed when the variant allele is carried by one chromosome of a pair, and recessive inheritance allele is expressed when both chromosomes of a pair carry the variant allele. Classically, the following four Mendelian patterns of the inheritance have been identified in single-gene disorders.

Autosomal Recessive

Recessive autosomal phenotypes account for approximately one-third of Mendelian phenotypes. Recessive disorders are only homozygotes, so a mutant allele must have been inherited from both parents. An autosomal recessive phenotype has a recurrence risk of one in four for each sibling of the proband. Parents may, in some cases, be consanguineous, and for most types, males and females are equally affected. When seen in more than one member of a kindred, the phenotype is found only in the sibling of the proband and not in their parents, their own children, or other relatives. An example of an autosomal recessive disorder is PKU, which if untreated may lead to developmental disability, seizures, behavioral disorder, and mental retardation. The basic defect is a mutation in the gene encoding phenylalanine hydroxylase. Build-up of phenylalanine damages the developing brain. The incidence of this disorder is 1:5,000–1:16,000 in Caucasians. The gene location is 12q22-q24, and there may be variation in expression.

Autosomal Dominant

Of the known Mendelian phenotypes, more than half are autosomal dominant traits (Nussbaum, McInnes and Willard, 2001). The phenotype appears in every generation, with each person having an affected parent (exceptions are fresh mutations and nonpenetrance); children of affected parents are at 50% risk of inheritance. Phenotypically normal individuals do not transmit the condition to their children. Male and females are equally likely to transmit to male or female offspring. Male-to-male transmission can occur and males may have unaffected daughters. An example that commonly involves the nervous system is neurofibromatosis (NF1); it occurs at an incidence of 1:3,000–1:5,000. This is a common autosomal dominant phenotype with full penetrance but with variation in expression from minimal to severe involvement. Gene location is 17q11.2.

X-linked Recessive

The incidence for X-linked recessive disorder is much greater in males than in females. The gene is transmitted from an affected male through all his daughters. The daughters' sons have a 50% chance of inheriting the disorder. It is never transmitted from father to son, but is transmitted by way of a series of females who are carriers. Ordinarily, heterozygous females are not affected, but in some disorders they may show the condition with varying degrees of severity. An example is Duchenne muscular dystrophy (DMD), which occurs in 1:3,000–1:3,500 male births. The basic defect, which leads to muscle degeneration, is an abnormality in the structural gene for the muscle protein dystropin. The gene location is Xp21. The dystropin gene was the first gene to be cloned based on knowledge of its chromosomal location.

X-linked Dominant

In this form of inheritance, in affected males with normal wives, all the daughters and none of the sons are affected. Each child, male or female, of an affected family member has a 50% chance of inheriting the phenotype just as in the autosomal dominant pedigree pattern. Although both sexes are affected, because of the severity of a condition, they may not reproduce. In very rare phenotypes, females are affected approximately twice as often as males, but often have a milder (although variable) form of the disorder. An example is X-linked hypophosphatemic rickets (vitamin D–resistant rickets), which affects the kidney tubules' ability to reabsorb phosphate. Both sexes are affected, but serum phosphate is less depressed and rickets less severe in heterozygous females.

Chromosomal Disorders (No Abnormal Gene or Gene Product)

Chromosomal abnormalities have been shown in more than 60 identifiable syndromes, represent 0.7% of live births, and account for half of spontaneous first trimester abortions. The major disorders of chromosomes are three autosomal trisomies (13, 18, and 21) and the four types of sex chromosomal aneuploidy: Turner's syndrome (ordinarily 45, X); Klinefelter syndrome (47, XXY); 47, XYY syndrome; and 47, XXX syndrome. There is no error in genetic information, that is, no mutation, but there is an excess or deficiency of genes in the whole chromosome or chromosomal segment. The chromosomal basis of a growing number of significant disorders has been demonstrated. These disorders occur in 7/1000 births and are responsible for approximately 50% of abortions. Down syndrome is an example of when an extra copy of chromosome 21 results in the most common intellectual disability syndrome, although no individual gene on the chromosome is abnormal.

Multifactorial Inheritance (No Single Error in Genetic Information; A Combination of Small Variations)

The greatest number of genetic phenotypes are found in families in which there is neither a single-gene mutation nor a chromosomal disorder; rather, these genetic phenotypes are multifactorial in origin. Multifactorial inheritance is defined as the inheritance of genetic factors and nongenetic factors, each of which is thought to have a small effect. In some instances, the role of environmental factors may be relatively large. In the multifactorial model, the disorder is familial, yet no distinctive pattern of inheritance is demonstrated in a family. Despite this, the recurrence risk is higher when more than one family member is affected in contrast to single-gene disorders in which the risk is unchanged from one child to the next. The risk is much lower for second-degree relatives than for first-degree relatives in contrast to autosomal dominant conditions in which the risk drops by half with each step of more distant relationship. In autosomal recessive conditions, it is the siblings and not other relatives who are at risk. In addition, more severely affected patients and their relatives are at greater risk. Finally, the risk to subsequent siblings is increased when the patients are consanguineous. A multifactorial threshold model that predicts that the risk for first-degree relatives is equal to the square root of the population incidence of a multifactorial trait has been developed. Such a relationship is not true for single-gene traits in which the risk for siblings is, for the most part, independent of population frequency.

Phenotypic Expression

Expression of abnormal genotype may be modified by other genetic loci and/or environmental factors. Differences in expression that are more often found in autosomal dominant conditions may lead to problems in diagnosis and in the interpretation of pedigrees. This is borne out in clinical experience where some disorders are not expressed at all in persons who are genetically predisposed. In other instances, there may be variability in clinical severity, age of onset, or both. Two important concepts in gene expression are penetrance and expressivity. Another variable in expression is age of onset. Some of the most severe neuropsychiatric disorders may have variable ages of onset. Finally, pleiotropy must be considered. Pleiotropy is a term used to describe multiple phenotypic effects of a single gene or gene pair.

Penetrance

Penetrance refers to the probability that a gene will have any phenotypic expression. It refers to all those who are actively affected. The term is used primarily for dominant traits in heterozygote carriers. It denotes the all-or-none expression of mutant genotypes. If less than 100% of the carriers of the responsible allele show the disorder, penetrance is reduced. If 60% of the carriers express it, it is 60% penetrant. It refers to the percentage of people who are actively affected. Failure of penetrance can lead to apparent skipping of generations in a family tree.

Expressivity

Expressivity indicates the degree or extent of expression of a genetic defect. A defect may show variable expressivity; the trait may vary in its expression from a mild to a severe form. In variable expressivity, the trait is expressed; it is never completely expressed in those who have that particular genotype. Many of the single-gene disorders show multiple characteristic effects. Differences may be seen in the range of abnormalities present and in the severity of the particular manifestation. Examples of gene disorders that show considerable variation in expression include Neurofibromatosis 1 and Marfan's syndrome.

Nonclassical Patterns of Inheritance

Recent genetic study has resulted in the description of non-Mendelian patterns of inheritance, for example, genomic imprinting (differential expression of chromosomal material depending on whether the material is inherited from the male or female parent) (Hodgson, 1991), uniparental disomy (UPD) (the presence of two chromosomes of a pair inherited from one parent with no representation of that chromosome from the other parent), mosaicism (the presence of two or more cell lines having the same origin in the same single zygote but being genetically different owing to postzygotic mutation or nondysjunction), transcriptional depression (gene-specific transcriptional repressors failing to properly regulate gene expression), and mitochondrial inheritance (inheritance of a disorder that is encoded in the mitochondrial genome). Of particular interest are the occurrences of genomic imprinting and mosaicism. Furthermore, studies of fragile X syndrome and Huntington's disease have provided insight into "heritable unstable elements" (Richards and Sutherland, 1992). In this situation, genes are disrupted by inherited unstable DNA elements.

Genomic Imprinting

Genomic imprinting challenges the fundamental assumption of Mendelian genetics that the effect of a gene is fully independent of whether it originally came from the offspring's mother or father. It has now been shown that genes at a chromosomal locus may be differentially inherited from the mother or the father. The parental origin of genetic material can have profound impact on clinical expression of defect. For example, deletion of the 15q11-q13 on one copy of chromosome 15 may be associated with difficulty in behavioral regulation in two different intellectual disability syndromes. In one instance, the deletion is in the maternal contribution, and in the other, in the paternal contribution. The Prader-Willi syndrome (paternal 15q11-13 absent) is characterized by hypogonadism and hyperphagia, leading to massive obesity. Angelman syndrome (maternal 15q11-13 absent) is characterized by motor clumsiness and problems in affect regulation with periodic bursts of unexpected laughter. Both Prader-Willi and Angelman syndrome conditions can be associated with sleep disturbances. These are contiguous gene syndromes that are due to the loss of a series of genes from a region of chromosome 15 termed 15q13-15.

Trinucleotide Repeat Expansion (Heritable Unstable Elements)

A type of genetic mutation in which genes are unstable and expand or grow larger in subsequent generations, resulting in increasingly more severe forms of disease in their progeny, has been described in myotonic dystrophy, in fragile X syndrome (the most common known inherited form of mental retardation), and in several other syndromes.

Prior to identification of heritable unstable DNA elements, the fragile X syndrome, which occurs in both sexes, was considered to be a dominant X-linked disorder with reduced penetrance in females. In fragile X syndrome, 80% of males who inherit the mutation have moderate-to-severe mental impairment, but other males with the mutation can have normal intelligence. Approximately 50% of females who inherit the disease from their mothers are cytogenetically positive, but only one-third have intellectual disability. To explain these findings, at least two distinct mutation types have been reported in fragile X syndrome. One, the premutation, consists of a 50- to 600-base pair insertion or amplification at the fragile X locus (normal range = 5–48; mean = 29). Individuals with the premutation do not show the most serious aspects of the clinical syndrome such as severe intellectual disability. In the full mutation, that is, the insertion of 600–3000 base pairs, both males and females are at greater risk for more severe neuropsychiatric disability related to inactivation of the adjacent candidate *FMR1* gene. This gene is characterized by an unstable CGG repeat sequence that may grow from generation to generation. In males, the degree of clinical involvement appears to correlate with the length of abnormal CGG repetitive sequence. When the premutation is passed from father to daughter, the premutation remains relatively unchanged in size. However, when it is passed through the mother, the premutation may increase in size and potentially convert to the full mutation in both sons and daughters. Children inheriting an X chromosome with the full mutation from their mother will also have the full mutation, and often it is even increased in size. Therefore, the premutation increases in size and potentially converts to a full mutation only when it is passed through a female. It has been hypothesized that this conversion occurs during female gametogenesis and that sex-specific imprinting is involved. In addition to the mechanism described above, the fragile X syndrome phenotype has now also been reported in a patient with a deletion of the *FMR1* gene (Meijer et al., 1994).

Although carriers of fragile X mental retardation 1 (*FMR1*) premutation alleles (55–200 CGG repeats) are ordinarily spared the more serious neurodevelopmental problems associated with the full-mutation carriers (>200 repeats), some adult male premutation carriers (55–200 repeats) develop a neurological syndrome involving intention tremor, ataxia, dementia, parkinsonism, and autonomic dysfunction, known as the fragile X-associated tremor/ataxia syndrome (FXTAS) (Hagerman and Hagerman, 2004). This may occur in over one-third of male premutation carriers older than 50 years of age. Moreover, one study found that female carriers of the *FMR1* premutation may also show the symptoms of FXTAS, although more subtly and less often than their male counterparts (Hagerman et al., 2004). In this study, unlike their male counterparts with FXTAS, none of the women had dementia. This syndrome represents a form of inclusion disease, with eosinophilic intranuclear inclusions found throughout the brain in both neurons and astrocytes.

Alteration of Repressor Activity (Transcriptional Derepression)

The specific properties of individual cells are determined by the selective expression and repression of genes (Gabellini, Green, and Tupler, 2004). The control of the expression of most genes takes place with the initiation of transcription (the synthesis of a single-stranded RNA molecule from a DNA template in the cell nucleus). The transcription of DNA into mRNA is a highly regulated process; this regulation of transcription occurs by both positive (transcriptional activation) and negative (transcriptional repression) mechanisms. Promoter-specific transcriptional activator proteins act to increase protein synthesis. However, gene-specific transcriptional repressors are involved in regulation of gene expression. Alteration of repressor activity has been linked to neurodevelopmental disorders. The first example of this mechanism was demonstrated in Rett's disorder.

The gene for Rett's disorder, the methyl-CpG-binding protein gene (*MECP2*) found on the X chromosome (Xq28), encodes a protein (MeCP2) that is involved in one of the biochemical switches controlling complex expression patterns of other genes (Amir et al., 1999; Shahbazian and Zoghbi, 2002). Methyl-CpG binding by *MeCP2* is essential for brain function. Lack of a properly functioning MeCP2 protein might result in other genes turning on or staying on at inappropriate stages in development, disturbing the precisely regulated pattern of development. The proposed mechanism is as follows: the MeCP2 protein binds to methylated CpG dinucleotides and silences gene expression by recruiting transcriptional corepressors. MeCP2 binds methylated DNA and in this way most likely regulates gene expression and chromatin structure; ultimately it may be a form of chromatin that represses gene expression.

Dynamic modulation of levels of MeCP2 protein within the nervous system mirrors neuronal maturation. The timing of the appearance of MeCP2 correlates with the ontogeny of the central nervous system, and its expression continues to increase with maturation (Neul and Zoghbi, 2004). It is proposed that MeCP2 is not required for proper development of neurons but rather required to maintain proper postmitotic function of neurons. This is consistent with the early apparent normal development during the first months of life in Rett's disorder that is followed by a rapid deterioration involving loss of acquired motor and speech skills, microcephaly, seizures, ataxia, intermittent hyperventilation, and characteristic midline hand stereotypical movements. Favorable skewing of X-inactivation patterns in a mother with mutation in *MECP2* can result in a normal phenotype, whereas in the daughter, a balanced inactivation results in Rett's disorder (Amir et al., 2000).

Inborn Errors of Metabolism

The inborn errors of metabolism include amino acid disorders, carbohydrate disorders, mucopolysaccharide disorders, mucolipid disorders, urea cycle disorders, nucleic acid disorders, copper metabolism disorders, mitochondrial disorders, and peroxisomal disorders.

The ethical considerations and the criteria for inclusion of newborns in a screening program for inherited disorders was initiated in the 1961 when newborn screening for PKU was introduced to prevent intellectual disability. The primary purpose is to screen all newborn infants for disorders in which symptoms are not clinically evident until irreversible damage has occurred and for which effective preventive treatments are available. The criteria for screening are treatability and a significant incidence to pose a public health risk. Technological advances in newborn testing, especially improved tandem mass spectrometry techniques that permits screening for multiple disorders in a single small blood sample and the increasing use of DNA testing for the specific gene mutations, have expanded our understanding of many inherited metabolic diseases (Rhead and Irons, 2004). These are mainly autosomal recessive disorders. Currently half of the states have implemented or are implementing tandem mass spectroscopy (MS/MS) screening for more than 20 fatty acid oxidation and amino acid disorders and organic acidemias.

Two tests, those for PKU and congenital hypothyroidism (CH), are universally mandated in the United States. The inclusion of other tests varies by state, but efforts are being made to increase screening. Without treatment (low phenylalanine diet), PKU results in vomiting, eczema, seizures, and eventually intellectual disability. The incidence of PKU in the United States is approximately 1 in 12,000 live births. Normal blood phenylalanine levels are below 2 mg/dL (120 μM); therefore, most screening programs request repeat specimens from any infant with a higher level. For the confirmation of this diagnosis, all plasma amino acids should be measured by a quantitative technique. A blood phenyl-alanine concentration of more than 20 mg/dL with a normal or reduced concentration of tyrosine carries a diagnosis of classic PKU. Treatment should be instituted by three weeks of age. Overall treatment prevents the intellectual and neurological abnormalities but must be maintained because of the risk of attentional and learning disabilities at school age.

Congenital hypothyroidism is a neonatal disorder that is caused by a prolonged loss of thyroid hormone, which is essential for early brain development. While congenital hyperthyroidism was once the leading cause of intellectual disability, newborn screening now allows for early identification and treatment. Congenital hyperthyroidism has been screened for since the mid-1970s. The incidence of congenital hyperthyroidism in the United States is approximately 1:3,600–1:5,000 live births. The metabolic consequences of untreated congenital hyperthyroidism lead to intellectual disability, abnormal growth, and neurological abnormalities. Newborn screening involves measuring the T4 or thyrotropin (thyroid-stimulating hormone) level of blood spots dried on filter paper. If the T4 level is under the laboratory's cutoff level or in the lowest tenth percentile for that day's assays, then a repeat analysis of T4 and thyroid-stimulating hormone is performed. Approximately 10% of all cases of congenital hyperthyroidism can be missed by these screening procedures, so ongoing clinical assessment is needed. Early treatment, begun in the first three months of life, can prevent intellectual disability and the other complications of the disorder; however, ongoing monitoring is needed for deficits in visuospatial processing, selective memory deficits, and attentional deficits (Rovet, 2002).

Although screening varies by region, other metabolic diseases screened for include galactosemia, maple syrup urine disease, homocystinuria, tyrosinemia, urea cycle disorders (e.g., argininemia), and biotinidase deficiency (Rhead and Irons, 2004). In each instance, when identified, early treatment should be initiated. Organic acid disorders identifiable with tandem mass spectroscopy include glutaric acidemia types I and II, isovaleric acidemia, methylmalonic acidemia, propionic acidemia, and some disorders of ketogenesis and ketolysis. Well-known organic acidemias, such as methylmalonic acidemia and propionic acidemia, should profit from early, premorbid detection and treatment with dietary management. A federal advisory panel has recommended newborn screening for 29 rare medical conditions.

Developmental Disorders of Brain Formation

Malformations of the central nervous system are associated with intellectual disability. These include neural tube defects, anencephaly, brain formation defects, cellular migration defects, and acquired brain defects. Neural tube closure defects and malformation of the human cortex are of particular importance. The traditional classifications of central nervous system malformations were based upon descriptive morphology. Current approaches integrate molecular genetic information to produce an etiological classification that is useful to the clinician who relies upon neuroimaging and tissue examination for diagnosis.

Neural tube defects, including spina bifida and anencephaly, are congenital malformations that occur when the neural tube fails to achieve appropriate closure during early embryogenesis. These are multifactorial defects whose etiologies have a significant genetic component that interacts with specific environmental risk factors. There is evidence that closure of the mammalian neural tube initiates and fuses intermittently at four discrete locations. Disruption at any of these four sites may lead to neural tube defects, possibly arising through closure site–specific genetic mechanisms. Candidate genes involved in neural tube closure include genes of the folate metabolic pathway, as well as those involved in folate transport. Maternal serum screening for neural tube defects is an essential component of antenatal care.

Cerebral malformations previously thought to be a single disorder are now known to be the end-result of several independent genetic mutations. Moreover, molecular genetic studies of malformations of the human cerebral cortex provide better understanding of the genetic control of cerebral cortical development. Such developmental disorders account for cases of epilepsy, intellectual disability, and other cognitive disorders.

The neurons of the cerebral cortex proliferate out from the ventricular zone, a region surrounding the ventricles. Postmitotic neurons exit the ventricular zone and migrate to form the cerebral cortex. This migration occurs on a scaffold of specialized glial cells called radial glia. As the neurons reach the cerebral cortex, recently arrived neurons pass beyond older neurons to form a normal six-layered cortex. Thus, the upper layers of the cerebral cortex are made up of later born neurons, resulting in an "inside-out" pattern of cortical layering. Migration of neurons into the cerebral cortex appears to peak between the 11th and 15th week of gestation in humans, with the majority of the neurons appearing to reach the cortex by the 24th week of gestation.

Genetic defects (Mochida and Walsh, 2004) involving these different steps of development lead to distinct disorders. Among these are genetic microcephaly (small head) syndromes in which the occipitofrontal circumference is less than two standard deviations below the mean. For example, primary autosomal recessive microcephaly results in microcephaly at birth, relatively normal early motor milestones, and intellectual disability of variable severity. The causative gene has recently been identified for two of the recessive microcephaly syndromes. Six genetic loci have been identified and named *MCPH1* through *MCPH6*; the gene for *MCPH1* is referred to as microcephalin. Disorders of neural migration include classical lissencephaly that is associated with severe developmental delay and epilepsy; these disorders are often associated with microcephaly. In classical lissencephaly, normal gyration of the cerebral cortex is absent or severely reduced, and the surface of the brain appears smooth. Pathologically, the cortex is greatly thickened and shows four layers instead of the normal six layers. Abnormalities of two genes—*LIS1* on chromosome 17p and *DCX* (doublecortin) on chromosome Xq—are involved. Both LIS1 and DCX proteins are considered to be regulators of microtubules. (Microtubules are dynamic components of the intracellular cytoskeleton and are important in regulating cell shape and motility). There is an X-linked form referred to as lissencephaly with abnormal genitalia. It is associated with agenesis of the corpus callosum and ambiguous or underdeveloped genitalia. Mutations in the aristaless-related homeobox transcription factor gene, *ARX*, have been found and identified. In mice, this gene is important for neuronal proliferation, as well as migration and differentiation of interneurons in the forebrain.

Holoprosencephaly is the most common major developmental defect of the forebrain in humans (Muenke and Cohen, 2000). Clinical expression is variable, ranging from a small brain with a single cerebral ventricle and cyclopia to clinically unaffected carriers in familial holoprosencephaly. Significant etiologic heterogeneity occurs with holoprosencephaly and includes both genetic and environmental causes. Defects in the cell-signaling pathway involving the sonic hedgehog gene (*SHH*), as well as defects in the cholesterol biosynthesis have been shown to cause holoprosencephaly in humans. More recently, holoprosencephaly genes from additional signaling pathways have been identified.

Besides these conditions, there are other brain malformation syndromes of unknown origin. With improved genetic methodology, the cause of these conditions may be delineated.

Environmental Influences

Environmental Etiologies

Among the etiologies of intellectual disability, the environmental causes offer an opportunity for prevention and preventive interventions. These include intrauterine malnutrition, toxic exposures (especially gestational substance abuse), prenatal maternal diseases (viral, metabolic, and genetic), and irradiation during pregnancy.

Maternal Infections

Although there have been major medical advances in interventions for maternal infections, such as the introduction of the rubella vaccine and prolonged postnatal therapy of infants with congenital toxoplasmosis, intrauterine infections remain important causes of deafness, vision loss, and behavioral or neurological disorders among children worldwide (Bale, 2002). Rubella infection during the first month of pregnancy affects organogenesis in 50% of embryos, with resulting risk for deafness, cardiovascular damage, and retinopathy. These problems can be prevented with appropriate immunization.

Congenital toxoplasmosis usually occurs as a result of primary maternal infection. Approximately 85% of women of childbearing age in the United States are susceptible to infection (Jones, Lopez, and Wilson, 2003). It may result in problems in approximately 20% of infected infants (intellectual disability, hydrocephalus, microcephaly, psychomotor retardations, vision, and hearing impairment). Toxoplasmosis is caused by the protozoan organism *Toxoplasma gondii*. Infection with this organism primarily results from contact with infected cats and from ingestion of improperly cooked meat (e.g., beef, pork, or lamb). Most adults with toxoplasmosis are asymptomatic. When symptoms are present, they resemble a mononucleosis or flu-like illness. The diagnosis of toxoplasmosis in the pregnant adult is best made using serological techniques to detect IgM antibody and to document significant changes in the IgG antibody titer. The most useful tests for confirmation of fetal infection are ultrasound examination, cordocentesis for detection of IgM-specific antibody, and amniocentesis for detection of toxoplasma DNA in amniotic fluid. Congenital toxoplasmosis can be treated with reasonable success by administration of antibiotics (spiramycin, sulfadiazine, and pyrimethamine) to the mother.

Congenital human cytomegalovirus (HCMV) infection is the leading infectious cause of intellectual disability and sensorineural deafness (Revello and Gerna, 2004). Intrauterine transmission and adverse outcome are mainly related to primary maternal infection. Mechanisms of intrauterine transmission are slowly being understood. In the absence of a vaccine or a specific antiviral therapy that could be safely administered to pregnant women with primary HCMV infection, the option of prenatal diagnosis is crucial in the management of pregnancy complicated by primary HCMV infection. In addition, the availability of different assays for detection of HCMV in both fetal blood and amniotic fluid samples will eventually reduce the risk of false-positive results. Drugs under development for treatment include those that act as DNA maturation inhibitors.

Congenital Human Immunodeficiency Virus (HIV) Infection

Human immunodeficiency virus type I (HIV-1) infection leads to penetration of the central nervous system in virtually all infected individuals and HIV-1-induced encephalopathy in a significant number of untreated patients. Infants born to HIV-seropositive mothers are generally at high risk for developmental impairments (Boos and Harris, 1987). HIV encephalopathy has been associated with microcephaly, intellectual disability, and neurological and behavioral symptoms. Congenital (or neonatal) transmission of the virus can result in an intellectual disability syndrome of delayed onset. Prenatal screening and rapid screening at the time of delivery may allow treatment with antiretroviral therapy to prevent infant infection at delivery.

Toxic Substances: Ethanol and Drug Exposure

The most important teratogenic substance affecting pregnancy is ethanol; it is the cause of fetal alcohol syndrome and fetal alcohol spectrum disorder. Fetal alcohol syndrome is a common cause of developmental disability, neuropsychiatric impairment, and birth defects (Burd et al., 2003). The disorder is recognized by growth impairment, central nervous system dysfunction, and a characteristic pattern of craniofacial features. The prevalence approaches 1% of live births. People with fetal alcohol syndrome have high rates of intellectual disability (15%–20%), attention deficit hyperactivity disorder (40%), learning disorders (25%), speech and language disorders (30%), sensory impairment (30%), cerebral palsy (4%), epilepsy (8%–10%), and behavioral disorders. Birth defects are common. The disorder is expensive to treat and most patients experience lifelong impairment. Early recognition and entry into appropriate long-term treatment programs improves outcome. Prevention efforts should involve screening for alcohol use prior to pregnancy and at the first prenatal care visit. Besides alcohol, drugs prescribed for illness must also be screened for adverse impact on the fetus.

PERINATAL CAUSES

The perinatal period refers to the time period from one week before birth to four weeks after birth.

Infections

Perinatal infections account for 2%–3% of all congenital anomalies. TORCH is an acronym for toxoplasmosis, other (syphilis, varicella-zoster, parvovirus B19), rubella, cytomegalovirus, and herpes infections, which are some of the most common infections associated with congenital anomalies. Most of the TORCH infections cause mild maternal illnesses but have serious fetal consequences. Treatment of maternal infection frequently has no impact on fetal outcome. Recognition of maternal disease and fetal monitoring once disease is recognized are critical. Knowledge of these diseases will help the practitioner to appropriately counsel mothers on preventive measures to avoid these infections. Counseling parents about the potential for adverse fetal outcomes when these infections are present should be part of routine care. Herpes simplex type 2 is of particular importance. Infection occurs at the time of delivery and may develop into encephalitis within two weeks. Early treatment with acyclovir may alleviate the poor outcome.

Problems at Delivery

During delivery, asphyxia is the most important risk factor for brain damage, especially for premature infants. Cerebral hypoxia-ischemia remains a major cause of acute perinatal brain injury, leading ultimately to neurological dysfunction manifested as cerebral palsy, intellectual disability, and epilepsy. Research in experimental animals has expanded our understanding of the cellular and molecular events that occur during a hypoxic-ischemic insult to brain, and recent discoveries have suggested that metabolic abnormalities arising in the recovery period after resuscitation contribute to the nature and extent of neuronal destruction. Neurochemical processes responsible for the maintenance of cellular homeostasis may fail in hypoxia-ischemia and culminate in brain damage (Vannucci, 1990). Knowledge of these critical events may lead to therapy for the fetus and newborn infant subjected to cerebral hypoxia-ischemia and prevent the serious delayed effects of perinatal brain injury.

Other Perinatal Problems

Extremely low birth weight infants are at risk for intracranial hemorrhage and hypoglycemia that are the consequence of limited hepatic glycogen storage.

Such problems have results similar to asphyxia. Untreated hyperbilirubinemia, resulting from Rh incompatibility, or decreased excretion of bilirubin, resulting from immature liver functioning, may lead to cerebral palsy, sensorineural hearing loss, and intellectual disability.

POSTNATAL CAUSES

Infections

Meningitis and encephalitis from bacterial or viral infections may lead to permanent brain damage with intellectual disability. These complications often can be prevented by immunization.

Toxic Substances

Lead poisoning is less common now than in the past, but it remains an important etiology for intellectual disability. It occurs most commonly after ingestion of lead-based paint. Lead exposure may also result from leaded gasoline, some pottery glazes, and fumes when automobile batteries are burned. Acute lead poisoning begins with gastrointestinal symptoms that may be followed by headache as intracranial pressure builds up. Without recognition and treatment (chelation), intellectual disability, attentional problems, ataxia, and changes in personality may occur.

Other Postnatal Causes

Traffic accidents with head trauma, drowning, and other accidents that result in loss of consciousness are strongly linked to developmental disability. Childhood brain tumors, particularly gliomas that make up to 70%–80% of these tumors, are especially devastating.

Psychosocial Risks

Poverty predisposes the child to several developmental risks. These include teenage pregnancy, malnutrition, abuse, and deprivation. Physical abuse may result in head trauma and result in developmental disability.

DETERMINING THE ETIOLOGY

Determining the etiology of intellectual disability is critical. If a genetic disorder is suspected, genetic testing may be used to confirm the diagnosis. Recognition of a genetic disorder may suggest additional evaluations for known associated medical or behavior features. A full diagnostic evaluation results in a treatment plan that is based on what is known about this particular condition. Appropriate treatment, interventions, genetic and psychological counseling, and referrals may proceed. An important referral is to the appropriate family support group (see appendix A) for this particular genetic disorder.

The search for a cause and a diagnosis also is essential because the effects of some progressive developmental disorders can be arrested or sometimes prevented through early diagnosis and treatment. For example, many of the clinical manifestations of several inborn errors of metabolism (e.g., PKU, galactosemia) can be prevented by recognition and dietary management. Accurate diagnosis can lead to important interventions, including genetic counseling and prenatal diagnosis, and possibly to corrective gene therapy in the future.

Accurate diagnosis is also important because specific syndromes may be associated with behavioral phenotypes. The Society for the Study of Behavioral Phenotypes, an international association, was established based on parents' concerns about the similarity of behaviors found in individuals with particular genetic forms of intellectual disability/developmental disability. Knowing about such behaviors is essential for families and caregivers so as to plan for current and future supports.

Knowledge about etiology assists with planning for the future life of the individual. It may also satisfy a personal need; knowing the cause may help to facilitate self-knowledge for the affected person and his family. Knowing, acknowledging, and accepting the diagnosis is the essential first step in moving toward life planning. Information about the etiology, knowledge about the natural history, and recognition of the behavioral features of the disorder may be used for planning throughout the life span. Moreover, knowledge of the condition and associated risk factors offers the opportunity to prevent or anticipate and ameliorate future disability. For example, in Down syndrome, hypothyroidism, hearing problems (otosclerosis), or depression may emerge as the individual grows older. Careful monitoring and early recognition may alleviate suffering from these conditions.

NEUROBIOLOGICAL AND ENVIRONMENTAL ETIOLOGIES

Neurobiological and sociocultural factors and their interaction contribute to the etiology of intellectual disability. Besides specific genes linked to known genetic syndromes, multiple genes that interact with environmental features, resulting in intellectual disability, may be involved. Genetic influences are important in mild intellectual disability, as well as the more severe forms (Rutter, Simonoff, and Plomin, 1996).

In the past, those intellectual disability disorders with known neurobiological causes ("organic mental retardation") were distinguished from those without known cause, often referred to as "sociocultural familial mental retardation," and presumed to be the result of environmental deprivation. This distinction is no longer meaningful as we learn more about brain functioning and behavior. Tarjan et al. (1972) used the terms "physiological" and "pathological" to describe forms of intellectual disability. Physiological referred to brain structures and functions that were quantitatively different from normal, suggesting possible multifactorial influences that involved both genetic and environmental experiences. The pathological forms potentially had an underlying neuropathology that was qualitatively rather than quantitatively different from normal. However, even this distinction—qualitative and quantitative differences—must now be reconsidered as we learn more about genetic factors in intellectual disability. Current evidence does not support the existence of two groups, one biological and the other non-biological. Even though severe deprivation may result in some cases of intellectual disability, it seems best to refer to those individuals where biological factors are not identified as nonspecific or idiopathic intellectual disability, rather than sociocultural, to indicate that the biological underpinnings, undetected genetic or neurobiological factors, are not yet identified. Severe environmental deprivation may affect brain development. It is expected that more refined diagnostic procedures will result in the identification of new genetic disorders and a better delineation of the biological factors that are linked to intellectual disability.

There may be differences in cognition, within the normal range, related to individual susceptibility or to environmental circumstances. Thus, causal influences linked to variations in the normal range of intelligence and pathological influences must be distinguished (Rutter, Simonoff, and Plomin, 1996). It has been established that severely intellectually disabled persons have limited life experiences and low reproductive rate, and that severe intellectual disability shows far less familial loading than mild intellectual disability. Severely intellectually disabled children show greater differences from their siblings than do persons with mild intellectual disability. Approximately one-third of severely intellectually disabled persons have a chromosomal abnormality, whereas demonstrated chromosomal abnormalities are less common, perhaps 1:10, in mildly intellectually disabled persons, although this percentage may increase as we learn more about genetic mechanisms. Still, even the distinction between pathological and physiological groups can be misleading (when this terminology is used) because there is so much heterogeneity within both groups. A substantial minority of those with mild intellectual disability has identifiable pathological causes. Thus, in systematic epidemiologic study of individuals with IQs in the 50–70 range, it is important to document cause and associated features.

EVALUATION PROCESS AND ETIOLOGY

The establishment of a diagnosis of intellectual disability may be made clinically or require more detailed laboratory assessment. In one study, 281 children (mean age = 7.4 years) referred to a tertiary care center were prospectively studied to establish the etiology of intellectual disability (van Karnebeek et al., 2002). The assessment involved a complete clinical history, three-generational pedigree, physical examination, and behavioral assessment. The extent of intellectual disability was as follows: 16% borderline, 39.2% mild, 31.3% moderate, 10.3% severe, and 3.2% profound. A diagnosis was made in 54% (150 individuals). One-third of the diagnoses were made based on clinical history and physical examination only, one-third were the result of clinical history and physical examination suggesting appropriate additional examinations, and, in the final one-third, the diagnoses were based only on additional investigations. The other cases were identified by clinical diagnosis as unknown etiology with monogenic inheritance, or clinical diagnosis with nonmonogenic or unknown inheritance.

Chromosomal anomalies were more common in individuals with a greater number of minor physical anomalies.

With the mapping of the human genome, new approaches to identifying the etiology of intellectual disability are becoming available. Among these are new approaches to X-linked forms of intellectual disability; these occur in 1 in 600 males and are usually genetically heterogeneous. New diagnostic strategies use a human X-chromosome-specific cDNA microarray analysis to identify candidate genes responsible for X-linked intellectual disability. Wang et al. (2002) have produced an X-chromosome-specific cDNA microarray that includes 70%–80% of the genes on the X chromosome and are using this approach to identify genetic defects on the X chromosome. Another approach to understand the genetics of intellectual disability is to study gene expression patterns as a way to understand gene function. This is now possible for those human chromosomes whose full nucleotide sequence is available. One group of investigators (Marigo et al., 2002) has sought to understand the gene expression on chromosome 21, the chromosome that is duplicated in Down syndrome (trisomy 21). Such an approach may allow the identification of clusters of coregulated genes in syndromes like Down syndrome in which there is an additional chromosome. These authors are studying all identifiable mouse orthologs of human chromosome 21 genes (161 of 178 confirmed human genes) and have observed patterned expression on tissues affected by trisomy 21 (central nervous system, heart, gastrointestinal track, and limbs). These findings are published on a website (http://homepages.go.com/xlmr/home.htm) to allow other investigators to study function and regulation of chromosome 21.

Regardless of the etiology of intellectual disability, the evaluation process considers biomedical, social, behavioral, and educational elements in treatment planning, as described in the AAMR Multidimensional Classification (see chapter 3), and the DSM-IVTR classification (see chapter 3) that uses a multiaxial approach to classification. Using these classifications allows consideration of each of the diagnoses that requires attention to establish a treatment plan. Both classifications are important. For diagnostic purposes, the DSM-IVTR system is used, but for the most comprehensive treatment planning, the AAMR multidimensional system should be implemented.

The complete implementation of the AAMR multidimensional system involves identification of biomedical, social, behavioral, and educational risk factors that influence the individual's current functioning and life course. These risk factors interact over the life span of the affected person. Recognition of risk factors allows the development of strategies to help the individual and family members through anticipatory guidance, preventive intervention, and direct treatment. For example, the AAMR lists ten issues for consideration:

1. Impact of biomedical problems on psychological outcome. Some intellectual disability syndromes may be associated with health-related problems that influence both physical and psychological functioning. For example, a biomedical problem, unrecognized hearing problems

in Down syndrome, may lead to psychological distress and misunderstanding.

2. Early biomedical diagnosis may minimize or prevent intellectual disability. Recognition of PKU at birth may prevent or minimize intellectual disability.
3. Individualized information that considers risk factors for a particular person is needed to design programs to prevent complications of intellectual disability.
4. Knowledge based on the study of homogenous groups of individuals with the same or similar causes of intellectual disability advances our understanding of the life span history of a disorder.
5. Recognition of behavioral phenotypes leads to anticipation of the types of supports needed over the life span.
6. Genetic counseling is facilitated by precise knowledge of biomedical etiology.
7. Knowledge of biomedical causes, support needs, and life course can be shared among families through family organizations.
8. Sharing causal information with the affected person enhances self-knowledge and allows that person to participate in his/her life plans.
9. Knowledge of biomedical causes is essential for service providers to plan interventions in crisis situations.
10. Recognition of outcome risk factors—biomedical, social, behavioral, and educational—offers opportunities for prevention of further disability.

COMPONENTS OF A COMPREHENSIVE EVALUATION

A comprehensive evaluation of an individual with intellectual disability must assess cognitive development, genetic and nongenetic causes of intellectual disability, associated medical conditions (e.g., cerebral palsy or a seizure disorder), mental, emotional, and behavioral problems that may influence cognitive functioning, and specific co-occurring problems such as major depression. The basic medical history, guidelines for clinical and genetic assessment, and the diagnostic process in genetics are described in the following section. The evaluation for behavioral, emotional, and psychiatric disorders is described in chapter 6.

Persons with mild and moderate intellectual disability may be evaluated using the same procedures, with slight modifications, as those that are used for typically developing persons. A comprehensive medical assessment includes a review of present concerns and symptoms, past and present developmental, medical, social, and family history, patient interview, and physical examination. The assessment leads to a diagnostic formulation and a treatment plan. Treatment plans are discussed in a meeting with the patient and family, with a review of follow-up plans (Deb et al., 2001; Szymanski, 1980). Both the individual and caregivers who know that person well are informants for the medical and behavioral health history. Disorders of interpersonal functioning, communication,

Table 5.3 Components of a Comprehensive History

Domain	Information Needed
Presenting symptoms	Behavioral description of symptoms in various settings, situations, from different caregivers; concrete examples; their evolution over time; antecedent events; management measures used and results
Assessments	Critical review of past cognitive tests and other tests; focus on profile of cognitive strengths and weaknesses rather than on IQ
Medical review	Review of past assessments; request new if past inadequate or out of date
Personality patterns	Premorbid and current patterns of behavior, personality, emotional style
Adaptive skills	Strengths and impairments in communication, self-care, social/interpersonal, community integration, self-direction, functional academic skills, work, leisure, health and safety
Mental health	Past diagnoses, psychotherapies, use of psychotropic drugs; their beneficial and adverse effects; behavioral and other treatments
Environmental supports and stressor	Past and present living; educational, habilitative, work settings: nature, consistency, ancillary therapies; their appropriateness; family events, school transfers, losses of important caregivers; possibility of physical and sexual abuse
Family/caregiving	Understanding of, and reaction to, the patient's intellectual disability; overprotection vs. encouraging growth; behavioral management and consistency; disability's effects on the family dynamics, lifestyle, and siblings; long-term plans; consideration of cultural factors

From Szymanski and King (1999). Reprinted by permission of the publisher, Lippincott, Williams & Wilkins, from Practice Parameters for the Assessment and Treatment of Children, Adolescents, and Adults with Mental Retardation and Comorbid Mental Disorders, *Journal of the American Academy of Children and Adolescent Psychiatry*, 38:12. American Academy of Child and Adolescent Psychiatry. Copyright© 1999.

emotion, and behavior are included in the assessment, and recommendations about them are an essential part of the treatment plan (see table 5.3).

Basic Medical History

A comprehensive medical history and a careful physical examination are essential to uncovering the etiology of intellectual disability. Following the history and physical examination, laboratory and diagnostic studies are chosen based on the clinical findings.

GUIDELINES FOR CLINICAL AND GENETIC ASSESSMENT

A genetic evaluation is central to understanding causation of intellectual disability syndromes. Such evaluation helps to answer questions about management, prognosis, recurrence risk, and the development of prevention strategies.

When families meet with a clinical geneticist, they ask a number of questions. For example: Why and how did this happen? Will it happen again? What is the long-term outcome? What are the usual and expected medical complications?

What can be done to treat or manage the condition? Can anything be done to prevent it from occurring or to detect its recurrence in another pregnancy? What reproductive options are available? What are the potent effects? What are the effects on the next generation? (Curry et al., 1997)

A clinical evaluation, including laboratory testing, is necessary to begin to answer these questions. The overall goal is to clarify the diagnosis and, if possible, to identify the cause and establish the pathogenesis of the disorder to help families deal with their concerns. An accurate diagnosis is essential for meaningful discussion of recurrence risk. Recurrence risk makes such evaluation critical. Moreover, early diagnosis may prevent costly and needless subsequent evaluations. With an accurate diagnosis and formulation, management and discussion of treatment options naturally follow. Planning for future consequences in the natural history of the condition throughout the life span is essential to counseling. Such anticipatory guidance is important for the family, the primary care physician, schools, medical and nonmedical treatment providers, and therapists. The benefits and the goals of the genetic evaluation are presented in table 5.4.

The cause for intellectual disability can be identified in 40%–60% of those undergoing an evaluation (Curry et al., 1997). The likelihood of finding the cause varies according to the severity of intellectual disability, the selection of the individuals who are studied, how the source was ascertained, and the age of the patient. Diagnostic accuracy is gradually increasing with advanced molecular cytogenetic techniques and improved neuroimaging techniques.

If the diagnosis is not known, not only families but also the relatives, referring physicians, and social agencies must be informed so that they may provide support in dealing with uncertainty. A diagnosis does bring relief from uncertainty even though it may involve an outcome that is difficult for family members to face. Moreover, a diagnosis allows identification of an appropriate support group and, in some instances, facilitates obtaining funding for special services,

---

Table 5.4 Benefits of Genetic Evaluation

I. For the individual patient
   1. Identification of appropriate medical and nonmedical therapies
   2. Presymptomatic screening for associated complications/functional disabilities
   3. Educational planning
   4. Elimination of unnecessary testing and evaluations

II. For parents
   1. Anticipatory guidance
   2. Education and advocacy
   3. Referral to appropriate medical and social service agencies
   4. Referral to support groups
   5. Reproductive counseling, carrier testing, prenatal diagnosis
   6. Family networking

From Curry et al. (1997). Reprinted by permission of author and publisher, Wiley-Liss, Inc., a subsidiary of John Wiley & Sons, Inc., from C. J. Curry et al., Evaluation of mental retardation: Recommendations of a consensus conference, *American Journal of Medical Genetics*, 72:468–477. Copyright © 1997.

such as counseling, assistive devices, or wheel chairs. An incorrect diagnosis is problematic and may result in counseling that is not appropriate and recommendations that are not specific to the needs of the person with intellectual disability. Therefore, it is preferable to wait to assign a specific diagnosis if there are questions about the designation.

A comprehensive assessment may involve serial evaluations of an affected individual over time. Diagnoses have been reported to increase in reliability by 5%–20% with return visits (Root et al., 1996). In addition, recognizable physical and behavioral phenotypes may evolve over time, leading to greater diagnostic certainty. Moreover, applying new diagnostic methods or repeating tests that were apparently normal may facilitate diagnosis, as does improved methodology. Such gradual and repeated diagnostic testing follows a step-wise approach with planned sequences of tests over time.

How often individuals with undiagnosed conditions should be reevaluated is based on several factors. These include (1) the age of the patient; (2) the severity and complexity of the clinical situation; and (3) the urgency about making decisions for having additional children. For those individuals who have complex undiagnosed conditions, at least two evaluations in the first year of life and subsequent yearly evaluations until school age may be necessary. An additional evaluation during puberty may be appropriate. New genetic or clinical information on the condition is discussed at follow-up. For clinical geneticists, diagnoses are often not achieved at the first visit; that visit is part of a process of gathering information about the individual's medical and behavior history, physical examination, and diagnostic testing. Family counseling is also an ongoing process and only is beginning at the first visit; such counseling cannot be accomplished in a single visit.

The Diagnostic Process in Genetics

The clinical geneticist utilizes a clinical history that includes prenatal and birth history, the family genetic pedigree (disease history in immediate family members), and a physical and neurological examination. The examination emphasizes the assessment of minor anomalies, growth, and physical development. This assessment is critical and cannot be replaced by laboratory testing and simple screening methods.

A review of pertinent medical records on the affected patient and selected relatives can be important, particularly in the assessment of neurodevelopmental and neurodegenerative processes. The record review may help to determine the causal role of perinatal complications and to assess the likelihood that the disorder is familial. The genetic pedigree chart focuses on three generations of immediate family members and, besides medical problems, searches for the presence of individuals with learning disorders, psychiatric disorders, autistic spectrum disorder, and intellectual disability. The measurement of head circumference is made and compared to normative charts. The head circumference measurement should be followed over a period of time and compared to normative information. The physical examination will focus on facial structures, particularly the midline of the face and the eye regions that may give clues to the clinical geneticist for specific syndrome diagnoses. The neurological examination should be comprehensive. The history should document evidence of behavioral phenotypes that may be helpful to establish a diagnosis. In some instances, such as tuberous sclerosis complex, Wood's light examination of the skin is needed. Dermatoglyphics (assessment of fingerprints) can also be a helpful diagnostic tool. In addition, hearing, eye, and psychometric assessments are appropriate adjuncts to the assessment procedure.

When abnormal physical findings are present, they must be carefully documented with measurements and description, including photographs. Videotaping may be utilized to document gait abnormalities, movement disorders, and certain behavioral characteristics. If minor congenital variance or anomalies are present in the affected person that are not found in family members, this information may be used in establishing when in prenatal life the problem may have begun. For minor congenital anomalies, efforts should be made to measure them accurately. For example, there are standards to measure thinness of the upper lip and the extent of the philtrum in FAS. Similarly, an increase in the distance between the eyes (hypertelorism), and small jaw (micrognathia), are important features in assessment. Such measurements need to take into account both ethnic and family variations in facial appearance. Thus, family resemblances need to be assessed by examining the patient and his or her parents, siblings, and half-siblings. When a child or adult with intellectual disability does not resemble other family members, this may be helpful evidence of aneuploidy, a chromosomal abnormality.

Diagnostic Tests

Diagnostic tests should be utilized selectively and focused on the suspected disorder. The tests used most commonly for intellectual disability assessment are general assessment, chromosomal analysis, fragile X testing, CT/MRI cranial neuroimaging studies, and metabolic testing (organic and amino acids).

Chromosome Analysis

Chromosome analysis in an individual with intellectual disability is the first step in an overall genetic evaluation process. Chromosomal anomalies are the single most common cause, in unselected individuals, of intellectual disability. Chromosomal anomalies are found in 4%–28% of individuals with intellectual disability, depending on the study. The severity of intellectual disability and the presence of congenital anomalies lead to the likelihood that a disorder will be diagnosed. Children who do not have physical features, referred to as "dysmorphic appearance," are less likely to have a chromosomal anomaly. Curry et al. (1997) found that 16 of 150 individuals (11%) with undiagnosed developmental delay had chromosomal anomalies. Of these 16, 4 were described as having no dysmorphic features; two of these had the XXY syndrome, one tetrasomy 15q, and the other had an unidentified marker that was found to be mosaic in his normal mother. Thus, chromosomal analysis in individuals with developmental delay, even in the absence of minor anomalies, can be diagnostic.

In studying microdeletion syndromes, targeted fluorescence in situ hybridization (FISH) studies may be utilized. This test should be performed by experienced examiners. In a study of three different genetic units, Curry et al. (1997) reported that19% of microdeletion syndromes were identified in one clinic, 10% in another, and 15% in a third. If a child with intellectual disability with no clear-cut diagnosis has a karyotype done, it is best that it be carried out at least the 500-band level. If a specific microdeletion syndrome is suspected, the clinical geneticist may turn to a FISH study, as this may be more diagnostically accurate. Children with known syndromic diagnoses without a documented chromosomal basis may require high-resolution chromosome studies, especially if there is an unusual clinical presentation or an atypical family history.

In the future, new molecular genetic techniques will become more widely available, such as those used to study uniparental disomy or screen for telomeric rearrangements. When these tests are more widely available, uniparental disomy studies can be carried out in patients with developmental disorder who have in utero growth retardation and minor anomalies, especially if chromosomes known to be commonly involved in uniparental disomy—for example, chromosome 7 and chromosome 14—are suspected. Finally, subtelomeric microsatellite screening and spectral karyotyping may be required when clinical findings or family history are suggestive of a chromosomal abnormality and the initial high-resolution studies show apparently normal results.

Fragile X Analysis

The fragile X syndrome is an example of an intellectual disability syndrome in which unstable trinucleotide repeats result in a worsening of the clinical presentation from one generation to the next. This phenomenon has been referred to as "anticipation." The initial description of fragile X syndrome by Martin and Bell in 1943 included a description of the physical features. Subsequently, Lubs (1969) described the marker X chromosome with the fragile site that resulted in its name. The gene, *FMR1*, has been isolated and mutational analysis has been standardized for fragile X syndrome. Fragile X syndrome is the etiology for approximately 40% of X-linked intellectual disability. Two-to-six percent of the males in residential and community programs have this diagnosis. Population prevalence ranges in estimates from 1:1,000 to 1:6,000 (Murray et al., 1996). Approximately one-half of all females with full mutations in the *FMR1* gene also test in the intellectually disabled range. Grandfathers who are premutation carriers are at risk for dementia in late life (Brunberg et al., 2002)

Despite the clear descriptions of the physical findings and its high prevalence, it may be difficult to decide which patients to test for fragile X syndrome. The condition may be inherited, but there also may be sporadic occurrence of the syndrome. The major difficulty in diagnosis is that there are several forms of X-linked intellectual disability that might be confused with fragile X syndrome (Lubs et al., 1996a, 1996b). The physical phenotype of fragile X syndrome and the behavioral phenotype gradually emerge during the developmental period, over several years, and may be less apparent in infancy and childhood. In addition, ethnic characteristics may make the facial characteristics more difficult to distinguish. To address the diagnostic issue, Giangreco et al. (1996) proposed a scoring system to determine who should be tested for fragile X syndrome. The scoring system includes the presence or absence of six historical and clinical characteristics. These include intellectual disability, a family history of cognitive deficits, an elongated face, large or prominent ears, attention deficit/hyperactivity syndrome, and autistic-like behavior. These authors propose that testing only subjects with scores of 5 or more on this index would eliminate 60% of the testing that was done at the time of their study without missing positive cases. Further evaluation of the long-term effectiveness of this scoring system is needed.

Laboratory confirmation in fragile X syndrome is based on molecular analysis of the *FMR1* gene. Laboratory analysis identifies the number of CGG repeat segments (trinucleotide repeats). A normal individual has approximately 50 repeats and premutation carriers 50–230 repeats; the full mutation is identified when there are 230 or more repeats. Fragile X syndrome may also result from deletions or point mutations of the *FMR1* gene, but these are rare. If the individual has the characteristic syndrome, thorough genetic analysis is necessary in addition to the CGG repeat analysis. Genetic approaches may be used to look for other fragile sites other than the one that is classically associated with fragile X syndrome. The molecular approach used to diagnose fragile X syndrome is increasingly more sophisticated. Because numerical and/or structural abnormalities of autosomes and sex chromosomes are most likely as common as fragile X syndrome, a banded karyotype may be necessary to clarify the diagnosis.

Laboratory testing for fragile X syndrome is relatively inexpensive. Thus, *FMR1* testing in males and females with unexplained intellectual disability should be routinely considered. *FMR1* mutations have been reported in 2%–6% of males and in 2%–4% of females with unexplained forms of intellectual disability. If there is a family history of fragile X syndrome, this test is most likely to find the abnormality, if present. Still, a family history of intellectual disability or the presence of nonspecific manifestations, such as a developmental disorder, speech delay, learning disability, behavioral disturbance, or seizure, do not increase the likelihood of finding a positive result for fragile X syndrome. However, the rates of diagnosis are higher in patients with macroorchidism (large testes) (15.6%) or autistic-like behavior (7.5%) (Sherman, 1996).

Details regarding the genetic analysis of other neurogenetic syndromes with behavioral phenotypes are discussed in chapter 7.

Neuroimaging Assessment

Individuals with intellectual disability syndromes have abnormal brain functioning. Such brain dysfunction may or may not be demonstrated in brain morphology or in histological brain studies. Structural brain abnormalities have been reported in from 34%–98% of samples of deceased, severely intellectually disabled individuals whose neuropathology was studied (Polednak, 1977). The likelihood of finding brain changes in neuroimaging in relatives of affected patients is substantially less, although results do range from 9% to 60%. The range of abnormalities in family members is linked to how restricted the selection criteria are for the study. Most commonly, neuroimaging abnormalities are seen in individuals with microcephaly (small head), macrocephaly (large head), or abnormalities of cranial contour. Still, neuroimaging deficits may also occur in individuals with a normal head size without non-central nervous system abnormalities (Bodensteiner and Chung, 1993).

What is the role of neuroimaging in the evaluation of a person with intellectual disability? Specifically, how does neuroimaging help in making a specific diagnosis in the determination of risk of occurrence in other family members or in improving individual case management? Brain imaging has an increasingly important role in the evaluation of children and adults with a variety of developmental disorders. Noninvasive imaging may be used to identify structural, and in some instances, functional abnormalities, such as abnormal metabolic activity, in persons with intellectual disability. Computerized transaxial tomography (CT), magnetic resonance imaging (MRI), functional MRI (fMRI), single photon emission computed tomography (SPECT), and positron emission tomography (PET) techniques may be used in the evaluation of intellectual disability syndromes, to study structure-function relationships, and to identify surgically correctable brain lesions associated with specific disorders.

The following guidelines are suggested for neuroimaging by the American College of Medical Genetics (Curry et al., 1997):

1. MRI scanning is generally superior to CT scanning in detecting abnormalities. MRI provides better anatomical definition, especially at the base of the cranium and in the posterior fossa of the brain. In addition, evaluation of myelination and gray-white matter differentiation is better demonstrated with MRI, especially after 6 to 9 months of age. Moreover, such subtle abnormalities as heterotopias and abnormalities of the cisterna magna and septus pellucidum are better demonstrated using MRI. The cost and the need for sedation/anesthesia are factors that result in less frequent use of MRI. Yet in a well-established imaging center, anesthesia/sedation should not be a major drawback even though there is some risk in using these sedation procedures. If there is an abnormal CT scan, the radiologist may request an additional MRI scan. In terms of cost, it may be more cost-efficient to do the MRI scanning first rather than subject the child to two procedures, especially if anesthesia/sedation is needed for both.

2. Age-related standards for relative size of major brain structures are increasingly available. Information on brain development over time in normally developing children is helpful in interpreting MRI findings (Durston et al., 2001).

3. The CT scan is the appropriate method for patients with suspected craniosynostosis or possible intracranial calcifications. Such calcifi-

cations may be seen with certain congenital infections and in tuberous sclerosis complex.

4. Findings on CT or MRI scans may assist in establishing the date of onset of the problem, that is, prenatal, perinatal, or postnatal. The identification of such abnormalities may also help target the diagnostic approach. Generally, but not in all cases, structural abnormalities in MRI suggest a nonprogressive or static process. Recognizing structural abnormalities may not affect prognosis but, in some instances, offers reassurance to a family. It may assist in long-term planning for the individual, particularly in disorders such as neurocutaneous disorders (Bodensteiner and Schaefer, 1995). Diagnostic imaging is essential in the evaluation and treatment of neurocutaneous disorders in which prognosis depends on the number, size, and location of associated neoplasms (e.g., neurofibromas, tubers, hamartomas, angiomas, and malignancies). This is especially important in tuberous sclerosis, where CT and MRI may reveal tubers, subependymal calcified nodules, cortical hamartomas, and migration defects. The number and size of the tubers may be correlated with the degree of intellectual disability, the extent and type of behavior problem, and the severity of the seizure disorder. In Sturge-Weber syndrome, MRI is used to detect the extent and distribution of angiomatosis in the meninges, skull, and brain, but CT is best for detecting cortical calcifications.

5. Long-term developmental studies of MRI in normal volunteers are being used (Durston et al., 2001; Gogtay, Giedd, and Rapoport, 2002) to confirm if there are minor morphological changes in the brain in the general population. If so, the risk of occurrence can be more usefully applied to individuals with intellectual disability. Developmental studies of variations in brain regions are helpful to clarify their pathological significance.

6. Long-term follow-up for individuals with isolated central nervous system abnormalities is needed to make comparisons and study the life course of the particular disorder. This is particularly the case for disorders that are estimated to have a very low prevalence. CT and MRI may be used to identify congenital malformations and/or brain changes related to infections of the central nervous system.

7. With microcephaly or macrocephaly, seizures, loss of psychomotor skills, and neurological signs (spasticity, seizures, dystonia, ataxia, loss of reflexes, or increase in reflexes, etc.), neuroimaging may have an important role in assessment. Ventricular enlargement, cyst formation, cerebral asymmetry, neuronal migration disorders (e.g., polygyria, lissencephaly, and schizencephaly), Chiari malformations, agenesis of the corpus callosum, and cerebral calcifications are among the abnormalities that may be recognized. CT is the preferred procedure for the visualization of calcifications, vascular lesions, and some tumors. MRI is superior to CT for specific identification of some structural anomalies (e.g., heterotopias), white matter abnormalities

(e.g., demyelinating disorders), abnormality of the gray-white matter junction, and masses in the posterior fossa of the brain. Individuals with clear-cut physical and neurological features more likely will show abnormalities on neuroimaging studies.

8. In patients with normal head circumference (normocephalic) who do not have focal neurological signs, the utility of a CT or MRI scan is unclear. For these patients, neuroimaging studies should not be mandatory as part of a diagnostic assessment.

9. Functional imaging, especially fMRI, may be used to evaluate some children with intellectual disability. FMRI allows assessment without the use of radioisotopes; however, it is difficult for some individuals to remain still for the time needed to carry out these procedures.

10. PET and SPECT scans are being used to localize seizure foci prior to surgery, determine the extent of malignancy of certain neoplasms, identify tubers in tuberous sclerosis, and evaluate the extent of intracranial hemorrhage in premature infants; they also may contribute to the early diagnosis of Huntington's disease and Sturge-Weber syndrome.

11. For children with most known syndromes or chromosomal abnormalities (e.g., fragile X syndrome, Down syndrome, and Williams syndrome) who do not have neurological signs that are inconsistent with the diagnosis, MRI and CT scans should not be necessary other than in research settings. For most children with such syndromes, neuroimaging abnormalities may be present, but this knowledge may contribute very little to patient management (Gabrielli et al., 1990).

In summary, when considering neuroimaging studies, the first step is a thorough assessment of the patient and an evaluation of his/her clinical presentation. After the assessment is completed, neuroimaging procedures may be considered. The MRI scan, when available and practical for that patient, is the imaging modality of choice, as noted; however, high-quality CT imaging is of value, particularly in those syndromes where intracranial calcification is suspected. Other neuroimaging studies, such as functional MRI, PET scanning, and diffusion tensor imaging, may be required in certain circumstances to assess an individual. These techniques allow clarification of functional deficits and neurochemical abnormalities in the individual and offer refinements in understanding pathways and structures.

Metabolic Testing

Inborn errors of metabolism play an important role in selected patients who have multiple congenital anomalies (e.g., Smith Lemli-Opitz syndrome). Testing for metabolic disorders is required in certain clinical presentations. These range from neonatal hypotonia to gradual coarsening of facial features and loss of developmental milestones.

Many abnormalities suggest metabolic investigation. These include failure of appropriate growth, recurrent unexplained illness, seizures, ataxia, loss of psycho-motor skills, hypotonia, coarse facial appearance, eye abnormalities (cataracts and corneal clouding), recurrent somnolence, abnormal sexual development, hepatosplenomegaly, metabolic acidosis, hyperuricemia, hyperammonemia, low cholesterol, unexplained deafness, bone abnormalities, skin abnormalities, (orange peel skin and ichthyosis) and abnormalities of hair. Testing is selected depending on clinical presentation. General assessment includes acid/base balance, plasma and urine amino and organic acid studies, thyroid screening tests, lysosomal enzyme analysis, plasma long-chain fatty acid assessment, and other tests for suspected syndromes.

What is the utility and frequency of positive findings regarding diagnosis from routine metabolic screening? The most common screening involves plasma amino acids and urine organic acids. How should these tests be used in the evaluation of individuals with intellectual disability who do not have specific signs or symptoms that suggest a particular metabolic abnormality? When children with general developmental delay or intellectual disability are assessed, the presence of identifiable metabolic disorders is low, ranging from 0% to 5% (Allen and Taylor, 1996). Some disorders are routinely tested with newborn screening, and these are not counted in these estimates. For example, PKU, congenital hypothyroidism, and galactosemia are all included in neonatal screening procedures. Besides this routine screening, there is a small-to-low identification of disorder for unselected metabolic screening unless the child has some signs or symptoms of a metabolic disorder. Moreover, the frequency of nonspecific, nondiagnostic abnormalities found in urine organic screens may result in more extensive, and often more expensive, laboratory procedures that still do not result in a diagnosis. Overall, infants and children with inborn errors of metabolism have signs and symptoms indicating a need for further assessment. Thus, metabolic screening should be selective and targeted at a category of disorder rather than used as an unselected screen. Metabolic screening, therefore, is not routinely performed in individuals with intellectual disability.

In summary, the following are recommendations of the American College of Medical Genetics (Curry et al., 1997) for the evaluation of intellectual disability:

1. The clinical assessment includes complete pre- and perinatal history, three-generational genetic pedigree, physical examination that includes gross physical features, physical examination and neurological findings, and documentation of minor abnormalities, as well as an evaluation for behavioral phenotype.
2. Longitudinal follow-up is critical following the initial assessment to establish the evolution of physical and behavioral phenotypes.
3. Most persons with intellectual disability should have a chromosome analysis. This involves high-resolution analysis at the 500-band level and above. Based on clinical signs, targeted FISH and molecular genetic studies are necessary. In long-term follow-up, if no abnormality was found in chromosomal screening and new clinical signs emerge, re-evaluation for repeated genetic testing should be carried out at ap-

proximately five-year intervals. Additional assessment for mosaicism may also be considered since somatic mosaicism may occur.

4. Molecular fragile X studies should be strongly considered in both males and females with unexplained intellectual disability. The identified case should also have a banded karyotype and fragile X molecular studies. A family history of female family members and grandfathers is needed in regard to the risk for fragile-X-associated tremor/ataxia syndrome.

5. Metabolic screening is directed by the individual's case presentation and history, with signs and symptoms suggestive of a particular disorder and is not a routine procedure.

6. Intracranial imaging should be considered for patients with microcephaly, macrocephaly, abnormalities of cranial contour, and neurological signs.

The Quality Standards Subcommittee of the American Academy of Neurology and The Practice Committee of the Child Neurology Society (Shevell et al., 2003) provide guidelines for the evaluation of global developmental delay in very young children. A specific etiology can be identified in the majority of children with global developmental delay. Specific routine screening tests are proposed, and depending on history and examination findings, additional specific testing may be carried out. Global developmental delay affects 1%–3% of children. In agreement with the genetics group, routine metabolic screening is not indicated in the initial evaluation; the yield is low: about 1% of children with global developmental delay are detected. Screening for fragile X syndrome is recommended because of the higher yield (3.5%–10%). This yield occurs in the absence of dysmorphic features or features suggestive of the specific syndrome; routine cytogenetic studies and molecular testing for the fragile X mutation are recommended. Rett's disorder should be ruled out in girls with unexplained moderate to severe developmental delay. For selected children with moderate to severe intellectual disabilities, additional genetic studies (e.g., subtelomeric chromosomal rearrangements) may also be considered. Such studies may use the FISH molecular methodology. Evaluation of serum lead levels is best restricted to those children with identifiable risk factors for excessive lead exposure. Thyroid studies are not carried out (unless clinically indicated) if the child underwent newborn screening. An EEG is not recommended as part of the initial evaluation unless there is clinical evidence that suggests epilepsy or a specific epileptic syndrome. Neuroimaging (MRI is preferred to CT) is recommended based on finding abnormalities on physical examination. There is an increased incidence of visual and auditory impairments in children with global developmental delay, thus appropriate visual and audiometric assessment should be considered at the time of diagnosis.

Finally, the evaluation of intellectually disabled persons is undergoing change as our understanding of the human genome develops with its mapping. This is resulting in better delineation of syndromes and the establishment of new cytogenetic and molecular techniques. For an individual child or adult who is being assessed for intellectual disability, there is no specific protocol that can replace an individual assessment of the individual and his or her family, and the clinical judgment of an experienced physician. A careful and thorough approach to the individual and family can be expected to lead to improved care and better prevention strategies.

KEY POINTS

1. There are multiple causes of intellectual disability and frequently there are associated features, such as language disorder and seizure disorders.
2. The causes reflect the interaction of genetic and environmental factors.
3. In determining the etiology, both genetic and epigenetic factors must be considered.
4. Environmental factors include nutritional status, exposure to endogenous and exogenous toxins, microorganisms, radiation, and other environmental factors; exposure may occur prenatally, perinatally, or postnatally during the developmental period.
5. A specific cause can be determined in approximately two-thirds of cases. The more severe the degree of impairment, the greater the likelihood of finding the cause.
6. The most commonly used etiologic classification focuses on the timing of the causative event or events: prenatal, perinatal, or postnatal.
7. Newborn screening for etiologies of intellectual disabilities can be critical in preventing impairment, lessening it, or modifying the extent of impairment.
8. Knowledge of the condition and associated risk factors provides an opportunity for prevention or anticipating and ameliorating future impairment.
9. The distinction between "organic intellectual disability" and "sociocultural/familial disability" is no longer a meaningful distinction with new knowledge about brain functioning and behavior.
10. A comprehensive evaluation includes cognitive assessment and consideration of genetic and nongenetic etiologies. Associated medical conditions and mental, emotional, and behavioral problems may influence cognitive functioning. A comprehensive evaluation may involve several assessment visits over time.

References

Allen, W.P., and Taylor, H. (1996). Mental retardation in South Carolina. VII. Inborn errors of metabolism. *Proceedings of the Greenwood Genetics Center,* 15:76–79.

Amir, R.E., Van den Veyver, I.B., Schultz, R., Malicki, D.M., Tran, C.Q., Dahle, E.J., Philippi, A., Timar, L., Percy, A.K., Motil, K., Lichtarge, O., Smith, E.O., Glaze, D.G., Zoghbi, H.Y. (2000). Influence of mutation type and X chromosome inactivation on Rett syndrome phenotypes. *Annals of Neurology,* 47:670–679.

Amir, R.E., Van den Veyve, I.B., Wan, M., Tran, C.Q., Francke, U., and Zoghbi, H.Y. (1999). Rett syndrome is caused by mutations in X-linked *MECP2*, encoding methyl-CpG-binding protein 2. *Nature Genetics,* 23:185–188.

Bale, J.F., Jr. (2002). Congenital inflections. *Neurology Clinics,* 20:1039–1060.

Bodensteiner, J B., and Chung, E.O. (1993). Macrocrania and megaloencephaly in the neonate. *Seminars in Neurology,* 13:84–91.

Bodensteiner, J B., and Schaefer, G.B. (1995). Evaluation of the patient with idiopathic mental retardation. *Journal of Neuropsychiatry and Clinical Neuroscience,* 7:361–370.

Boos, J., and Harris, S.A. (1987). Neurology of Aids virus infection: A clinical classification. *Yale Journal of Biology and Medicine,* 60:537–543.

Brunberg, J.A., Jacquemont, S., Hagerman, R.J., Berry-Kravis, E.M., Grigsby, J., Leehey, M.A., Tassone, F., Brown, W.T., Greco, C.M., and Hagerman, P.J. (2002). Fragile X premutation carriers: Characteristic MR imaging findings of adult male patients with progressive cerebellar and cognitive dysfunction. *American Journal of Neuroradiology,* 23:1757–1766.

Burd, L., Cotsonas-Hassler, T.M., Martsolf, J.T., and Kerbeshian, J. (2003). Recognition and management of fetal alcohol syndrome. *Neurotoxicology and Teratology,* 25: 681–688.

Curry, C.J., Stevenson, R.E., Aughton, D., Byrne, J., Carey, J.C., Cassidy, S., Cunniff, C., Graham, J.M., Jr., Jones, M.C., Kaback, M.M., et al. (1997). Evaluation of Mental Retardation: Recommendations of a consensus conference: American College of Medical Genetics. *American Journal of Medical Genetics,* 72:468–477.

Deb, S., Matthews, T., Holt, G., and Bouras, N. (2001). Practice guidelines for the assessment and diagnosis of mental health problems in adults with intellectual disability. (European Association for Mental Health in Mental Retardation). Pavilion, UK.

Durston, S., Hulshoff Pol, H.E., Casey, B.J., Giedd, J.N., Buitelaa, J.K., van Engeland, H. (2001). Anatomical MRI of the developing human brain: what have we learned? *Journal of the American Academy of Child and Adolescent Psychiatry,* 40:1012–1020.

Egger, G., Liang, G., Aparicio, A., and Jones, P.A. (2004). Epigenetics in human disease and prospects for epigenetic therapy. *Nature,* 429:457–463.

Evans, P.D., Anderson, J.R., Vallender, E.J., Choi, S.S., and Lahn B.T. (2004). Reconstructing the evolutionary history of microcephalin, a gene controlling human brain size. *Human Molecular Genetics,* 13:1139–1145.

Gabellini, D., Green, M.R., and Tupler, R. (2004). When enough is enough: genetic diseases associated with transcriptional derepression. *Current Opinon in Genetic and Development,* 14:301–307.

Gabrielli, O., Salvolini, U., Coppa, G.V., Catassi, C., Rossi, R., Manca, A., Lanza, R., and Giorgi, P.L. (1990). Magnetic resonance imaging in the malformative syndromes with mental retardation. *Pediatric Radiology,* 21:16–19.

Giangreco, C.A., Steele, M.W., Aston, C E., Cummins, J.H., and Wenger, S.L. (1996). A simplified six-item checklist for screening for fragile X syndrome in the pediatric population. *Journal of Pediatrics,* 129:611–614.

Gogtay, N., Giedd, J., and Rapoport, J.L. (2002). Brain development in healthy, hyperactive, and psychotic children. *Archives of Neurology,* 59:1244–1248.

Hagberg, B., Hagberg, G., Leverth, A., and Lindberg, U. (1981). Mild mental retardation in Swedish school children. *Acta Pediatrica Scandinavia,* 70:444–452.

Hagerman, P.J., Hagerman, R.J. (2004). Fragile X-associated tremor/ataxia syndrome (FXTAS). *Mental Retardation and Developmental Disability Research Reviews,* 10: 25–30.

Hagerman, R.J., Leavitt, B.R., Farzin, F., Jacquemont, S., Greco, C.M., Brunberg, J.A.,

Tassone, F., Hessl D, Harris SW, Zhang L. et al. (2004). Fragile-X-associated tremor/ataxia syndrome (FXTAS) in females with the *FMR1* premutation. *American Journal of Human Genetics.* 74:1051–1056.

Hodgson, S. (1991). Genomic imprinting. *Developmental Medicine and Child Neurology,* 33:552–556.

Holliday, R. (2002). Epigenetics comes of age in the twenty-first century. *Journal of Genetics,* 81:1–3.

Jones, J., Lopez, A., and Wilson, M. (2003). Congenital toxoplasmosis. *American Family Physician,* 67:2131–2138.

Kaufmann, W.E., and Moser, H.W. (2000). Dendritic anomalies in disorders associated with mental retardation. *Cerebral Cortex,* 10:981–991.

Lamont, M.A., and Dennis, N.R. (1988). Aetiology of mild mental retardation. *Archives of Diseases of Children,* 63:1032–1038.

Lederberg, J. (2001). The meaning of epigenetics. *The Scientist,* 15:6.

Lubs, H.A. (1969). A marker X chromosome. *American Journal of Human Genetics,* 21: 231–244.

Lubs, H.A., Chiurazzi, P., Arena, J.F., Schwartz, C., Tranebjaerg, L., and Neri, G. (1996a). XLMR genes: Update 1996. *American Journal of Medical Genetics,* 64: 147–157.

Lubs, H.A., Schwartz, C.E., Stevenson, R E., and Arena, J.F. (1996b). Study of X-linked mental retardation (XLMR): Summary of 61 families in the Miami/Greenwood Study. *American Journal of Medical Genetics,* 64:169–175.

Luckasson, R., Borthwick-Duffy, S., Buntinx, W.H.E., Coulter, D.L., Craig, E.M., Reeve, A., Schalock, R.L., Snell, M.E., Spitalnik, D.M., Spreat, S. and Tasse, M.J. (2002). *Mental retardation: Definition, classification, and systems of supports,* 10th ed. American Association on Mental Retardation, Washington, DC.

Luckasson, R., Coulter, D.L., Polloway, E.A., Reiss, S., Schalock, R.L., Snell, M.E., Spitalnik, D.M., and Stark, J.A. (1992). *Mental retardation: Definition, classification, and systems of supports,* 9th ed. American Association on Mental Retardation, Washington, DC.

Marigo, V., Reymond, A., Yaylaoglu, M.B., Leoni, A., Ucla, C., Scamuffa, N., Cacciopoli, C., Dermitzakis, E.T., Lyle, R., Banfi, S., et al. (2002). *Human chromosome 21 gene expression atlas in the mouse.* Abstracts, Meeting of the American Society of Human Genetics, No. 1309, October 16–19, 2002, Baltimore, Maryland.

Martin, J.P. and Bell, J. (1943). A pedigree of mental defect showing sex linkage. *Journal of Neurology and Psychiatry,* 6:154–157.

Matzel, L.D., Han, Y.R., Grossman, H., Karnik, M.S., Pate, D., Scott, N., Specht, S.M., Gandhi, C.C. (2003). Individual differences in the expression of a "general" learning ability in mice. *Journal of Neuroscience,* 23:6423–6433.

McKusick, V.A. (1998). *Mendelian inheritance in man. A catalog of human genes and genetic disorders,* 12th ed. Johns Hopkins University Press, Baltimore.

Meijer, H., de Graaff, E., Merckx, D.M., Jongbloed, R.J., de Die-Smulders, C.E., Engelen, J.J., Fryns, J.P., Curfs, P.M., and Oostra, B.A. (1994). A deletion of 1.6 kb proximal to the CGG repeat of the FMR1 gene causes the clinical phenotype of the fragile X syndrome. *Human Molecular Genetics,* 3:615–620.

Mochida, G.H., and Walsh, C.A. (2004). Genetic basis of developmental malformations of the cerebral cortex. *Archives of Neurology,* 61:637–640.

Muenke, M., Cohen, M.M. Jr. (2000). Genetic approaches to understanding brain development: Holoprosencephaly as a model. *Mental Retardation and Developmental Disability Research Reviews,* 6:15–21.

Murray, A., Youings, S., Dennis, N., Latsky, L., Linehan, P., McKechnie, N., Macpherson, J., Pound, M., and Jacobs, P. (1996). Population screening at the FRAXA and FRAXE loci: Molecular analyses of boys with learning difficulties and their mothers. *Human Molecular Genetics,* 5:727–735.

Neul, J.L., and Zoghbi, H.Y. (2004). Rett syndrome: a prototypical neurodevelopmental disorder. *Neuroscientist,* 10:118–128.

Nussbaum, R.L, McInnes, R.R., and Willard, H.F. (2001). *Genetics in medicine.* 6th ed. W.B. Saunders Company, Philadelphia.

Plomin, R., and Craig, I. (2001). Genetics, environment and cognitive abilities: Review of work in progress towards a genome scan for quantitative trait locus associations using DNA pooling. *British Journal of Psychiatry,* Supplement 40:S41–48.

Polednak, A.P. (1977). Post-mortem neuropathology in a mentally retarded population. *Lancet,* 1(8009):492–493.

Ramakers, G.J. (2002). Rho proteins, mental retardation and the cellular basis of cognition. *Trends in Neuroscience,* 25:191–199.

Revello, M.G., and Gerna, G. (2004). Pathogenesis and prenatal diagnosis of human cytomegalovirus infection. *Journal of Clinical Virology,* 29:71–83.

Rhead, M.J., and Irons, M. (2004). The call from the newborn screening laboratory. *Pediatric Clinics of North America,* 51: 803–818.

Richards, R.I., and Sutherland, G.R. (1992). Heritable unstable DNA sequences. *Nature Genetics,* 1:7–9.

Root, S., Viskochil, D., Leonard, C.O., and Carey, J.C. (1996). Genetic evaluation of children with developmental delay. *Proceedings of the Greenwood Genetics Center,* 14:32 (Abstract).

Rovet, J.F. (2002). Congenital hypothyroidism: an analysis of persisting deficits and associated factors. *Neuropsychology, Development and Cognition, Section C, Child Neuropsychogy,* 8:150–162.

Rutter, M., Simonoff, E., and Plomin, R. (1996). Genetic influences on mild mental retardation: Concepts, findings, and research implications. *Journal of Biosocial Science,* 28:509–526.

Shahbazian, M.D., and Zoghbi, H.Y. (2002). Rett syndrome and *MeCP2*: linking epigenetics and neuronal function. *American Journal of Human Genetics,* 71:1259–1272.

Sherman, S. (1996). *Epidemiology in fragile X syndrome: Diagnosis, treatment, and research,* 2nd ed., pp. 165–192. R.J. Hagerman and A. Cronister (eds.). Johns Hopkins Unversity Press, Baltimore, MD.

Shevell, M., Ashwal, S., Donley, D., Flint, J., Gingold, M., Hirtz, D., Majnemer, A., Noetzel, M., Sheth, R.D. (2003). Practice Parameter: Evaluation of the child with global developmental delay: Report of the Quality Standards Subcommitee of the American Academy of Neurology and the Practice Committee of the Child Neurology Society. *Neurology,* 60:367–380.

Stromland, K., Nordin, V., Miller, M., Akerstrom, B., and Gillberg, C. (1994). Autism in thalidomide embryopathy: A population study. *Developmental Medicine and Child Neurology,* 36:351–356.

Szymanski, L.S. (1980). Individual psychotherapy with retarded persons. In L.S. Szymanski and P.E. Tanguay (eds.), *Emotional disorders of mentally retarded persons.* University Park Press, Baltimore.

Szymanski, L.S., and King, B.H. (1999). Practice parameters for the assessment and treatment of children, adolescents, and adults with mental retardation and comorbid mental disorders. American Academy of Child and Adolescent Psychiatry Working

Group on Quality Issues. *Journal of the American Academy of Child and Adolescent Psychiatry*, 38 (suppl. 12):5S–31S.

Tarjan, G., Tizard, I., Rutter, M., Bergab, M., Brooke, E., de la Cruz, F., Lin, T-Y, Montenegro, H., Strotzka, H., and Sartorius, N. (1972). Classification and mental retardation: Issues arising in the Fifth WHO Seminar on Psychiatric Diagnosis, Classification and Statistics. *American Journal of Psychiatry*, 128:34–35.

van Galen, E.J., and Ramakers, G.J. (2005). Rho proteins, mental retardation and the neurobiological basis of intelligence. *Progress in Brain Research*, 147:295–317.

van Karnebeek, C.D., Scheper, F.Y., Abeling, N.G., Alders, M., Barth, P.G., Hoovers, J.M., Koevoets, C., Wanders, R.J., and Hennekam, R.C. *Etiology of mental retardation in 281 children referred to a tertiary care center: A prospective study.* Abstracts, Meeting of the American Society of Human Genetics, No. 117, Baltimore, Maryland, October 16–19, 2002.

Vannucci, R.C. (1990). Experimental biology of cerebral hypoxia-ischemia: Relation to perinatal brain damage. *Pediatric Research*, 27:317–326.

Waddington, C.H. (1939). *An introduction to modern genetics.* Allen and Unwin, London.

Wang, T., Zhang, L., Obie, C., Mousses, S., Trent, J., and Valle, D. *Identification of genes responsible for X linked mental retardation (XLMR) using a human X chromosome specific cDNA microarray.* Abstracts, Meeting of the American Society of Human Genetics, No. 125, Baltimore, Maryland, October 16–19, 2002.

6

Understanding and Evaluating Emotional and Behavioral Impairment

MENTAL ILLNESS AND INTELLECTUAL DISABILITY

In English property law, intellectual disability and mental illness were differentiated in the thirteenth century. By 1690, John Locke's *An Essay Concerning Human Understanding* had clarified differences between intellectual disability and mental illness. Locke wrote:

> The defect in [intellectual disability] seems to proceed from want of quickness, activity, and motion in the intellectual faculties, whereby they are deprived of reason; whereas mad men seem to suffer by the other extreme. For they do not appear to me to have lost the faculty of reasoning: but having joined together some ideas very wrongly . . . they argue right from wrong principles. . . . But there are degrees of madness as folly; the disorderly jumbling of ideas together is in some more, and some less. In short, herein seems to lie the difference between [intellectually disabled] and mad men, that mad men put wrong ideas together, and so make wrong propositions, but argue and reason right from them: but [those with intellectual disability] make very few or no propositions, but argue and reason scarce at all. (Scheerenberger, 1983, p. 41)

Thus, Locke is often credited with establishing the dichotomy between mental illness and intellectual disability that influenced social policy for people with intellectual disability. But he did not appreciate the capacity persons with intellectual disability do have to reason with adequate supports, nor did he consider that persons with intellectual disability are also at risk for mental illness and behavior disorders.

Historically, intellectual disability and mental illness were regarded to be mutually exclusive conditions. Affective and behavioral disturbances in individuals with intellectual disability generally were regarded as manifestations of maladaptive learning and adverse psychosocial experiences rather than as indications of a psychiatric disorder. This view has been shared by both intellectual disability and mental health professionals. Health professionals typically fail to consider the diagnosis of a psychiatric disorder among persons with intellectual disability despite the presence of signs and symptoms that would be readily ascribed as psychiatric disturbance among typically developing persons within the general population. This diagnostic bias may be an outgrowth of several factors. First, the development of valid and reliable tests of intelligence and adaptive functioning early in this century enabled professionals to diagnose intellectual disability. This resulted in more specific and more appropriate treatment interventions and remediation programs for intellectual disability and the assumption that such treatment would, in itself, reduce associated behavioral and emotional problems that were thought to be linked to it. Second, professionals wished to protect individuals with intellectual disability from the unfortunate stigma sometimes associated with the label of mental illness and ensure that their primary diagnosis of intellectual disability received appropriate intervention. Third, professionals believed that because of cognitive impairment, psychological structures and processes underlying the expression of psychopathology did not develop. For example, it was thought that a cognitively impaired person could not express self-blame and guilt, which were essential for the diagnosis of a major depression. Therefore, it was thought that the diagnosis of depression could not be applied to a person with intellectual disability. Fourth, it was believed that individuals with intellectual disability benefit more from educational and behavioral interventions. However, interpersonal psychotherapy and, in some instances, insight-oriented methods of psychotherapy and/or pharmacotherapy are needed for co-occurring mental disorders.

How might mental and behavioral disorders be linked to intellectual disability? There are at least four possible causal links that might account for the association between intellectual disability and psychiatric disorder (Goodman and Scott, 1997). First, the same neurobiological factors that result in intellectual disability may lead independently to psychiatric disorder. For example, a child with an IQ of 45 and tuberous sclerosis complex has a high risk of an autistic disorder, but a child with an IQ of 45 and cerebral palsy is not at the same risk for an autistic disorder. IQ does not account for the difference; rather, the neurobiological underpinnings of the autistic disorder (i.e., tuberous sclerosis complex) and cerebral palsy are different. Second, intellectual disability may predispose a child to a psychiatric or behavioral disorder. This might occur when cognitive impairment and poor academic achievement result in lower self-esteem following negative interpersonal experiences with classmates and/or teachers. Moreover, children who are cognitively impaired may find it more difficult to cope with day-to-day stressors and may be more prone to show impulsive and aggressive behavior when stressed. Thus, due to a stress response, a person with intellectual disability might show greater anxiety or anger. Such stress may lead to antisocial behaviors. In this way, lower IQ may become associated with conduct disorder due to environmental conditions. Third, severe psychosocial deprivation results in lower intelligence and/or psychiatric/behavioral problems. Stressful circumstances that contribute to lower intelligence, such as malnutrition and severe environmental deprivation are different from the usual social factors that increase the psychiatric risk, suggesting that this possible link is rare, occurring only in extreme cases. Fourth, psychiatric and behavioral problems themselves result in lower IQ. Even though psychiatric or behavioral problems may interfere with school performance, there is no direct evidence that psychiatric disorders reduce intelligence itself. Thus, the most likely causes for psychiatric disorder are underlying neurobiological factors that contribute both to intellectual disability and, separately, to mental illness and severe psychosocial stressors in a cognitively vulnerable person.

Finally, there are difficulties in applying diagnostic criteria for psychiatric disorders to persons with intellectual disability. Such criteria must take into account the presence of developmental disabilities that make assessment more complex. For typically developing persons, the individual provides a full description of experiences and feelings, but individuals with cognitive impairments may have difficulties in receptive and expressive language. Limitations in cognitive and verbal skills may make such communication difficult or impossible. Individuals with mild levels of intellectual impairment may try to hide their disability or respond falsely or inaccurately to please the evaluator. This has been referred to as "the cloak of competence" (Edgerton, 1993). Sovner (1986) has proposed that the following four issues may influence the diagnostic process for persons with intellectual disability: (1) *Intellectual distortion.* This term refers to impaired communication skills and concrete thinking (limited ability to abstract) that impact on communicating one's own life experiences in responding to diagnostic interviewing. (2) *Psychosocial masking.* This term refers to limited social skills and restricted life experiences that may result in difficulty for the evaluator in interpreting psychiatric symptoms. For example, nervousness or "silliness" during an interpersonal interview might be mistaken for psychiatric symptoms. (3) *Cognitive disintegration.* This term refers to disrupted thinking, poor information processing and odd behavior when experiencing stress. Such thinking or behavior may suggest psychotic symptoms to the evaluator rather than a temporary stress-related cognitive disorganization. (4) *Baseline exaggeration.* This refers to an exaggeration of pre-existing cognitive deficits and maladaptive behaviors that may worsen in demand situations or under stress, making interpretation of symptoms difficult unless the evaluator knows the individual well.

The National Association for the Dually Diagnosed (NADD), working with the American Psychiatry Association (APA), has developed more suitable diagnostic criteria to use for the classification of disorders in persons with intellectual disability as a supplement to DSM-IVTR. The NADD/APA Classification modifies the DSM-IVTR Diagnostic Manual to optimize its use with intellectually disabled persons. It is an evidence-based adaptation of DSM-IVTR. It provides detailed instructions about how to apply DSM-IVTR diagnostic criteria for people with intellectual disability and offers modified criteria where appropriate. Because unmodified diagnostic criteria can often be used for persons with mild intellectual disability, its emphasis is on making diagnoses in those with moderate to severe intellectual disability. Chapters in the manual focus on the general issues of assessment and diagnostic procedures and the presentations of behavioral phenotypes of genetic disorders in addition to discussion of the DSM-IVTR disorders themselves. For each disorder, a summary of the relevant literature and tables of proposed modified diagnostic criteria accompany descriptive text reviewing the DSM-IVTR criteria and their limitations. Finally, issues related to Etiopathogenesis, risk factors, and genetic syndromes are discussed.

The DSM approach includes operational definitions of symptoms, rules for cut-off criteria, and rules for inclusion or exclusion of the diagnosis. However, other than the diagnostic criteria for Pervasive Developmental Disorder, people with intellectual disability were excluded from the DSM field trials. The NADD supports field trials on NADD/APA criteria for each of the categories in DSM-IVTR. Such trials, using stratified random sampling, should include participants diagnosed in the mild range of intellectual disability, the moderate range of intellectual disability, severe intellectual disability, and those with profound intellectual disability.

The Royal College of Psychiatrists (2001) in UK has published a classification system that provides operationalized diagnostic criteria for psychiatric disorders intended for use with adults with moderate to profound intellectual disability. This classification is available for the adult population with intellectual disability. The Diagnostic Criteria for Psychiatric Disorders for Use with Adults with Learning Disabilities/Mental Retardation [Intellectual Disability] (DC-LD) also was designed to be used in conjunction with the ICD-10 and DSM-IVTR manuals when assessing persons with mild intellectual disability; for mild intellectual disability less adaptation is needed in utilizing ICD-10 and DSM-IVTR diagnostic criteria. In one study (Cooper, Melville, and Einfeld, 2003), there was 96.3% concordance with clinical opinion in diagnosis using the DC-LD.

RISK FACTORS ASSOCIATED WITH PSYCHIATRIC DIAGNOSIS

Overall, individuals with intellectual disability have an increased vulnerability to emotional and behavioral disorders, so emotional and behavioral disorders should be routinely asked about and assessed. In addition, rates of psychiatric and behavior disorder are higher in individuals with mild-to-moderate intellectual disability than they are in the general population, and are highest in those who test in the severe-to-profound range of intellectual disability when behavioral problems are included. However, Cowley et al. (2004) found that specific ICD-10 psychiatric diagnoses were made at a higher rate in those in mild intellectual disability when compared with those who were severely involved. This inconsistency may be linked to the definition of psychiatric disorder used and the diagnostic criteria used that may not be appropriate across the IQ range.

Vulnerability for mental disorder is related to a reduced capacity to deal with complex social and cognitive demands, difficulty in problem-solving ability, especially in the resolution of conflicts, poor social judgment, and sensorimotor and language disorders that affect communication. Moreover, persons with intellectual disability may be further handicapped by the unwillingness of some professionals to provide treatment for them.

In community settings, risk factors associated with a psychiatric diagnosis must be considered. As noted, the level of IQ is a major variable associated with a psychiatric diagnosis. Certain psychiatric diagnoses, such as schizophrenia spectrum disorder, personality disorder, and depressive disorder, have been identified more frequently in those with mild intellectual disability when compared with moderate and severe intellectual disability. Gender has been associated with anxiety disorder and depressive disorder (Hurley, Folstein, and Lam, 2003); both disorders are more prevalent in women. With increasing age, those with intellectual disability have increased rates of dementia, and Deb, Thomas, and Bright (2001) found that dementia presents at an earlier age in persons with intellectual disability than in the general population. Cowley et al. (2004) collected data from 752 individuals referred to a specialty intellectual disability mental health service. They found that older age, mild intellectual disability, admission to an inpatient unit, detention under mental health legislation, and referral from mental health facilities were associated with high rates of psychopathology.

Severe intellectual disability, epilepsy, and residence in the family were associated with lower rates; however, behavioral disorders were not included and other diagnoses, such as schizophrenia spectrum disorder, are difficult to diagnose in those with severe intellectual disability because those diagnoses rely on reporting subjective symptoms. Reports of dementia were highest in persons with moderate intellectual disability, suggesting that middle-aged adults in this intelligence range be monitored for dementia. The use of DC-LD criteria may provide a better measure of rate of disorder in the severely intellectually disabled group.

The causes of self-injury vary with the syndrome. In some incidences, self-injurious behavior is a stress-related behavior disorder and not specific to the syndrome (e.g., skin picking and head banging) and, in others, it is a characteristic behavioral phenotype (e.g., Lesch-Nyhan disease). In evaluating the etiology, an individual assessment is required.

Psychological Factors

Children and adults with intellectual disability may show problems with self-esteem and personality development. Unlike individuals who are not developmentally disabled, children and adults with intellectual disability may show less differentiated self-concept and less idealized views of themselves (Dykens, 2000; Evans, 1998). These self-attitudes may set the stage for unrealistic and perhaps negative self-appraisals. Such predisposing negative self-esteem may be worsened by constant exposure to daytime failure. Failure experiences are important in the learning histories of children and adults with intellectual disability. Such uncertainty that comes from failure may result in learned helplessness that has been linked to depression and other difficulties (Weisz, 1990). Although an emphasis on positive behavioral supports and inclusion is thought to help with these vulnerabilities, it is unclear to what extent the risks are offset by these positive interventions; nevertheless, they are an important part of treatment.

Specific personality styles may be linked to psychopathology (Dykens, 1999). These include an outwardly directed orientation in which children look to others instead of themselves for solutions to difficult problems. Inappropriate social styles such as excessive wariness or disinhibition with others and reduced expectancy of success (Zigler and Bennett-Gates, 1999) may be maladaptive sequelae to these personality styles that result in low self-esteem, sadness, dependency, social withdrawal, helplessness, and impulsivity.

Family Issues

Stress in the family and work place has frequently been considered a factor in the adjustment difficulties of children and adults with intellectual disability. It was initially assumed that families with family members who had disabilities experienced stress and developed psychological problems, and that this would be expected from everyone who had a handicapped child (Solnit and Stark, 1961). Family stress, indeed, is higher among families who have family members with disabilities, including intellectual disability. However, with family support, positive outcomes are common (Hodapp, 1995). The current understanding is that how the family adapts is related to factors in the impaired family member, such as age, the cause of the intellectual disability, and the extent of the intellectual disability. Other issues that affect adaptation are the degree of support family members receive from one another, the coping style of the parents, parental maladjustment that preceded the birth of an affected child, and the parents' perception of their child (Minnes, 1998) or adult family member. Positive supports make a difference; additional supports are needed when the parents themselves are intellectually disabled (Feldman, Leger, and Walton-Allen, 1997; Feldman and Walton-Allen, 1997).

The best predictors of family adjustment tend to be factors involving the disabled family member, including behavioral and psychiatric problems. This has been shown in specific syndromes, such as Prader-Willi syndrome, Smith-Magenis syndrome, and the 5p-syndrome. The behavioral and psychiatric problems tend to be more stressful for the family than the age or intellectual level (Hodapp, Fidler, and Smith, 1998). It has been proposed (Dykens, 2000) that it is the disabled person's predisposition to particular kinds of emotional and behavioral difficulties that elicits stressful parental responses. The parents' response may facilitate the disabled family member's adjustment or potentially worsen the problem, if the parent is not familiar with the appropriate strategies to help with development. Still, there are problems within the family, such as marital discord and psychiatric disorder in the parent, that may trigger behavioral and psychiatric problems in the child or adult. This has been demonstrated in families with a member affected by Down syndrome (Gath, 1990). Thus, both family and child or adult features play a role in adaptation to a handicapping condition. The earlier view of inherent family stress primarily related to intellectual disability is not sufficient to deal with the complexity of dealing with a child or adult with intellectual disability or other developmental disabilities.

Psychosocial Issues

Children and adults with intellectual disability are at greater risk for exploitation and for abuse, both physical and sexual (Ammerman et al., 1994). The exact frequency of abuse among those with intellectual disability is unknown. However, it is established that poor interpersonal treatment may worsen both behavioral and emotional difficulties. Moreover, adults, particularly those with milder cognitive impairment, may experience social stigma that affect their self-esteem and adjustment in the community and at work (Reiss and Benson, 1985). Social intelligence may also be diminished in individuals with intellectual disability who have problems in social pragmatics, show poor social understanding, and may misunderstand social cues in interpersonal interactions. This is particularly the case in those with social communicative problems who have both intellectual disability and pervasive development disorder diagnoses.

New relationships are frequently problematic and rejection by peers is an ongoing concern. Children with intellectual disability have difficulty making compromises and working through conflict with peers. They may be seen as different by others, which contributes to their exclusion from the group (Freeman and Kasari, 1998). If friendships are established, the friendships tend to be atypical because of difficulties that the person with intellectual disability may have with sharing and participating in play, making joint decisions, and understanding interpersonal roles (Siperstein, Leffert, and Wenz-Gross, 1997). The etiology of the intellectual disability may contribute to the type of peer difficulty that is experienced. For example, children or adults with Lesch-Nyhan disease may become aggressive following a positive interaction with others if the other person gets too close physically. The child or adult may then pinch or hit the other person and then profusely apologize. With Prader-Willi syndrome, the obesity and behavioral features may result in teasing and negative responses from peers (Dykens and Kasari, 1997). In other syndromes, such as Williams syndrome, in which sociability is a feature, affected individuals may have difficulty making friends despite their innate sociability owing to anxiety and indiscriminate responses to others (Dykens and Rosner, 1999). Peer relationships are critical in development, so understanding the genetic syndrome and the person's interactional style is critical as to when to provide emotional supports.

Associated Neurobiological Risk Factors

Besides the genetic risk for behavioral and psychiatric problems when contrasted to the general population, persons with intellectual disability have neurobiological vulnerabilities that may result in problems in physiologic self-regulation. Associated disorders, such as seizure disorder, sensory impairment, impulse control problems, and self-injury, must be taken into account in addition to the extent of intellectual disability. From 30% to 50% of persons with the more severe and profound levels of intellectual disability may have a seizure disorder (Bird, 1997). Children with seizure disorder may show dysphoria following their seizures and various types of behavioral dyscontrol. Moreover, certain syndromes, like fetal alcohol syndrome and fetal alcohol spectrum disorder, may be associated with antisocial behavior.

Self-injurious behavior is present in 4%–16% of individuals with severe forms of intellectual disability (Rojahn, 1994). Up to 17% of children with intellectual disability are deaf, and intellectual disability is found in approximately 30% of children with visual impairments and in 60% of those with cerebral palsy (Hodapp, 1998). Children who are deaf have a greater likelihood to develop psychiatric disorders, particularly problems with anxiety and conduct (Hindley, 1997). Motor impairments, such as spina bifida/hydrocephalus and cerebral palsy, have been linked to inattention and overactivity (Wills, 1993). Blindness is particularly problematic in regard to psychosocial adjustment and pragmatic language understanding. Those children who have both intellectual disability and sensory handicaps have a greater vulnerability to emotional and behavioral problems.

In summary, many factors—psychosocial, psychological, physiological, and neurobiological—are linked to various intellectual disability syndromes. Because both behavioral and psychiatric problems frequently accompany intellectual disability and do so in approximately a third of those with this diagnosis, the term "dual diagnosis" has been used to describe individuals with both intellectual disability and a behavioral or psychiatric disorder. However, rather than focus on terminology, it is best to look at the multiplicity of factors that affect these children and adults throughout their lives. Each of the genetic, environmental, psychosocial, and biological factors listed here needs to be addressed for an individual child or adult to develop a specific treatment program for that person.

To understand the individual child or adult, it is important to appreciate the natural history or life course of the known causes of intellectual disability so that one may plan for interventions at each phase in the developmental life cycle. One must consider what might be anticipated in the future based on the child or adult's age, intelligence level, genetic diagnosis, socioeconomic status, gender, peer relationships, and the extent of family adjustment. Research in these areas may help to predict the best approaches to intervention. When one monitors the disabled person's development from early life through middle childhood and adulthood, it is critical to consider both risk and protective factors that may worsen the condition or prevent difficulties as the child or adult and the parents grow older together. Ongoing research is essential to establish why children, adolescents, and adults with intellectual disability are at greater risk for behavioral and psychiatric problems and how their treatment can best be accomplished.

SPECTRUM OF PSYCHIATRIC AND BEHAVIORAL DISORDERS

There is increasing interest in studying the pattern of psychopathology manifested by children, adolescents, and adults with intellectual disability (NIH, 2001). Systematic investigations indicate that the full spectrum of recognized psychiatric disorders can be identified among those with intellectual disability.

Chart reviews of clinical diagnoses, however, indicate that psychotic disturbances are overdiagnosed and anxiety, affective, and personality disorders are
underrecognized.

When evaluating persons with intellectual disability, it is important to keep
in mind that persons with severe intellectual disability are generally multiply
disabled. Some are mobile and some are nonmobile. Community surveys will
frequently demonstrate two or more additional disabilities. These disabilities are
not simply additive but rather multiplicative in their effects. When persons with
intellectual disability express psychiatric disorders, these may present as maladaptive behavior. The origin of psychopathology is multiply determined. Moreover, acute psychiatric diagnosis or behavioral disorder may initially present as
an increase in the rate of a previously established maladaptive behavior.

Children and adults with mild-to-moderate intellectual disability manifest a
profile of psychiatric symptoms and disorders similar to that of the typically
developing persons. Preliminary studies using standardized methods of assessment reveal similar rates of attention deficit/hyperactivity disorder, conduct disorder, anxiety disorders (phobias, obsessive compulsive disorder, and generalized
anxiety), affective disorders, personality disorders, and schizophrenia, although
these rates may vary in those with more extensive brain dysfunction and severe
intellectual disability (Dekker and Koot, 2003). Some symptoms occur with
particular frequency among community residents, including feelings of social
inadequacy, dependency, and sensitivity to criticism (affecting one-quarter to
one-half), anxiety (affecting one-third), and aggressive behavior (affecting one-
fifth to one-fourth).

Mood Disorders

Mood disorders (e.g., major depression, bipolar disorder, and dysthymia) occur
commonly; they are responsible for a significant degree of morbidity and are
underdiagnosed. Approximately 2%–10% of intellectually disabled individuals
manifest major affective disorders; as many as 25% suffer from dysthymia. Thus,
affective disorders are common and often chronic. Preliminary investigations
have reported the successful use of assessment instruments developed for the
general population (e.g., Beck Inventory of Depression. Schedule for Affective
Disorders and Schizophrenia, Children's Depression Inventory). However, studies are needed to confirm adequate reliability and validity of these diagnoses in
adults with intellectual disability (Powell, 2003). The DC-LD field trials found
101 of 709 clinical cases had an affective disorder (Cooper, Melville, and Ein-
field, 2003). In persons with mild intellectual disability, the symptoms are similar
to those in individuals with typical development. However, the complaints may
be simpler and expressed more concretely; for example, feeling sick rather than
feeling sad. DSM-IVTR allows observer ratings of mood change in place of
self-reports. The diagnosis is then based on subjective change in mood, loss of
pleasure in usual activities and associated features, change in concentration,
sleep pattern and general interest. Symptoms are assessed in context, to the life

situation, and over time. Depression may lower the threshold for aggressive and self-injurious behavior and be associated with irritability, agitation, or increased rates of pre-existing routines or rituals. Thus, depression may reduce the threshold for other behaviors. Biological markers have been sought in an attempt to improve diagnostic accuracy. The dexamethasone suppression test (DST) has been piloted as an indicator of major depression in approximately 150 adults with intellectual disability. Results are similar to those reported for the general population, including a sensitivity of 40%–50% and a specificity of 75%–85%. Further study may clarify if the DST will be useful as a corroborative tool in the diagnosis of major depression among persons with intellectual disability. Environmental events have a greater likelihood of triggering depression because of limited cognitive adaptational strategies; for example, an unexpected change in housing or an awareness of difference from siblings.

Bipolar disorder can be distinguished from behavioral and psychiatric diagnoses in adults with intellectual disability, using DSM-IVTR criteria. Those individuals with clinical symptoms of bipolar disorder had significantly more mood-related and non–mood-related symptoms and also greater functional impairment than those with major depression (Cain et al., 2003). Rapid cycling bipolar disorder in people with intellectual disability (Vanstraelen and Tyrer, 1999) may differ from its occurrence in typically developing individuals with relative preponderance of males, increased likelihood of rapid cycling with pre-pubertal onset, and different response to medication. Rapid cycling bipolar disorder is characterized by significant changes in mood, behavior, and sleep, shifting frequently every few days. Finally, the issue of behavior as depressive equivalents in severe/profound intellectual disability has been examined (Tsiouris et al., 2003). These authors suggest that challenging behaviors (aggression or self-injury), were not closely associated with depression and recommend focusing on the core DSM-IVTR symptoms of depression in these individuals.

Suicide

Suicidal behavior is not generally emphasized in persons with intellectual disability, but suicides do occur and suicide threats must be taken seriously. Suicide attempts are most likely to occur in persons with mild intellectual disability. As is the case with typically developing persons, it is essential to consider an underlying psychiatric diagnosis when suicide ideation or behavior occurs. The major diagnosis associated with suicide is depressive disorder. Suicidal ideation and attempts are more common in mild intellectual disability and attempts have been reported in those with moderate-to-severe intellectual disability. Thoughts and gestures are similar to people without intellectual disability; however, certain means, such as guns, tend not to be available. For example, Hurley (1998) reported suicide attempts in a 26-year-old man and a 25-year-old woman with Down syndrome. The 26-year-old male had a supportive family and attended a community vocational program. His full-scale IQ was 62. He attempted suicide by jumping from a second-story window after several months of agitation and expressed sadness following rejection by a young woman. The 25-year-old woman lived with her mother and attended a vocational program. When her mother refused to allow her to attend social programs and other activities, she became agitated and inattentive, cried often, and appeared sad. She talked about feeling hopeless. She ran away from home, went to the town square and attempted to throw herself in front of a car. Her full scale IQ was 56. In both instances, these young adults were mildly intellectually impaired and distressed about social issues. Life event stresses, such as the loss of a loved one, trauma, physical and sexual abuse, and interpersonal or family discord, are correlated with suicide in the general population and in adolescents and adults with intellectual disability.

In inpatient settings, half of admissions for intellectually disabled persons to one unit were because of suicidality, and psychosocial stress was the main triggering event (Hardan and Sahl, 1999). The most common diagnoses on this inpatient unit were oppositional defiant disorder, depressive disorders, and posttraumatic stress disorder. Lunsky (2004) interviewed 98 adults with intellectual disability in the community setting, with collaborative information from caregivers. One in three reported that life was not worth living, 11% reported previous suicide attempts, and 23% reported thinking of killing themselves. Suicidal ideation was present in those with borderline IQ, as well as mild and moderate intellectual disability. Caregivers were aware of suicidal ideation for three-quarters of the group but not aware for almost one-quarter.

Death of a family member, abuse, and interpersonal distress were the most common precursors. Those with suicidal ideation were more likely to be unemployed and have a co-occurring psychiatric diagnosis. They reported more loneliness, stress, depression and anxiety. Suicidal thoughts or behavior were not limited to the higher functioning group; rates were high for those with moderate intellectual disability. In the inpatient setting (Hardan and Sahl, 1999), hanging was the most common method. In the community setting, overdose, self-cutting, and jumping were most commonly mentioned.

Finally, Patja et al. (2001) investigated suicidal mortality among people with intellectual disability over a 35-year period in a nationwide population cohort study in Finland. Women with intellectual disability had an equal suicide rate to Finnish women in general, while men had only one-third of the general population risk. Risk factors were similar to those in the general population. Most cases were mildly intellectually disabled and hospitalized for co-occurring mental disorders. Overall, the authors conclude that suicide prevention should focus particularly on family bereavement, abuse, and comorbid mental disorders, especially depressive disorder.

Suicidal behavior and deliberate self-harm are more common in mildly intellectually disabled persons than self-injurious behavior, which occurs most often in severely intellectually disabled persons. Self-injurious behavior and deliberate self-harm have been referred to as stress-related behavior disorders (Verhoeven et al., 1999).

Anxiety Disorders

Anxiety disorders are common in persons with intellectual disability overall and have an increased prevalence in specific neurogenetic syndromes. In a survey involving 10,438 children between ages 5 and 15 in the United Kingdom, the occurrence of any anxiety disorder was 8.7% (Emerson, 2003). The following diagnoses were identified using the Development and Well Being Assessment and a computer assisted diagnostic rating for DSM-IV and ICD-10 diagnoses: post traumatic stress disorder (0.8%), separation anxiety (2.7%), social phobia (0.8%), specific phobia (1.9%), panic disorder (0.4%), generalized anxiety disorder (1.5%), and other anxiety disorder (1.9%). In each instance, the rates for these disorders were substantially higher than population norms in the comparison group. Rates of over 20% have been noted in a referral population to specialty clinics (Feinstein and Reiss, 1996). Care should be taken evaluate for anxiety symptoms following physical and sexual abuse and bereavement.

Other instruments available for the diagnosis of anxiety in intellectually disabled persons include the Developmental Behavioral Checklist (Dekker et al., 2002) (where anxiety is one of the five subscales identified), Psychopathology Instrument for Mentally Retarded Adults (PIMRA), Zung Self-rating Scale for Anxiety, the internalizing scales on the CBCL, and the Glasgow Anxiety Scale for people with Intellectual Disability (GAS-ID). The GAS-ID measures state anxiety and includes 27 self-report items (Mindhan and Espie, 2003). Anxiety disorders are associated with several neurogenetic syndromes; among them are fragile X syndrome, Turner syndrome (Lesniak-Karpiak, Mazzocco, and Ross, 2003), and Williams syndrome. Social withdrawal, avoidance of social interaction, and gaze aversion, are reported in fragile X syndrome. Anxiety, shyness, and difficulty in understanding social cues have been reported in Turner Syndrome. Anxiety, fears, and phobias are reported in Williams syndrome. In one study (Dykens, 2003), individuals with Williams syndrome were compared with a mixed population of individuals with intellectual disability. Those with Williams syndrome had more generalized and anticipatory anxiety (51% and 60%, respectively), increases in specific phobia, and fearfulness. The majority of the group, 84%, expressed fearfulness and avoided fear-provoking situations. Cognitive behavior and psychopharmacologic treatments have been introduced to treat anxiety disorders. When medication is used, careful monitoring for side effects is essential.

Obsessive Compulsive Disorder

Obsessive compulsive disorder occurs at a higher rate in persons with intellectual disability, but must be distinguished from perseverative behaviors, stereotypies, self-stimulatory behaviors, and compulsions. In nonverbal persons, there is particular difficulty because of the inability to describe obsessional thoughts or to recognize compulsive behaviors as a response to obsessions. Repetitive behaviors, such as hoarding objects and arranging and rearranging items, have been considered evidence of obsessive compulsive disorder, in addition to classic contamination and cleaning rituals. A general population survey (Emerson, 2003) suggested a prevalence of 0.4% versus 0.2% in this population-based study. However, the rates are substantially higher in several neurogenetic synrdromes. In velocardiofacial syndrome, obsessive compulsive–like behavior, such as contamination, somatic worries, hoarding, repetitive questions, and cleaning, were noted, and 36% of a sample of 43 subjects who met DSM-IV criteria for obsessive compulsive disorder led the authors to propose early onset obsessive compulsive disorder in this condition (Gothelf et al., 2004). In Prader-Willi syndrome, nonfood obsessions and compulsions were investigated in 91 people aged 5 years to 47 years (mean age = 19 years). Prominent symptoms seen in 37%–58% of the sample included hoarding; ordering and arranging; concerns with symmetry and exactness; rewriting; and needs to tell, know, or ask (Dykens, Leckman, and Cassidy, 1996).

Schizophrenia and Psychotic Disorders

Although schizophrenia and schizophrenia spectrum disorders were once a controversial diagnosis in intellectually disabled persons, they are now well accepted. Careful studies have documented the presence of such symptoms as hallucinations, delusions, and thought disorder. The expression of these symptoms is generally more concrete and less elaborated than their occurrence in the general population. Comparisons of intellectually disabled and non–intellectually disabled persons with schizophrenia reveal that the former group has an earlier age of onset and a less favorable premorbid history. However, both groups exhibit a very similar profile of psychotic symptoms (e.g., hallucinations, delusions, or thought disorder). To make this diagnosis, a certain level of language development is required, and where that is present, the diagnosis is similar to those without intellectual disability.

Historically, Emil Kraeplin distinguished schizophrenia from mood disorders in 1896. He suggested that the disease had its onset early in life, thus referring to it as "dementia praecox" (premature deterioration of the brain). In 1911, Bleuler introduced the term "schizophrenia" and reported that the onset could occur in the later years and that most of those affected, after an initial deterioration in function, tended to stabilize for extended periods of time. The term "schizophrenia" (split mind) referred to the splitting of affective and cognitive functioning. Schizophrenia is increasingly considered to be a neurodevelopmental disorder rather than a neurodegenerative disorder.

Kraeplin identified cases in which low intellectual functioning existed before the onset of psychosis and did not worsen with the onset of psychosis. Thus, he recognized a type of schizophrenia that resulted from disrupted neurodevelopment. He referred to these cases as "pfropfschizophrenie." (Kraeplin, 1919). He described 3.5%–7% of cases of dementia praecox (schizophrenia) as "engrafted" (in German, pfropf, "to engraft") upon or the result of intellectual disability. Thus, Kraeplin accepted a model of schizophrenia that was not neurodegenerative and may be compatible with current neurodevelopmental models (Mack, Feldman, and Tsuang, 2002).

Kraeplin's focus on pfropfschizophrenie was subsequently obscured by varying diagnostic criteria (Turner, 1989). Recent studies are consistent with an increased incidence of psychotic illness among those with intellectual disability. Moreover, lower IQ is associated with an increased risk for schizophrenia, schizoaffective disorder, and nonaffective psychoses, but not bipolar disorder (Zammit et al., 2004.) Reid (1982) reported that schizophrenia occurs in intellectually disabled persons at a rate 2–3 times higher than in the general population, and subsequent studies have agreed. In one study (Deb, Thomas, and Bright, 2001) that used ICD-10 criteria, 4.4% of those with mild-to-moderate intellectual disability were identified as being affected by schizophrenia. The reason for the increased prevalence of schizophrenia in those with mild intellectual disability is not clear. Sanderson et al. (2001) carried out neuroimaging studies in 3 groups: comorbid mild intellectual disability and schizophrenia (23 cases), schizophrenia alone (25 cases), and mild intellectual disability alone (20 cases). With structural MRI, there was no clearly predictive inter- or intragroup difference; however, the authors report small amygdalo-hippocampal size associated with nervous system injury, especially meningitis. They propose that cognitive impairment and comorbid psychosis may result from a common etiology, for example, meningitis or obstetrical complications possibly interacting with family genetic factors. The authors further propose that those with comorbid intellectual disability and schizophrenia resemble patients with schizophrenia and no intellectual disability.

In regard to symptomatic presentation, Doody et al. (1998) compared 39 persons with mild intellectual disability and schizophrenia, 34 control subjects with schizophrenia, and 28 persons with mild intellectual disability alone. The comorbid group had more negative symptoms, episodic memory deficits, soft neurological signs, and seizure disorders; they received more community services. In addition, there was a trend for the comorbid group to be members of multiply affected families and show higher rates of chromosomal variants. These findings suggest that persons with premorbid intellectual disability be viewed as a discrete group; the authors suggest that this group may provide valuable genetic clues to the disorder.

One syndrome, velocardiofacial syndrome (22q11 deletion), has been linked to schizophrenia. It is a relatively common genetic disorder that results in malformation of the heart, face, and limbs. One in four affected persons develops a psychotic disorder with features of schizophrenia or schizoaffective disorder, and one in six a mood disorder. There is a range of other neuropsychiatric phenotypes, including intellectual disability, attention deficit disorder, rapid cycling bipolar disorder, and personality traits of shyness and impulsivity. The deleted region, 22q11.2, contains at least three genes (*COMPT, PRODH2, ZDHHC8*) implicated in schizophrenia risk (Jablensky, 2004). Bassett et al. (2003) report that those with the diagnosis of schizophrenia with 22q11.2 deletion show the same core clinical schizophrenia phenotype as those without the deletion. Because patients with different genomic deletions within the 22q11 region have similar phenotypes even though their deletions do not comprise the same set of genes, it may be that the full spectrum of anomalies may result from the disruption of numerous genes in this region that are linked to developmental or cellular processes. Thus, studying these syndromes may not only benefit persons with intellectual disability, who have an increased risk of schizophrenia, but also provide new genetic knowledge as to the mechanisms involved in psychosis for those who do not have this syndrome.

Those with severe and profound intellectual disability show a different profile of psychopathology than those who are moderately or mildly intellectually disabled. Certain symptoms occur less frequently, primarily because of limitations in cognitive and symbolic processes. These include delusions, hallucinations, referential ideation, obsessions, and guilty ruminations. Other symptoms must be used to make the diagnosis of psychosis; that is, change in behavior and mental state, onset of catatonic symptomatology, and deterioration in functioning linked to abnormal responses to the environment. Stereotyped behaviors, such as finger flicking and hand flapping, are present in 15%–50% of individuals with severe intellectual disability; self-injurious behaviors (SIB), such as eye gouging and head banging, are present in 10%–20% of these individuals.

Social Impairments/Pervasive Developmental Disorder

A particularly common association with intellectual disability is social impairment. Wing and Gould (1979) conducted an epidemiologic study of severely intellectually disabled children in London and concluded that more than half were socially impaired. Social impairment in children with brain dysfunction consisted of a triad of impairments encompassing social interaction, nonverbal and verbal communication, and imaginative development, accompanied by an increase in repetitive and stereotyped behaviors. These problems are broadly grouped under the ICD-10 category of "pervasive developmental disorder." Although some persons in the Wing and Gould study met diagnostic criteria for autistic disorder, the majority had less severe social impairments. Of these, three subgroups of social impairment were identified: (1) aloof and indifferent to others; (2) passive acceptance of social approaches; and (3) active, but with odd and inappropriate interaction. In other studies, the prevalence of social impairment has ranged from 25% to 42%.

Approximately 75% of children and adults with autistic disorder are diagnosed with intellectual disability. Intellectually disabled persons should be evaluated for the broader designation, DSM-IVTR pervasive developmental disorder. These disorders are more common among children and adults with severe-to-profound intellectual disability. The Scale of Pervasive Developmental Disorder in Mentally Retarded Persons (PDD-MRS) has been developed to aid in this assessment. Overall, 4%–8% of intellectually disabled children meet criteria for autistic disorder, or approximately 10–20 times the general population prevalence; however, the prevalence varies greatly among the neurogenetic syndromes.

Autistic disorder, atypical autistic disorder, or autistic features have been described in several neurogenetic disorders including tuberous sclerosis and following infection with the rubella virus in the first trimester. If autistic features are present there are significant impairments in reciprocal social interaction, social communication (verbal and nonverbal), and restricted repertoire of activities or interests (characteristic stereotypies) along with the intellectual disability. The modal IQ for persons with autistic disorder is in the moderate-to-low mild range of intellectual disability. Care should be given in making this diagnosis for individuals who are severely or profoundly intellectually disabled. Those with severe intellectual disability may have limited language, especially verbal language, limitations in social understanding, and exhibit stereotypies and self-stimulation. The diagnosis of pervasive developmental disorder should not be made unless there is evidence of significant impairment of social skills and communication and stereotypes typical of autistic disorder. Moreover, if there is a known syndrome, the behavioral phenotype and its natural history must be taken into account. For example, in fragile X syndrome, when autistic features occur, the evolution of these behaviors over time differs from classic autistic disorder. The same is the case for congenital rubella syndrome. The pattern of symptoms may change over time so that the diagnosis may be more difficult to confirm in adulthood. It is best to consider the developmental trajectory or natural history of the disorder in addition to the diagnostic criteria. Ascertaining, to the extent possible, whether an individual met criteria for a pervasive developmental disorder in childhood is part of the diagnostic assessment for adults with intellectual disability.

Anatomical and genetic studies are ongoing to understand the biological basis of autistic disorder and its relationship to intellectual disability syndromes. Classic neuropathological findings in autistic disorder are consistent regarding the limbic system (9 of 14 studied cases show increased cell packing density and smaller neuronal size), the cerebellum (21 of 29 studied cases showed a decreased number of Purkinje cells; in all 5 cases that were examined for age-related morphological alterations, these changes were found in cerebellar nuclei and inferior olive) and the cerebral cortex (>50% of the studied cases showed features of cortical dysgenesis). Approximately 70% of these cases have co-occurring intellectual disability (Palmen et al., 2004). There are ongoing efforts using neuroimaging techniques to clarify how brain morphology functioning is linked to autistic behaviors. For example, one study compared children with intellectual disability with and without the diagnosis of autistic disorder. Children with autistic disorder, with and without intellectual disability, had a larger right hippocampal volume than typically developing controls. The amygdala in typically developing children increases substantially in volume from 7.5 to 18.5 years of age; however, the amygdala in children with autistic disorder is initially larger but does not undergo the age-related increase observed in typically developing children. Thus, there may be an abnormal early amygdala development in autism and an abnormal pattern of hippocampal development that persists through adolescence (Schumann et al., 2004).

Attention Deficit Disorder

Intellectual disability is frequently associated with short attention span and overactivity. Overall, the prevalence of ADHD is at least as common, 4%–11%

(Feinstein and Reiss, 1996), if not more common in those with intellectual disability than in the general population. The rate of hyperactivity is increased with increasing severity of intellectual disability. The prevalence of ADHD varies by syndrome, with rates far higher than the general population rate in several syndromes. Among these are fragile X syndrome, phenylketonuria, velocardiofacial syndrome, Williams syndrome, and neurofibromatosis. Rating scales completed by teachers provide valid information for the assessment of ADHD in children with intellectual disability and DSM-IVTR criteria may be utilized. One study compared rating scales and found the best support for the Aberrant Behavior Checklist-Community Version (ABC-C) in the assessment of children with ADHD and intellectual disability (Miller, Fee, and Jones, 2004). The diagnosis of ADHD in adults with intellectual disability may also be assessed, using the Diagnostic Criteria for Learning Disabilities/Mental Retardation [DC-LD] (Seager and O'Brien, 2003). Overall, children who test in the intellectually disabled IQ range with the diagnosis of ADHD definitely respond to stimulant treatment with methylphenidate, but their rate of beneficial response appears to be well under that found for those testing in the normal IQ range and their response to treatment shows greater variability (Aman, Buican, and Arnold, 2003). Different attentional mechanisms may moderate the response to psychostimulants in specific intellectual disability syndromes to account for these differences. In the evaluation, whether attention deficits and hyperactivity are situation-specific or pervasive is an important consideration in making the diagnosis.

Disruptive Behavior Disorders and Antisocial Behavior

Disruptive behavior disorders are the common psychiatric disorders in childhood and occur ranging from 4% to 9% in various surveys. The prevalence of conduct disorder, as well as other disruptive behavior disorders (oppositional behavior disorder or disruptive behavior disorder not otherwise specified) is higher among children with intellectual disability, with rates more than double those found in the general population. For those affected with severe intellectual disability, the term challenging behavior is used to describe aggression and self-injurious behavior. Challenging behaviors present major problems in management. In one survey, data was collected on multistage, stratified, random sample of 10,438 children between 5 and 15 years of age in England, Scotland, and Wales. Conduct disorder was found to be significantly greater among children with intellectual disability than among their typically developing peers. The rate for any conduct disorder was 25% in the intellectually disabled group and 4.2% in the control group. Among these, the rates were the following: oppositional defiant disorder (13.3% vs. 2.2%), unsocialized conduct disorder (3.3% vs. 0.3%), and socialized conduct disorder (3.8% vs. 0.8%) (Emerson, 2003). The major factors associated with an increased risk of psychopathology among children and adolescents with intellectual disability included age, gender, social deprivation, family composition, number of potentially stressful life events, the mental health of the child's primary caregiver, family functioning, and child management practices. Psychosocial intervention is required to ensure that support services are responsive to both the needs of child and the needs of the family. For those with severe disruptive behavior, medication treatment may be indicated (De Smedt et al., 2002). A double-blind placebo controlled study involving 118 children (aged 5–12 years) with IQs between 36 and 84 found that risperidone was effective and well tolerated for treatment of severely disruptive behaviors. (Aman et al., 2002).

Low Overall Risk for Criminal Behavior

Because of concerns regarding increased criminality in intellectually disabled persons, intellectual disability has been regarded as a risk factor for criminal behavior. Studies carried out in special schools for youth with behavioral problems and prisons find that a significant number of their residents have intellectual and developmental disabilities. Even though a disproportionately higher number of adults with intellectual disability are found in correctional facilities, criminal offenders account for only a small fraction of the entire population of persons with intellectual disability. It is difficult to determine the rate of antisocial behavior in intellectual disability because crime often goes unreported, intelligence may not be measured properly, and studies investigate only those in the criminal justice system (Holland, Clare, and Mukhopadhyay, 2002). Factors to consider in rates of crime include the following: (1) those with intellectual disability may be more likely to be apprehended when they are involved in antisocial behavior, (2) the person with intellectual disability may lack the life experience to understand what appropriate community behavior is and get into trouble for that reason, and (3) persons with intellectual disability may confess to crime, thinking they are pleasing those in authority by doing so.

One study identified two broad groups of individuals with antisocial behavior and intellectual disability. The larger of these was made up of individuals with mental disorders (often substance abuse) or severe psychosocial disadvantage. The smaller group had challenging, usually aggressive behavior or difficult behavior characterized as antisocial. The authors (Holland, Clare, and Mukhopadhyay, 2002) call for greater emphasis on the mechanisms that lead from difficult behavior to antisocial ones.

Self-Injurious Behavior (SIB)

Self-injurious behavior is perhaps the most extreme and dangerous form of behavior seen in persons with intellectual disability (NIH, 1990; Schroeder, Oster-Granite, and Thompson, 2002). Self-injury presents therapeutic, economic, and ethical problems. Acts of self-injury by persons with intellectual disability indicate failure in community treatment and necessitate the return of the person to more restrictive settings. It occurs in many syndromes and is multiply determined. There are multiple etiologies that involve both psychosocial stress and genetic vulnerability. In the DSM-IVTR diagnostic system, it is classified as stereotypical movement disorder with self-injurious behavior. The criteria list behaviors that are (1) repetitive, driven, nonfunctional motor behavior, (2) interfere with normal activities, (3) result in self-inflicted bodily injury/or wound (4) are severe and a focus of treatment, and (5) persist for 4 weeks or longer. Self-injury has been reported in 10%–70% of institutionalized persons with intellectual disability: The lower the IQ, the higher the prevalence rate. It occurs most often in severely and profoundly intellectually disabled individuals, and in younger children who have associated language disabilities, visual impairments, or seizures. The peak rate is in adolescence and frequency of occurrence is greater in males than females (3.5 to 1). In a community sample, Griffin et al. (1987) documented the prevalence of self-injury in 2,663 intellectually disabled, autistic, or multiply disabled children and adolescents in a large community metropolitan school district. They found 69 cases, or 2.6%, demonstrated self-injury during the 12-month period chosen for this study; 59% were male and 41% were female. The majority of this group (83%) was severely or profoundly intellectually disabled. The mean age of those surveyed was 10 years and the majority, three-quarters of the group, demonstrated the behavior daily. For those ages 14 and above, the prevalence was lower, perhaps related to community placement for older individuals. The most common symptoms were hand hitting, head hitting, and head banging. Other forms of self-injury include eye gouging, hair pulling, and nail picking, as well as multiple forms of self-injury in one individual.

The following must be considered in assessment: normal self-stimulatory behavior, self-stimulation in the blind, tic behaviors, factitious disorder and deliberate self-harm, obsessive compulsive disorder with self-injury, impulse control disorders such as trichotillomania, and self-injury associated with mood dysregulation and mood disorders. In normal development, the head-banging rate from ages 8 months to 36 months is 3.6%–6.5%. For infants and preschool children, it is linked to teething and otitis media. It may be preceded by self-stimulation or tantrums and generally terminates without treatment by age 36 months. Several models have been proposed to understand self-injury. These include animal models of isolation rearing, opioid/nonopioid stress-induced analgesia, and issues involving neuromaturation, particularly development of the cerebellum. Other models include altered anatomy/physiologic state, neurotoxic lesions, and drug-induced changes in physiologic state (Harris, 1995).

Neurogenetic disorders with associated self-injurious behavior include Lesch-Nyhan disease (hand and lip biting), Rett's disorder (hand injury with hand-to-mouth behavior), congenital insensitivity to pain (chewing fingers and tongue and accidental physical injury), Smith-Magenis syndrome (hand/wrist biting, head banging, onychotillomania, and polyembolokoilamania), Tourette syndrome (head banging, body punching, tooth pulling, and body piercing), Prader-Willi syndrome (skin picking), fragile X syndrome, pervasive developmental disorder, Riley-Day syndrome (biting mouth, lips, and tongue; deliberate self-harm). The treatment of self-injurious behavior is described in chapter 9.

Specific behavioral difficulties linked to specific syndromes are discussed in other chapters describing specific neurogenetic conditions and fetal alcohol spectrum disorder.

Dementia and Delirium

Dementia may occur in persons with intellectual disability. When both diagnoses are present, both should be recorded. This has been studied most often in individuals with Down syndrome, but is also reported as a risk factor with aging, particularly in persons with moderate intellectual disability. It is important to provide monitoring so that cognitive decline is recognized. Standard screening instruments, such as the Mini-Mental State Examination, do not distinguish between intellectual disability and developing dementia. The diagnosis is based on functional decline in five areas: memory, general mental functioning (e.g., planning and thinking), higher cortical functions, including language (e.g., dysphasias and dyspraxias), skills (community or home living and work), and personality (onset of apathy, disinhibited behaviors, and stubbornness). But memory is the most critical element. To assess for dementia, the informant must know the person for at least six months and must have the knowledge to probe for functional decline in each of these five areas. Informant-based questionnaires are recommended for diagnosis (Deb and Braganza, 1999) along with repeat neuropsychological assessments. There should be no clouding of consciousness, and the disorder must be progressive over time to rule out delirium. Depression and physical illness that might be linked to decline should be ruled out since they may be responsive to treatment.

In Down syndrome and in fragile X carriers, a dementia syndrome occurs, and these disorders require careful observation.

Alcohol and Substance Abuse

Substance abuse among persons with intellectual disability following deinstitutionalization is now a greater concern because of greater exposure to alcohol and other substances of abuse. Intellectually disabled persons do appear to use and abuse alcohol at similar or lower rates than noncognitively impaired peers and illicit drugs at a moderately lower rate (Burgard et al., 2000). By the mid-1990s, over 50% of intellectually disabled persons lived in noninstitutional settings with six or fewer residents. Abuse of alcohol and other substances occurs, particularly in mildly intellectually disabled individuals. Of the two, alcoholism and alcohol misuse are the more common problems. One study (Westermeyer et al., 1988) compared 40 mildly intellectually disabled persons with substance abuse to 40 mildly intellectually disabled persons without substance abuse. Similarities with substance abusers who are not intellectual disabled were demonstrated. Demographic characteristics, family and childhood history, substance use patterns, and substance-related problems were reviewed.

A survey of older individuals (DiNitto and Krishef, 1983/1984) found that 52% of 214 people with intellectual disability had ever consumed an alcoholic beverage, with 7% drinking daily and 33% at least once a week. These authors found that alcohol use contributed to job-related problems including absenteeism, tardiness, and poor relations with coworkers. Another survey of 596 adults with intellectual disability living semi-independently in the community found

56% drank alcohol and 3% used marijuana. These rates for alcohol used were lower than general population exposure of 88% for alcohol use and 41% for marijuana. When drug use among special education students and those in regular education was compared, approximately 55% of students with developmental disabilities reported using alcohol compared to 72% in the general population (Gress and Boss, 1996). Moreover, marijuana (27%), cocaine (3%), and amphetamine (8%) exposure were noted in the special education group; these values were lower than those found in the regular education students. For adults, alcohol use affected family relationships (Westermeyer, Phaobtong, and Neider, 1988) and relationships outside the family. Seven percent of alcohol users reported legal problems, including warnings and being taken to jail. One-third of the total sample of alcohol users reported having seizures and taking medications. The interaction of medications with alcohol use requires careful monitoring.

Persons with intellectual disability may be at risk for substance abuse owing to impulsivity and problems in self-regulation or a desire to gain social attention and "fit in" with others; however, this has not been carefully studied. Individuals whose mothers abused alcohol during pregnancy (gestational substance abuse) are at increased risk for alcohol abuse themselves. Early signs of alcohol use are irritability, loss of self-help skills, socially inappropriate behaviors, and aggression. Slurred speech, unsteady gait, and poor coordination must be distinguished from movement disorders and dysarthria that may be related to intellectual disability (Rivinius, 1988). Screening for drug use is appropriate in evaluations for independent living and supportive employment. More effective assessments and interventions and modifications in existing intervention programs are needed when problems are identified. Staff in chemical dependency programs may lack training in intellectual disability and medical conditions associated with intellectual disability. Barriers to treatment include diminished skills in reading and in abstract reasoning, as well as social skills deficits. However, inadequate detection, lack of funding for programs, and lack of outreach are all barriers to effective treatment. Best practice guidelines for detection, treatment, and prevention are needed (Christian and Poling, 1997).

Eating Disorders

Nutrition, weight-related health issues, and eating disorders must be considered in persons with intellectual disability. Weight surveys suggest that up to one-third of institutional adults with intellectual disability are obese or significantly underweight, with somewhat lower rates in community settings, suggesting that eating problems are more common than in the general population. The ingestion of nonnutritive substances, pica, and rumination are particularly associated with severe intellectual disability. Adults with severe and profound intellectual disability may be significantly underweight, especially if there is not adequate supervision of their eating behaviors. Those with severe intellectual disability who are immobile, unable to self-feed, have difficulty tolerating solid foods, or have problems with chronic vomiting, rumination, and regurgitation are of particular concern.

Overall, specific eating problems that have been recognized include pica, rumination, regurgitation, psychogenic vomiting, and food faddiness or food refusal. The ICD-10-MR guide indicates that diagnostic guidelines for childhood onset rumination/regurgitation, food faddiness/food refusal, and pica may be used when these disorders occur in adults with intellectual disability. However, there are difficulties in making eating disorder diagnoses in persons with limited communication and abstract reasoning abilities. Anorexia nervosa and bulimia nervosa are rare in persons with intellectual disability, especially those in the moderate-to-severe range. Eating disorders may be associated with physical disorders, behavioral disorders, behavioral phenotypes in certain syndromes, and other psychiatric diagnoses (Gravestock, 2000). A cardinal feature of the Prader-Willi syndrome is hyperphagia, which, if left untreated, leads to extreme obesity. Food foraging and pica also occur in Prader-Willi syndrome. Pica and rumination have been described in tuberous sclerosis and Rett's disorder. Eating disturbances are reported in Down syndrome, Klein-Levin syndrome, Turner syndrome (anorexia nervosa), and phenylketonuria.

EVALUATION OF BEHAVIORAL AND PSYCHIATRIC DISORDER

The assessment process in developmental neuropsychiatric disorders involves a comprehensive evaluation of the individual child and his family. Three approaches are involved: (1) clinical assessments, which include the history, individual and family clinical interviews, and mental status examination of the child, adolescent, or adult; (2) structured interviews, questionnaires, behavior checklists, and rating scales; and (3) standardized tests including psychological and neurological examinations. Background knowledge in normal development, psychopathology, classification, knowledge of the genetic disorder, and the specific tests used is a prerequisite. In dealing with developmental psychopathology in persons with intellectual disability, knowledge of the specific syndromes and their natural history is essential. The establishment of a diagnosis based on clinical assessment is complicated by difficulties in adapting the mental disorders classification system to children and adults with developmental disorders and acquired neurological dysfunction. Because of the complexities of each case, familiarity with a variety of assessment approaches and instruments is important. Guidelines for assessment are provided by the American Academy of Child and Adolescent Psychiatry in their "Practice parameters for the assessment and treatment of children, adolescents, and adults with mental retardation and comorbid mental disorders" (Szymanski and King, 1999) and for adults by the European Association for Mental Health in Mental Retardation through their "Practice guidelines for the assessment and diagnosis of mental health problems in adults with intellectual disability" (Deb et al., 2001).

The interview must take into account the person's cognitive and adaptive limitations. Consequently, interviews frequently need to be more structured, directive, and shorter than those conducted with typically developing persons. After establishing rapport, the interviewer should provide overt support and ongoing social reinforcement so that the interview is not perceived as a test that might be failed. Care must be taken to avoid leading questions. When findings are discussed with an intellectually disabled person, the interpretation about emotional and behavioral functioning should be presented so as to be understood at the individual's overall developmental level.

The Psychiatric Interview

Informants

Children, adolescents, and adults with intellectual disability and neuropsychiatric problems are most often referred because of parental or staff concerns about their development and behavior. The assessment aims at establishing a clear account of behavior and its effects on the individual and others. Since many persons with intellectual disability do not live alone and attend school, activities, or vocational programs, their development can be influenced by interpersonal relationships and the attitudes of those with whom they come in contact. The assessment, then, involves not only interviewing and observing the person with intellectual disability, but also the attitudes and behavior of others (parents, siblings, teachers, peers, staff members, and other significant adults) that are directed toward the affected person in the context of the developmental disorder. Moreover, because of limitations of the intellectually disabled person to provide a detailed account of the presence of behavioral difficulties, informants who can describe behavior at home, at school, at workshops, in supportive employment, and in the community are essential in the assessment process. One may then compare accounts of the behavior in each of these settings to clarify whether the behavioral problem is situational, that is, only occurring at home, at school, or in community programs; or pervasive, that is, occurring in each of these settings. It is not uncommon for there to be major differences between reports that come from school, home, and community settings.

The assessment process must take into account that intellectually disabled persons are continually developing, although at a rate commensurate with their disability, so that their expressed behavior and psychological symptoms must be evaluated in the context of the developmental phase. For assessment purposes, it is best to consider the intellectually disabled person and family or surrogate together as a unit and to take into account the milieu in a community setting. Background information about the family will assist in understanding how development has proceeded for this particular person. In addition, an understanding of the strengths and weaknesses of the family unit and/or milieu in a community setting are essential for treatment planning. The response of parents and siblings, peers, and teachers to the difficulties—the impact of the behavior on others—must always be considered.

In conducting the assessment, observations of the person with intellectual disability, both alone and in his interactions with family members or staff, must be arranged. The examiner observes the intellectually disabled person in both structured and unstructured settings. The assessment begins in the waiting area, with observations of the intellectually disabled person's interactions with his parents and/or siblings or staff members, and continues with observations of the manner of separation when leaving the family or staff to enter the examining room. Observation in structured settings, such as neuropsychological testing, is also important.

A flexible approach is most helpful whether the person with intellectual disability is seen separately or as part of a family or community group. One approach is for the interviewer to see both together to clarify the intellectually disabled person's understanding of the reason for the consultation, to clarify whether the reason for the visit has been discussed between the informant and the person with intellectually disability, and to establish the confidential nature of the interviews with both the informant and the person with intellectual disability.

A complete assessment of the family includes a phase of interviewing the whole family, which allows information to be gathered about hierarchical relationships within the family, communication patterns, affective tone among family members, and alliances between them. Individual interviews are then conducted with each parent to establish their perspective on the intellectually disabled person's difficulties. While interviews with parents are conducted, the person with intellectual disability generally waits outside to be interviewed until after the interview is completed, although this varies with the age and developmental level of the person being evaluated.

Before leaving his family or staff, the person is informed about what will take place during his absence, and he is then taken to a waiting section where adequate supervision is available. Special arrangements may be necessary for preschool children who may have difficulty separating from parents in a strange setting and for persons with intellectual disability and brain injury who have severe behavioral problems.

Interview with Parents or Caretakers

It is always best to see both the mother and the father. The role of both parents in the life of the intellectually disabled person is essential and, although the extent of involvement may differ between the parents at different ages, each parent is intimately involved in the individual's psychological experience whether they are physically present or not. For those with developmental disorders, involvement of both parents is of particular importance since it is not uncommon for one parent to have borne the burden of primary care, which may have precluded the other parent's developing a realistic attitude regarding the individual's abilities. Moreover, an interview with both parents together often provides an excellent opportunity to observe parental interaction and their relationships. When parents are divorced or separated and the person with intellectual disability spends time with each of them, it may be best and more appropriate to see each parent on a separate occasion. For adults living in a group home setting, the same recommendations apply to guardians and staff members.

Information from Other Sources

Parental consent must be obtained to contact agencies, primary physicians, and other referral sources. For adults, permission must be sought through community programs. Obtaining permission to contact the school and other agencies is essential to establish a well-rounded view of the current life situation. The teacher or community staff's account of the behavior at school, workshop, or supported employment is critical. Knowledge about the type of classroom and the specific individualized educational program for developmentally disordered children and the workshop or work setting must be reviewed as part of the assessment process. In addition, information on school, workshop, or work attendance, particular academic strengths and weaknesses, nonacademic skills, such as artistic and musical ability, behavior in the classroom or work place, and relationships with peers and with teachers or staff are important. Moreover, rating scales completed by teachers or work place staff are gathered at the time of the initial assessment and on an ongoing basis. For an older adolescent or young adult enrolled in a workshop program, information from the job coach or supervisor will be needed.

Developmental Aspects of Interviewing

Persons with intellectual disability are developing, so the diagnostic assessment must maintain a developmental perspective that considers the following: (1) individuals behave differently at different ages, so knowledge of age-appropriate behavior is necessary; (2) the disorder may interfere with the normal course of development; (3) different phases of development are associated with different stresses, thus a preschooler is most likely to be affected by separation experiences, and a stressed adolescent may exhibit frequent mood swings; and (4) developmental tasks vary with age.

The interview with the intellectually disabled person must take into account both the individual's developmental level and his ability to communicate. The purpose of the initial interview is to make contact with the person with intellectual disability, to establish confidence and cooperation, to know the person, to learn his responses to his current difficulties and his perception of them, and to assess his ability to cooperate in treatment. The person with intellectual disability may experience anxiety in encountering the interviewer and will concurrently be "sizing up" the interviewer during the interview process.

When examining infants or severely and profoundly intellectually disabled children who have not established expressive language milestones, the initial observations must focus on social milestones. During the first year, the most important of these are the establishment of eye contact, attachment, stranger anxiety, and the reciprocal use of language in babbling and jargon. With infants, one uses the infantile form of language called "motherese," which involves extending vowel sounds and speaking more slowly to the infant. An infant responds to the adult's mood and gestures in an active and perceptive way, which emerges from his own experience with familiar caregivers. The response to change or newness is more intense after a mental age of six months, when selective attachments and stranger anxiety have emerged as developmental mile-stones.

In examining an infant, the approach is indirect, almost casual. The inter-viewer may be still and quiet but close enough to observe. Initially, the inter-viewer makes no gesture or threat and does not use direct eye contact until the infant has had the opportunity to observe the interviewer from a safe and com-fortable distance. In approaching an infant or a withdrawn intellectually disabled child, an outstretched hand may be offered to encourage the child to reach out. For infants and nonverbal intellectually disabled children, it is generally best for them to make the first move. In making infant observations, it is important to observe the parents' preferred holding posture and imitate it.

With many intellectually disabled children, one should keep in mind that although they may not be speaking, their receptive language might be adequate to understand what is said about them. Since language comprehension precedes verbal expression, words they hear may be misinterpreted by them.

For those with mental ages between 2 and 4 years who are able to talk and have a better understanding of what is said to them, the interviewer may proceed verbally and with the use of play materials. At this mental age, individuals are very literal in their understanding of the words they use and those that they hear from others. Since thinking is concrete, actions may be understood in a concrete way. Descriptions should avoid the use of analogies, and it is important to be aware that abstractions should be used cautiously when discussing problems with the person with intellectual disability. Learning to speak at the language level of the person interviewed will facilitate communication in future visits. In ad-dition to literalness, at a mental age between 2 and 4 transductive, reasoning is apparent, leading to giving inanimate objects human attributes. The individual may attribute feelings and motives to household objects or at least speak as if they have them. For example, he may say that a machine that has stopped has gone to sleep and may practice putting toys to sleep and waking them up. During this mental age period, individuals tend to be active and may be difficult to please or satisfy in a new office setting. Feelings such as sadness, anger, fear-fulness, and jealousy are poorly modulated. Moreover, the individual may have difficulty controlling anger and show unpredictability in behavior related to emo-tions.

During an examination, an initial period of warming up and talking to a person about his interests and successes may alleviate this initial anxiety. Younger individuals communicate their feelings through their behavior or through imaginary play. During play interviews, the individual may show themes that are conflictual in home or community settings.

From mental age 7, individuals are better able to express fears and feelings verbally but may be unclear about the nature of their concerns. They may ask questions in a veiled fashion, so it is essential to clarify the meaning of their questions before responding to them. A frequent and persistent question may indicate a hidden concern.

Individuals whose cognitive function is at a mental age above 7 may be interviewed more directly about their concerns and life experiences. For the older individual, the interview is semistructured, as described in the following section.

Interview with the Person with Intellectual Disability

The person with intellectual disability can be the most important source of information and during the assessment should be seen separately unless severe separation anxiety or the extent of behavioral difficulty does not allow this. The person's view of the presenting problem should be sought out, although the quality of this report will vary according to developmental age. For those who are nonverbal, specific adaptations of the interview are necessary and specific devices, such as letter boards and speech aids, may be necessary to facilitate communication.

In the past, there has been reluctance to use a formalized mental status examination with intellectually disabled persons because of concerns about the reliability of verbal information from them and a sense that their language and thought are too elusive for clinical description. Concerns have been expressed regarding the person's developmental level, the age when verbal approaches could be used, and the possible transient nature of psychopathology. There have been concerns that directed interviewing would lead to anxiety and hostility, and questions have been raised about phenomenology, psychodynamics, and their usefulness in determining causation in persons with intellectual disability. Because of these considerations, interview behavior has varied with some interviewers using direct questioning and observation and others using less formal approaches, such as play, drawings, and other imaginative methods. Yet both approaches are needed, the formal direct interview to elicit symptoms needed to make a diagnosis and the imaginal methods to establish contact and conduct treatment.

Because of past concerns about the nature of the mental status examination in persons with intellectual disability, considerable effort has gone into improving psychiatric interviewing procedures. The establishment of structured and semistructured interviews has been motivated by dissatisfaction with reliability and validity of traditional diagnostic procedures. The development of structured interview schedules for persons with intellectual disability followed the development of such interview schedules with typically developing persons (Endicott and Spitzer, 1978; Robins et al., 1981). Moreover, the development of a more comprehensive classification of psychiatric disorders with more explicit diagnostic criteria has required a more standardized approach to the assessment of symptoms (APA, 2000; WHO, 1992). However, the use of the standard interview must be modified for persons with intellectual disability because descriptions of symptoms are affected by the extent of cognitive impairment, as well as receptive and expressive language deficits.

Face-to-face interviews are important to establish rapport and to focus on symptoms of concern, which help maintain the individual's interest during the interview. Such interviews help to clarify misunderstandings about the parents' or staff's interpretation of the individual's behavior and provide an opportunity to document the context and chronicity of symptoms. Although the assessment of psychopathology requires data from parents and other informants, persons with intellectual disability are essential informants regarding their own feelings, behaviors, and social relationships. Symptom-oriented interviews are effective means for establishing diagnoses in individuals who may be too young to complete verbal self-reports.

The earliest structured interviews for children are those of Lapouse and Monk (1958) and Rutter and Graham (1968). However, detailed evaluation of structured and semistructured interviewing was developed in the ensuing years. These interviews are used for both clinical and research purposes and have involved conceptual, methodological, and technical problems in their development. All these instruments provide a list of target behaviors, symptoms, and life events that must be covered together with guidelines for conducting the interview and recording the child or adolescent's responses. The degree of structure imposed on the interview varies from the semistructured approach in which only general and flexible guidelines for conducting the interviewing and recording the information are given, to highly structured interviews that specify the exact order, wording, and coding of each item. Because they can be individualized to the person and provide greater range in phrasing questions and following alternative lines of inquiry and interpreting responses, semistructured interviews are usually conducted by clinically sophisticated interviewers. The highly structured interview, which is used most commonly in epidemiologic studies, reduces the role of clinical inference made by a more experienced examiner and can be administered by lay interviewers. The development of appropriately structured interviews of adaptation for older persons is an ongoing issue for persons with intellectual disability.

Although there are differences in the type of information gained from structured and semistructured interviews, the majority produce information about the presence, absence, and severity of onset and/or duration of specific symptoms. Some interviews produce a quantitative score regarding symptom profiles or a global index of psychopathology.

The use of semistructured approaches to elicit the nature and extent of abnormalities of emotions, behavior, and interpersonal relationships is the most appropriate method in a clinical setting. Specific probes related to particular diagnostic criteria are incorporated into the clinical interview.

The Psychiatric History

After establishing demographic and other background information and clarifying the reliability of the person referred, then the parent or other informant, the person with intellectual disability, or staff are asked about their specific concerns. The reason for referral, as well as a statement about the onset of the current difficulties and the family life situation or community situation at the time the difficulties began, are elicited. The interviewer specifically asks about why the individual is being referred at this particular point in time. Precipitating stressful events that may contribute to the behavioral, emotional or interpersonal problem are reviewed and the individual's, parents', or staff's specific concerns are addressed. Among the specific concerns to be considered are academic, school problems and/or work behavior, emotional conflicts, regressive behavior, and interpersonal difficulties with others. The individual's previous treatment should be reviewed, and the effects of the person's current behavior on family functioning addressed and clarified. Following these questions, a reclarification of the goals in seeking help at this time is elicited.

The family history is reviewed, clarifying what the individual's current status is in regard to step-parenting, adoption, foster care, group home, or community placement. The family background for both parents is obtained, including information about their childhood experiences, with particular emphasis on the family atmosphere in their homes as they grew up, stresses related to emotional and economic issues, and deaths or separation from close relatives. Information about the grandparents and others closely affiliated with the person with intellectual disability is elicited along with a developmental family history of how the parents' marriage evolved. The quality of relatedness in the current marriage, including the frequency of disagreements and how disagreements are expressed, coping mechanisms, how conflict is dealt with in the family, and the relationship to the family of origin, are reviewed. The siblings are described in regard to age, school placement, history of significant illness, personality, and relationship to other family members.

A family history of executive dysfunction in parents and extended family members is sought, as is family history of developmental milestones, learning disability, and problems in school achievement. The family history should include specific questions about alcoholism, drug abuse, abnormal personality, suicide/homicide, manic-depressive disease, and schizophrenia.

A review of past and personal history should include the date and place of birth, birth weight, attitude of both parents toward the pregnancy, and whether the pregnancy was planned or unplanned. If there were difficulties with the pregnancy or delivery, the response of the parents to those events should be included.

Developmental milestones should emphasize the social developmental milestones, which include eye contact, social smile, language communication, and interpersonal attachment. Interpersonal issues that relate to feeding and illness must be considered, as are the parents' attitudes toward child rearing. Rearing practices and attitudes about permissiveness and limit setting are reviewed. For adults and adolescents, the current relationship with the family is discussed.

A behavioral review of systems, which includes information on temperament, early development, emotional responsiveness, antisocial behavior, attentional difficulties, self-stimulation, and imaginative behavior, is then carried out.

This is followed by an assessment of school activities including the age of beginning school, the current grade, schools attended, types of class placement, and emotional adjustment to beginning school. Separation problems at the time of entry into preschool or elementary school or the work place are discussed. If there were prolonged absences from school or if school years were repeated, this information along with specific difficulties in reading, writing, math, and spelling are noted. Study habits and academic goals for the person are discussed, and the person's peer relationships are clarified. If the person is teased or is a bully, this information is included, as is information about particular friendships. Attitudes toward his teachers, peers, schoolwork, and work place are obtained, as appropriate. For adults, attitudes toward staff and colleagues in the workplace are reviewed.

An assessment of the individual's awareness of his sexual identity, which includes questions regarding curiosity about his own body and about reproduction, as well as his sexual interest and activities, is made. For the adolescent, the interview includes information regarding the mastery of adolescent developmental tasks and the young person's attitude toward entry into adolescence, as appropriate for mental age. One looks for mature versus pseudomature behavior and attitudes toward peers, family members, and those in authority. Rebelliousness, drug taking, periods of depression and withdrawal, and the adolescent's fantasy life are discussed with the parents. How the young person has responded to puberty with accompanying voice changes, hair growth, and menarche, as well as masturbation and sexual concerns, are raised. Similar questions are posed, as appropriate, for adults with intellectual disability.

Previous mental health history, which includes details of any disturbances for which treatment was received and the type of treatment that was carried out, is gathered. This is followed by a description of the life situation at present, which includes current housing, social situation, parents' work and financial circumstances, the composition of the household, the relationship with neighbors, recent stresses, bereavement, losses, or disappointments and how both parents and the individual have reacted to them. A typical day in the individual's life, which includes getting off to school or work, activities during the school or workday, returning home, and evening activities, is described.

In the parent interview, questions about personality are addressed. This includes habitual attitudes and patterns of behavior that distinguish him as an individual. Among the personality characteristics reviewed are attitudes toward others, including ability to trust others and to make and sustain a relationship with them. Whether the individual is secure or insecure in interpersonal relationships and is a leader or a follower are established. The attitude toward interpersonal relationships, whether it is friendly, warm, and demonstrative or reserved, cold, or indifferent is considered. Other characteristics discussed include aggressiveness, quarrelsomeness, sensitivity, and suspiciousness. The interviewer asks about the individual's attitude toward himself, including self-dramatizing behavior, egocentric behavior, self-consciousness, and ambition. Moreover, attitudes toward personal health and bodily functions are included in the assessment to establish whether or not the individual's self-appraisal is realistic.

An assessment of personality also includes appraisal of moral and religious attitudes, an assessment of whether the individual is easygoing, permissive, overly conscientious, perfectionistic, or conforming. Mood is considered in regard to lability and general attitude and whether the individual is optimistic or pessimistic. The presence of anxiety, irritability, excessive worrying, and apathy are noted. The ability to express and control feelings of anger, sadness, pleasure, and disappointment is reviewed.

Leisure-time activities and interests, including interest in books, pictures, music, sports, and creative activities, are noted. Determining how the person with intellectual disability spends leisure time, including descriptions of whether the individual is alone or with others during free time, is essential.

Finally, questions are asked about daydreams, nightmares, and reactions to stress. This involves the ability to tolerate frustration, loss, or disappointment and includes a description of circumstances that arouse anger, anxiety, or depression. Evidence of excessive use of particular psychological defenses, such as denial, rationalization, and projection, is obtained.

Since executive dysfunction interferes with adaptive behavior both at home and at school, the parent interview asks about both settings; however, teacher or staff interviews may be necessary to cover school or work place matters. Individuals with executive dysfunction have difficulty in regulating their behavior regarding their schoolwork and in their interpersonal activities. To clarify these problems, the history identifies the frequency and severity of target symptoms in each of these settings.

The Psychiatric Examination (Mental State Examination)

Appearance

The first part of the interview relies on the interviewer's powers of observation. It takes skill and experience to understand the implications of what has been observed.

The individual's appearance, stature, and nutritional status are observed to determine his medical well-being. The examiner should note his reaction to the person with intellectual disability. Extremes in height and weight have implications metabolically and in regard to emotional development. The examiner observes whether the individual is clumsy or ataxic, shows disinhibited movements, has a strabismus, or shows rigid or floppy muscle tone. Skin coarseness or rash and hair abnormalities that might suggest metabolic disorders may be easily visible. Bruises should prompt thinking regarding abuse, accident proneness, or clumsiness.

Behavior

Behavior is observed under the categories of relatedness and motor behavior.

Relatedness. How does the individual relate to his parents (or staff) and the interviewer? Does he maintain reserve with the interviewer and only gradually warm up, or never warm up? Is he overly friendly? Does he make eye contact with the interviewer and show turn-taking as the dialogue progresses? Is he sullen, angry, oppositional, aggressive, or is he totally withdrawn and preoccupied by his own thoughts and actions? Relatedness varies from the autistic person who may constantly ignore others, including his parents or staff, or only make fleeting glances at them, to the shy individual who may show no initial eye contact but gradually warms up over time, to the disinhibited individual who hugs total strangers.

Motor behavior. How active and impulsive is the individual? Is he moving all over the room and getting into everything? Does he respond to every passing stimulus? Does he maintain interest in a task or does he lose interest quickly? Will he pay attention and inhibit his disruptiveness when verbal limits are placed on him? Does he squirm and fidget in the chair, is he immobile, or does he move normally in response to what is said to him? Does he have nervous tics or repetitive behaviors? Are his movements graceful and coordinated? Since different degrees of activity may be appropriate at different ages, a 4-year-old and a 10-year-old may show the same activity level with very different implications.

Speech and Language

The assessment of speech and language is based not only on what is said but how it is said. The quality of speech gives some clues about the individual's mood. Does the person speak clearly, slur his words, stutter, or substitute letters (e.g., *w* for *r*)? How verbal is he? Does he become frustrated trying to communicate his ideas? Does he know words but have difficulty with conceptual communication? Is the rate of speech fast or slow? Does he whine, whisper or shout? Does he speak spontaneously or in monosyllabic grunts? Are the rate, rhythm, and prosody of speech appropriate? Is the volume loud or soft? Finally, can the individual hear what is said and understand at a normal conversational tone? Hearing deficits for certain frequencies may make words virtually unintelligible to the listener.

Thought Process and Content

How a person thinks and the content of those thoughts can be assessed both indirectly and directly. The first part of the interview entails getting to know the individual, for example, what he like or dislikes, who his friends are, what they do together, what school or work is like, how he does in school or at work, how he gets on with parents, sibs, and others. What are this person's preoccupations; are there intrusive thoughts? What does the individual talk about with interest and affective investment?

The second part of the interview is specifically related to why the person is being evaluated, what his parents or staff told him about coming to the interview, what he sees his problems to be, and how he feels about the problems presented and about family relationships. In those with mental age over 7, thought content as it relates to mood, fears, somatic problems, hallucinations, and delusions is elicited.

For those with mental age over 11 or 12 years, the mental status examination is similar to the adult mental status examination. Content items also focus on drug and alcohol use, difficulties with antisocial behavior, and attitudes toward dating, peers, sex, menarche, growing up, and parents.

From interchanges in the interview, the interviewer assesses the coherence of the child, adolescent, or adult's thought process and whether his concerns are age-, sex-, and situation-appropriate.

Mood and Self-Concept (Emotional Feeling, Tone, and Its Outward Manifestations)

This is ascertained directly and indirectly. Does the person look happy, sad, tense, or angry? Does he smile or seem tearful? Does he speak dejectedly or assertively or with excess bravado? How does he respond to questions about feelings like "When were you the most angry, happy, frightened or sad?" And what does he do when he feels those ways? What are his specific fears and worries? Does he like himself, or is he self-blaming? Does he think others like him? Does he feel picked on, does he "fight back"? Is he comfortable with his gender identity? Does he blame himself or others for his problems? Is he dramatic in talking about his problems, or does he minimize them? Is he guarded and suspicious, irritable, and volatile? Does he see himself as evil, bad tempered? What has he done that he is proud of doing? How does he feel about his future?

Abnormal Beliefs and Interpretation of Events

Are there ideas of persecution or special treatment? Are there delusional beliefs? Does the individual believe that others can read his mind?

Abnormal Experiences Referred to the Environment, Body, or Self

Does the individual report sensory or somatic hallucinations or recurrent dreams? These areas may be addressed indirectly by asking the individual if his eyes or ears ever play tricks on him, causing him to see things that others do not see or hear things others do not hear. Are there feelings of depersonalization?

Cognition (Orientation, Memory, Attention and Concentration, and General Intelligence)

How alert is the person with intellectual disability? Is he oriented to time, place, and person in an age-appropriate manner? Does he seem to know what is happening around him, or does he appear distracted or inattentive? How does his history account compare to that of his parents in regard to past significant events? Depending on his mental age, he should be able to copy the Gesell figures (circle, square, diamond, Maltese cross, and cylinder) or draw a human figure in some detail. The interviewer observes how the person draws, how he holds the pencil, how he plans the task. How is his memory? Does the person know where he lives and how he got to the site where the interview is taking place? Are there problems with attention and concentration? Can he perform basic arithmetic (addition, subtraction, multiplication, and division)? Can he carry out subtraction of serial 3s from 30 and serial 7s from 100? How is his reading comprehension? What is his level of intelligence? In play, what is his choice of toys, how does he approach them and use them in imaginative ways? Does he show curiosity about how things work?

Insight and Judgment

Does he appreciate his role in the current difficulties? Does he take responsibility for his behavior? What is his capacity to reflect on his behavior? Does he link current difficulties with life stresses?

Assessment Instruments

The use of standardized assessment instruments and procedures may improve the reliability and validity of the behavioral and mental symptoms evaluation for intellectually disabled persons. Because of variability in cognitive functioning, caution is needed in interpreting results. The use of multiple informants (physicians, psychologists, educators, and direct care providers who see the person in different settings) must be considered in regard to the reliability and validity for these instruments. Still, several behavior checklists and semistructured interview schedules have been developed for use with intellectually disabled persons and other informants (e.g., caregivers) (O'Brien et al., 2001). Some instruments focus on making a specific diagnosis; others are used to assess the range and severity of affective and behavioral symptoms or adaptive abilities.

O'Brien et al. (2001) provided a comprehensive listing of available instruments to assess developmental disability. They include the following: (1) schedules for the detection, diagnosis, and assessment of autism spectrum disorder; (2) schedules for the detection, diagnosis, and assessment of psychiatric disorder; and (3) schedules for the assessment of problem behaviors. Aman (1991a,b) systematically reviewed instruments for assessing emotional and behavioral disorders in individuals at all levels of intellectual disability. The following items are commonly included in measurement, using factor analytic methodology: (1) aggressive, antisocial behavior; (2) withdrawal; (3) stereotypic behavior; (4) hyperactivity; (5) repetitive verbalization; (6) anxiety, tension, and fearfulness; and (7) self-injurious behavior. Rating scales for younger children also have been validated that deal with similar items. There is no one screening instrument that can be recommended for preschool children. The Reiss Scales for Children's Dual Diagnosis (Reiss and Valenti-Hein, 1990) should be considered for school-age children. For the assessment of broad behavioral dimensions, the Aberrant Behavior Checklist (ABC) (Aman, 1991a) and the Developmentally Delayed Child Behavior Checklist (DDCBCL) (Einfeld and Tonge, 1990) should be considered. For the assessment of older adolescents, the instruments that are shown in table 6.1 may be used.

The ABC is an informant-based questionnaire that assesses the severity of 58 maladaptive behaviors. It is appropriate for use with individuals with moderate-to-profound levels of intellectual disability. Extensive psychometric analyses of the ABC have been carried out in several different countries, utilizing subjects of varying ages and IQ levels. Factor analysis identifies five factors: irritability, lethargy/social withdrawal, stereotypic behavior, hyperactivity/

Table 6.1 Tests of Cognitive, Intellectual, and Adaptive Behavior Skills

Test Name/Publisher	Age Range (Years)
Tests of Cognitive and Intellectual Functioning	
Wechsler Intelligence Scale for Children-III (WISC-III) (The Psychological Corporation) IQ (verbal IQ, performance IQ, full-scale IQ); yields subtest scores enabling specific skill assessment, as well as overall IQ and percentiles. One note of caution is that with intellectually disabled children below the age of 10, floor effects may restrict the range of scores obtained.	6–16
Wechsler Preschool and Primary Scale of Intelligence-Revised (WPPSI-R) (The Psychological Corporation) Revised; yields the same IQ scores as the WISC-R.	4–6
Stanford-Binet, 4th ed. (Riverside Publishing Company) Revised; provides scores for verbal reasoning, abstract/visual reasoning, quantitative reasoning, and short-term memory; IQ score, standard age score, percentiles. The use of this instrument with the intellectually disabled does not appear to be as useful as the previous version of the Stanford-Binet L-M, in part because of floor effects.	2 ½–adult
Kaufman Assessment Battery for Children (K-ABC) (American Guidance Service) Based on a theoretical model of information processing; separates problem solving from acquired knowledge; scaled scores, mental processing composite (IQ equivalent); standard scores for sequential and simultaneous processing, achievement standard score, age equivalents, percentiles. Children who are intellectually disabled tend to score higher on sequential as opposed to simultaneous processing.	2½–12 ½
Hiskey-Nebraska Test of Learning Aptitude (H-NTLA) (Hiskey, 1966) A nonverbal measure of intelligence that assesses verbal labeling, categorization, concept formation, and rehearsal; can be administered through pantomimed instruction; standard scores; norm sample of hearing-impaired and non–hearing-impaired children.	3–17
Adaptive Behavior Scales	
AAMR Adaptive Behavior Scales: Residential/Community and School Versions (American Association on Mental Retardation) Personal independence and maladaptive behavior; percentiles; norms are based on institutionalized intellectually disabled. Based on information provided by a primary caregiver.	3–69
Vineland Adaptive Behavior Scales (American Guidance Service) Global adaptive behavior, communication, daily living skills, socialization, motor (below age 5), and maladaptive (above age 5); standard scores, percentiles, age equivalents, developmental scaled scores; normed for normal, visually handicapped, learning impaired, emotionally disturbed, and intellectually disabled. Based on an interview with primary caregiver.	Normal: 0–19 Retarded: All ages

Adapted from Sparrow and Carter, (1992). Reprinted from *Handbook of Neuropsychology, Vol. 6, Child Neuropsychology* (I. Rapin and S. J. Segalowitz, eds). Adapted from S. S. Sparrow and A. S. Carter, Mental retardation: Current issues related to assessment. Copyright © 1992 with permission from Elsevier and author.

noncompliance, and inappropriate speech. The factors have high internal consistency, and the instrument itself possesses good reliability. Internal consistency has been found to be satisfactory, but interrater reliabilities were relatively low.

The Psychopathology Instrument for Mentally Retarded Adults (PIMRA), developed by Matson (1988), is a 56-item scale with both self-report and informant versions that are designed to assess psychopathology among mildly and moderately mentally retarded persons. The individual items were derived from the symptom lists based on several DSM-III disorders and organized into seven clinical subscales. The subscales include the following diagnoses: schizophrenia, affective disorder, psychosexual disorder, adjustment disorder, anxiety disorder, somatoform disorder, and personality disorder. Factor analysis yielded two factors for the self-report version (termed "anxiety and social adjustment") and three factors for the informant version (termed "affective, somatoform, and psychosis"). The psychometric properties of the PIMRA have been evaluated in a number of studies. Initial analysis shows high internal consistencies of the subscales and total scores, and good interrater and test-retest reliabilities. However, follow-up analyses by several investigators have raised questions about this instrument's internal consistency and reliability. Other concerns raised about it include a low correspondence between the factor structure and the clinically derived scales and the limited number of disorders represented. Despite these shortcomings, the PIMRA is a useful instrument for the assessment of psychopathology.

The Reiss Screen for Maladaptive Behavior (1988) is an informant-based rating scale that assesses the frequency, circumstances, and intensity of various symptoms of psychiatric disorders in intellectually disabled persons. The instrument is organized into seven clinical scales, which include aggressive disorder, psychosis, paranoia, depression (behavioral signs), depression (physical signs), avoidant disorder, and dependent personality disorder. There are six maladaptive behaviors: drug abuse, overactivity, self-injury, sexual behavior, suicidal tendencies, and stealing. Its validity has been documented in conjunction with clinical psychiatric diagnoses. Other instruments from which preliminary psychometric analyses are available are the Emotional Disorders Rating Scale for Developmental Disabilities (EDRSDD) (Feinstein, Kaminer, and Barrett, 1988) and the Diagnostic Assessment for the Severely Handicapped (DASH) Scale (Matson et al., 1990).

The Developmental Behaviour Checklist, (DBC) is an instrument for the assessment of behavioral and emotional problems of children and adolescents with developmental disabilities. The DBC (Aman, 1991b; Einfeld and Tonge, 1995, 1996a,b) is a 96-item instrument that is completed by parents or other primary caregivers or teachers, reporting problems over a six-month period. The DBC shares the structure of the Child Behaviour Checklist (Achenbach and Edelbrock, 1981). The items are completely independently derived from a study of the medical files of 7000 intellectually handicapped children and adolescents seen in a developmental assessment clinic.

Two versions of the checklist are available. These are the Parent/Carer Version (DBC-P), and the Teacher Version (DBC-T). The instrument has a high interrater reliability between parents and between teachers. The DBC-P has also been demonstrated to be sensitive to change over time. There is also a high correlation between a total score on the checklist and two other measures of behavior disturbance in children with intellectual disability that require professionals to administer them. These are the AAMD Adaptive Behaviour Scales (Lambert, Nihira, and Leland, 1993) and the Scales of Independent Behaviour (Bruininks et al., 1996). The instrument has high criterion group validity in distinguishing psychiatric cases from noncases (t = 7.8, $p < 0.001$). Five subscales were derived from factor analysis. The subscales have documented content, construct, and concurrent and/or discriminant validity. It is both specific and sensitive with regard to expert clinician judgment of the subject as a psychiatric case or not having a psychiatric disorder. Community norms for the DBC are derived from an extensive multicenter epidemiological study in New South Wales and Victoria, Australia (Einfeld and Tonge 1996a,b). Norms are available for boys and girls and for the mild, moderate, and severe intellectually disabled groups. A revised factor structure is based on parent and teacher ratings on the DBC in a combined sample of 1536 Dutch and Australian children and adolescents (ages 3–22) with mild-to-profound intellectual disability. Principal components analyses produced five subscales: Disruptive/Antisocial, Self-Absorbed, Communication Disturbance, Anxiety, and Social Relating, explaining 43.7% of the total variance. Internal consistencies of these subscales ranged from 0.66 to 0.91 (Dekker et al., 2002).

The DBC can be scored at three levels. The first is the Total Behaviour Problem Score, which gives an overall measure of behavioral/emotional disturbance. The second level is that of the subscale scores, which measure disturbance in five dimensions. The third level is for scoring of individual items. The norms provide community prevalence rates for 96 individual disturbed behaviors and emotions.

Assessment instruments developed for typically developing children and adolescents also have also been used to evaluate psychopathology among children and adults with intellectual disability. These instruments generally have good test-retest reliability, yet vary in terms of their interrater reliability, internal consistency, and validity. These tests include the Child Behavior Checklist, the Rutter Behavioral Scales, the Beck Depression Inventory, the Zung Self-Rating Depression Inventory, and the Standardized Assessment of Personality. Further investigation is needed to provide information on their applicability to persons with intellectual disability. Moreover, structured or semistructured interviews with the individual are needed to elicit symptoms of mental disorders. Face-to-face contact with the individual is critical for every clinical assessment.

DSM-IVTR PSYCHIATRIC DIAGNOSTIC CRITERIA FOR PERSONS WITH INTELLECTUAL DISABILITY

The DSM-IVTR classification attempts to provide more objective diagnostic criteria. It provides operational definitions of symptoms, cut-off rules in regard to criteria, rules for inclusion and exclusion, and describes criteria related to the duration of a disorder, the extent of the impairment, and its relationship to other diagnoses. However, with the exception of the diagnostic criteria for pervasive developmental disorders, most specifically autistic disorder, persons with intellectual disability were not specifically included in the DSM-IVTR field trials. The National Association for the Dually Diagnosed (NADD), in association with the American Psychiatric Association, has reviewed the diagnostic criteria for DSM-IVTR and clarified how criteria can be applied to those with intellectual disability and other developmental disabilities. A variety of diagnostic questionnaires and some structured and semi-structured interviews have been established to assess, screen, and diagnose psychopathology in persons with intellectual disability. Moreover, and more complicated, a range of behavioral equivalents has been suggested in making the diagnosis from observation. Here, it is proposed that certain maladaptive behaviors that are not part of DSM-IVTR diagnostic criteria may be substituted for them. Yet objective assessment of behavioral equivalents is limited, particularly in regard to interrater reliability, retest reliability, internal consistency, and validity. This requires a field trial to assess these behavioral equivalent criteria.

Efforts to clarify the application of DSM-IVTR criteria in persons with intellectual disability are underway. For example, Tsiouris et al. (2003) evaluated whether or not depression, one of the more common forms of psychopathology in persons with intellectual disability, could be assessed in regard to a behavioral equivalent of challenging behavior, such as self-injury or aggression. These authors found that such behaviors as self-injury and aggression were not necessarily associated with depression.

Psychiatric Assessment: Special Considerations for Severe and Profound Intellectual Disability

The clinical presentation of mental disorders in people with borderline-to-moderate intellectual disability is, in general, similar and not qualitatively different from that in persons who are typically developing. However, adaptations do need to be made in the interview procedure for these individuals. Interview schedules such as the Psychiatric Assessment Schedule for Adults with Developmental Disability (PAS-ADD) (Moss et al., 1993) provide an approach to interviewing individuals with intellectual disability. The interview schedule provides probes if further exploration of symptoms is warranted. On the PAS-ADD, items are reworded to break them down into components that may be easier to understand. For example, in eliciting symptoms of guilty ideas of reference, the PAS-ADD includes the following component questions: Do you think you are blamed for something? If the answer is "yes," the probes continue with "Has anyone said you have done something bad?" "What do you think you have done?" "Is it your fault?" "Do you feel guilty?" "Do other people say it is your fault?" "Do you think you should be punished?" Although these items have only face validity, the simplification in questioning allows the interviewer to take into account the language ability of the intellectually disabled person and increases the possibility that the questions will be understood and that the answers will be more valid.

Table 6.2 Use of DSM-IVTR Criteria for Major Depression in Persons with Severe and Profound Intellectual Disability.

Criteria	Potential Problems
1. Depressed mood by either subjective report or observations of others	The individual may not be able to provide a subjective report. Others may have to infer mood from behavior, which can be unreliable.
2. Diminished interest or pleasure by subjective report or observations of others	The individual may not be able to provide a subjective report. The person has a restricted range of interests, and autistic characteristics may be responsible for the restricted range of interests rather than a depressive disorder.
3. Significant weight loss when not dieting, weight gain, or decreased/increased appetite	Medical etiologies of weight gain or loss must be ruled out. The evaluation of appetite, which is a subjective experience, has sometimes been inferred from food refusal or excessive intake. However, dislike, food preferences, or adversive experiences in eating need to be eliminated. However, food refusal may be a subjective symptom in an intellectually disabled person that meets this criterion.
4. Insomnia or hypersomnia	Insomnia may be linked to parent or staff routines expected of the individual. Noise, need to toilet, or other factors may keep the individual awake. Day-time sleepiness may be linked to lack of appropriate activity to stimulate the individual, sedation, or physical problems.
5. Observable psychomotor agitation	Agitation may be linked to other psychiatric disorder, such as mania, attention deficit disorder, or anxiety. It may be learned behavior that is maintained by parents, staff, or peers.
6. Fatigue or loss of energy every day	It may be difficult to evaluate and to infer the meaning of this symptom from observable behavior.
7. Feelings of worthlessness, excessive or inappropriate guilt	The individual may not be able to subjectively report guilt. Depending on cognitive level, he or she may not be able to sufficiently abstract to understand the questions posed.
8. Diminished ability to think or concentrate	Problems in thinking and concentration may be baseline problems. Since subjective experience may not be reported, it is hard to infer, although observations of interest in previously preferred tasks may be observed and a lack of interest in them linked to the symptom. Sedation and side effects of medications, particularly seizure medications, must be considered.
9. Recurrent thoughts of death, suicide, or a suicidal plan	The individual may not understand the permanence of death, or the meaning of suicide or be able to prepare such a plan.

Adapted from Sturmey (1999). Reprinted by permission of publisher, adapted from P. Sturmey, Classification: Concepts, progress and future. *Psychiatric and behavioral disorders in developmental disabilities and mental retardation* (N. Bouras, ed.). Cambridge University Press, Cambridge, UK. Copyright © 1999.

In contrast, the diagnosis of psychiatric disorders in individuals with severe and profound intellectual disability presents particular difficulties. The person's pre-illness behavior may be quite restricted. Maladaptive behaviors such as stereotypies, poor social skills, odd language usage and social withdrawal may have been evident to others for most of that person's life. Moreover, the person may have little or no ability to communicate his or her mental state. Thus, observation of behavior and reports of staff and family members of behavior and inferences made from observations about behavior must be incorporated into the assessment. Consequently, many people with severe and profound intellectual disability cannot meet the DSM-IVTR criteria for mental disorders as written. In addition, medical problems, changes in program, and learning ability may need to be considered in assessing a symptom. In the DSM-IVTR, the criteria for major depression require five of nine symptoms concurrently for at least two weeks. To make the diagnosis, depressed mood and loss of interest must be present. Moreover, physical conditions and bereavement must also be excluded in making the diagnosis. Finally symptoms must lead to significant distress or impairment. A review of the DSM-IVTR criteria and potential problems in its use are shown in table 6.2.

Thus, assessing the mental health needs of persons with intellectual disability is particularly complex for those with severe and profound deficits. Diagnostic classification is one partial guide to the extent of illness and the quality of life experienced by the individual. The problem-based rather than the strictly diagnostic approach as proposed by the AAMR may facilitate a better description of the individual than using the DSM-IVTR criteria alone. Complete and thorough evaluation, both from a mental health point of view that considers the individual's history in the context of the illness and from a functional assessment perspective that evaluates behavior, is needed as a baseline and for continued long-term maintenance of mental health.

SUMMARY

A comprehensive evaluation of a person with intellectual disability includes assessment of genetic, medical, mental and behavioral disorders. Familiarity with the assessment process is critical for both parents and professionals. With the mapping of the human genome, it is expected that genetic assessment will become more refined. As we learn more about development across the life span for persons with an intellectual disability syndrome, anticipatory guidance and planning will improve. The further delineation of behavioral phenotypes will enhance our understanding of how presentation of psychiatric disorders (e.g., attention deficit disorder and anxiety disorders), may vary across syndromes. Finally, advances in classification and more refined interview techniques and functional behavioral assessment may result in a better delineation of mental and behavioral disorders. Advances in case evaluation are expected to result in more individualized treatment planning and interventions.

KEY POINTS

1. Historically, intellectual disability and mental illness were thought of as mutually exclusive conditions.
2. In the past, affective and behavioral disturbances in persons with intellectual

disability were attributed to maladaptive learning and adverse psychosocial experiences rather than indications of a psychiatric disorder.

3. Psychiatric disorder may occur in a person with intellectual disability when any of the following are present: (1) underlying neurobiological factors that contribute to both intellectual disability and, separately, mental disorder; (2) exposure of a cognitively vulnerable person with intellectual disability to severe psychosocial stressors; (3) underlying genetic vulnerability to a psychiatric disorder in the family; or (4) a neurogenetic disorder unmasks an underlying vulnerability to psychiatric disorder.

4. The overall rate of psychiatric disorder is greater in persons with moderate-to-severe intellectual disability.

5. Risk factors for psychiatric disorder include the following: (1) reduced capacity to master complex social and cognitive demands; (2) difficulty in resolving emotional conflicts; (3) limited social judgment; and (4) associated language and sensorimotor disorders that affect interpersonal communication.

6. The causes of behavioral and psychiatric disorders vary with the syndrome. In some instances, behavioral phenotypes are associated with a neurogenetic syndrome (see chapter 7).

7. Individuals with intellectual disability may show a less differentiated self-concept and are at greater risk for negative self-appraisals and problems in self-esteem and personality development.

8. Although there is increased family stress, with appropriate family support, positive outcomes are to be expected. However, the type of impairment, its cause, and the extent of the intellectual disability and its associated features all impact on the degree of family stress.

9. Persons with intellectual disability are at risk for both physical and sexual abuse.

10. The full spectrum of psychiatric disorders can be diagnosed in persons with mild-to-moderate intellectual disability, although adaptations are needed in some criteria.

11. The diagnostic process for those with severe and profound intellectual disability is more problem-focused and reveals more behavioral problems, especially challenging behavior, such as self-injury, aggression, and property destruction.

12. The interview process utilizes a developmental perspective; both the intellectually disabled person and the parent or caregiver should be included in the diagnostic assessment.

References

Achenbach, T.M., and Edelbrock, C.S. (1981). Behavioral problems and competencies reported by parents of normal and disturbed children aged four through sixteen. *Monographs of the Society for Research in Child Development,* 46(1).

Aman, M.G. (1991a). *Assessing psychopathology and behavior problems in persons with mental retardation: A review of available instruments.* DHHS Publication No. (ADM) 91–1712. U.S. Department of Health and Human Services, Rockville, MD.

Aman, M.G. (1991b). Review and evaluation of instruments for assessing emotional and behavioural disorders. *Australia and New Zealand Journal of Developmental Disabilities,* 17:127–145.

Aman, M.G., Buican B., Arnold L.E. (2003). Methylphenidate treatment in children with borderline IQ and mental retardation: Analysis of three aggregated studies. *Journal of Child and Adolescent Psychopharmacology,* 13:29–40.

Aman, M.G., De Smedt, G., Derivan, A., Lyons, B., and Findling, R.L. (2002). Double-blind, placebo-controlled study of risperidone for the treatment of disruptive behaviors in children with subaverage intelligence. *American Journal of Psychiatry,* 159: 1337–1346.

American Academy of Child and Adolescent Psychiatry. (1999). Practice parameters for the assessment and treatment of children, adolescents, and adults with mental retardation and comorbid mental disorders. *Journal of the American Academy of Child and Adolescent Psychiatry,* 38(12):5–31.

American Psychiatric Association, Committee on Nomenclature and Statistics. (2000). *Diagnostic and statistical manual of mental disorders,* 4th ed., Text Revision, Author, Washington, DC.

Ammerman, R.T., Hersen, M., van Hasselt, V.B., Lubetsky, M.J., and Sieck, W.R. (1994). Maltreatment in psychiatrically hospitalized children and adolescents with developmental disabilities: prevalence and correlates. *Journal of the American Academy of Child and Adolescent Psychiatry,* 33:567–576.

Bassett, A.S., Chow, E.W.C., Abdel Malik, P., Gheorghiu, M., Husted, J., and Weksberg, R. (2003). *American Journal of Psychiatry,* 160:1580–1586.

Bird, J. (1997). Epilepsy and learning disabilities. In O. Russell (ed.), *Seminars in the psychiatry of learning disabilities,* pp. 223–244. Gaskell, London.

Bleuler, E. (1950). *Dementia praecox oder die Gruppe der Schizofrenien* (J. Zinkin, Trans.). International Universities Press, New York. (Original work published 1911).

Bruininks, R.H., Woodcock, R.W., Weatherman, R.F., and Hill, B.K. (1996). *Scales of Independent Behavior-Revised.* Riverside Press, Ithica, IL.

Burgard, J.F., Donohue, B., Azrin, N.H., and Teichner, G. (2000). Prevalence and treatment of substance abuse in the mentally retarded population: An empirical review. *Journal of Psychoactive Drugs,* 32:293–298.

Cain, N.N., Davidson, P.W., Burhan, A.M., Andolsek, M.E., Baxter, J.T., Sullivan, L., Florescue, H., List, A., and Deutsch, L. (2003). Identifying bipolar disorders in individuals with intellectual disability. *Journal of Intellectual Disability Research,* 47:31–38.

Christian, L., and Poling, A. (1997). Drug abuse in persons with mental retardation: a review. *American Journal of Mental Retardation,* 102:126–136.

Cooper, S.A., Melville, C.A., and Einfeld, S.L. (2003). Psychiatric diagnosis, intellectual disabilities, and diagnostic criteria for psychiatric disorders for use with adults with learning disabilities/mental retardation ((DC-LD). *Journal of Intellectual Disability Research,* 47 (suppl. 1):3–15.

Cowley, A., Holt, G., Bouras, N., Sturmey, P., Newton, J.T., and Costello, H. (2004). Descriptive psychopathology in people with mental retardation. *Journal of Nervous and Mental Disorders,* 192:232–237.

Deb, S., and Braganza, J. (1999). Comparison of rating scales for the diagnosis of dementia in adults with Down's syndrome. *Journal of Intellectual Disability Research,* 43:400–407.

Deb, S., Matthews, T., Holt, G., and Bouras, N. (2001). *Practice guidelines for the assessment and diagnosis of mental health problems in adults with intellectual disability*. European Association for Mental Health in Mental Retardation. Pavilion, UK.

Deb, S., Thomas, M., and Bright, C. (2001). Mental disorder in adults with intellectual disability. 1: Prevalence of psychiatric illness among a community based population aged between 16 and 64 years. *Journal of Intellectual Disability,* 45:495–505.

Dekker, M.C., and Koot, H.M. (2003). DSM-IV disorders in children with borderline to moderate intellectual disability. II: Child and family predictors. *Journal of the American Academy of Child and Adolescent Psychiatry*, 42:923–931.

Dekker, M.C., Nunn, R.J., Einfeld, S.E., Tonge, B.J, and Koot, H.M. (2002). Assessing emotional and behavioral problems in children with intellectual disability: Revisiting the factor structure of the developmental behavior checklist. *Journal of Autism and Developmental Disorders,* 32:601–610.

De Smedt, G., Derivan, A., Lyons, B., and Findling, R.L. (2002). Disruptive behavior study group. Double-blind, placebo-controlled study of risperidone for the treatment of disruptive behaviors in children with subaverage intelligence. *American Journal of Psychiatry,* 159:1337–1346.

DiNitto, D.M., and Krishef, C.H. (1983/84). Drinking patterns of mentally retarded persons. *Alcohol, Health, and Research World*, 8:40–42.

Doody, G.A., Johnstone, E.C., Sanderson, T.L., Owens, D.G., and Muir, W.J. (1998). "Pfropfschizophrenie" revisited. Schizophrenia in people with mild learning disability. *British Journal of Psychiatry,* 173:145–153.

Dykens, E.M. (1999). Personality-motivation: New ties to psychopathology, etiology, and intervention. In E. Zigler and D. Bennett-Gates (eds.), *Personality-motivation in individuals with mental retardation,* pp. 249–270. Cambridge University Press, New York.

Dykens, E.M. (2000). Psychopathology in children with intellectual disability. *Journal of Child Psychology and Psychiatry,* 41:407–417.

Dykens, E.M. (2003). Anxiety, fears, and phobias in persons with Williams syndrome. *Developmental Neuropsychology,* 23:291–316.

Dykens, E.M., and Kasari, C. (1997). Maladaptive behavior in children with Prader-Willi syndrome, Down syndrome, and nonspecific mental retardation. *American Journal of Mental Retardation,* 102:228–237.

Dykens, E.M., Leckman, J.F., and Cassidy, S.B. (1996). Obsessions and compulsions in Prader-Willi syndrome. *Journal of Child Psychology and Psychiatry,* 37:995–1002.

Dykens, E.M., and Rosner, B.A. (1999). Refining behavioral phenotypes: Personality-motivation in Williams and Prader-Willi syndromes. *American Journal of Mental Retardation,* 104:158–169.

Edgerton, R.B. (1993). *The cloak of competence.* University of California Press, Berkeley, CA.

Einfeld, S.L., and Tonge, B.J. (1990). *Development of an instrument to measure psychopathology in mentally retarded children and adolescents.* Unpublished manuscript. University of Sydney, Australia.

Einfeld, S.L., and Tonge, B.J. (1995). Developmental behaviour checklist: The development and validation of an instrument to assess behavioural and emotional disturbance in children and adolescents with mental retardation. *Journal of Autism and Developmental Disorders,* 25:81–104.

Einfeld, S.L., and Tonge, B.J. (1996a). Population prevalence of behavioural and emotional disturbance in children and adolescents with mental retardation: I Rationale and methods. *Journal of Intellectual Disability Research*, 40:91–98.

Einfeld, S.L., and Tonge, B.J. (1996b). Population prevalence of behavioural and emotional disturbance in children and adolescents with mental retardation: II Epidemiological findings. *Journal of Intellectual Disability Research*, 40:99–109.

Emerson, E. (2003). Prevalence of psychiatric disorders in children and adolescents with and without intellectual disability. *Journal of Intellectual Disability Research*, 47: 51–58.

Endicott, J., and Spitzer, R.L. (1978). A diagnostic interview: The schedule for affective disorders and schizophrenia. *Archives of General Psychiatry*, 35:837–844.

Evans, D.W. (1998). Development of the self-concept in children with mental retardation: Organismic and contextual factors. In J.A. Burack, R.M. Hodapp, and E. Zigler (eds.), *Handbook of mental retardation and development*, pp. 462–480. Cambridge University Press, New York.

Feinstein, C., Kaminer, Y., and Barrett, R. (1988). *Emotional Disorders Rating Scale: Developmental Disabilities.* Unpublished document. Emma Pendleton Bradley Hospital, East Providence, RI.

Feinstein, C., and Reiss, A.L. (1996). Psychiatric disorder in mentally retarded children and adolescents: the challenges of meaningful diagnosis. *Child and Adolescent Clinics of North America*, 5:827–852.

Feldman, M.A., and Walton-Allen, N. (1997). Effects of maternal mental retardation and poverty on intellectual, academic, and behavioral status of school-age children. *American Journal of Mental Retardation*, 101:352–364.

Feldman, M.A., Leger, M., and Walton-Allen, N. (1997). Stress in mothers with intellectual disabilities. *Journal of Child and Family Studies*, 6:471–485.

Freeman, S.F.N., and Kasari, C. (1998). Friendships in children with developmental disabilities. *Early Education and Development*, 9:341–355.

Gath, A. (1990). Down syndrome children and their families. *American Journal of Medical Genetics*, 7:314–316.

Goodman, R., and Scott, S. (1997). *Child psychiatry*, p. 15. Blackwell Science, London.

Gothelf, D., Presburger, G., Zohar, A.H., Burg, M., Nahmani, A., Frydman, M., Shohat, M., Inbar, D., Aviram-Goldring, A., Yeshaya J., et al. (2004). Obsessive-compulsive disorder in patients with velocardiofacial (22q11 deletion) syndrome. *American Journal of Medical Genetics.* 126B:99–105.

Gravestock, S. (2000). Eating disorders in adults with intellectual disability. *Journal of Intellectual Disability Research*, 44:625–637.

Gress, J.R., and Boss, M.S. (1996). Substance abuse differences among students receiving special education school services. *Child Psychiatry and Human Development*, 26: 235–246.

Griffin, J.C., Ricketts, R.W., Williams, D.E., Locke, B.J., Altmeyer, B.K., and Stark, M.T. (1987). A community survey of self-injurious behavior among developmentally disabled children and adolescents. *Hospital and Community Psychiatry*, 38:959–963.

Hardan, A., and Sahl, R. (1999). Suicidal behavior in children and adolescents with developmental disorders. *Research in Developmental Disabilities*, 20:287–296.

Harris, J. (1995). *Developmental neuropsychiatry: Assessment, diagnosis, and treatment of developmental disorders, Vol. II*, pp. 3–16. Oxford University Press, New York.

Hindley, P. (1997). Psychiatric aspects of hearing impairments. *Journal of Child Psychology and Psychiatry*, 38:101–117.

Hodapp, R.M. (1995). Parenting children with Down syndrome and other types of mental retardation. In M. Bornstein (ed.), *Handbook of parenting, Vol. 1*, pp. 232–253. Lawrence Erlbaum, Mahwah, NJ.

Hodapp, R.M. (1998). *Development and disabilities: Intellectual, sensory, and motor impairments.* Cambridge University Press, New York.

Hodapp, R.M., Fidler, D.J., and Smith, A.C.M. (1998). Stress and coping in families of children with Smith-Magenis syndrome. *Journal of Intellectual Disability Research,* 42:310–340.

Holland, T., Clare, I.C., and Mukhopadhyay, T. (2002). Prevalence of criminal offending by men and women with intellectual disability and the characteristics of offenders: Implications for research and service development. *Journal of Intellectual Disability Research,* 1:6–20.

Hurley, A.D. (1998). Two cases of suicide attempt by patients with Down's syndrome. *Psychiatric Services.* 49:1618–1619.

Hurley, A., Folstein, M.D., and Lam, N. (2003). Patients with and without intellectual disability seeking outpatient psychiatric services: Diagnoses and prescribing pattern. *Journal of Intellectual Disability,* 47:39–50.

Jablensky, A. (2004). Resolving schizophrenia's CATCH 22. *Nature Genetics,* 36:674–675.

Kraeplin, E. (1896). *Psychiatrie, Ein Lehrbuch fur Studirende und Aerzte. Funfte, vollstandig umgearbeitete Auflage.* Barth Verlag, Leipzig.

Kraeplin, E. (1919). Dementia praecox and paraphrenia. Translated by R.M. Barclay from G.M. Robertson (ed.), *Text-Book of Psychiatry,* 8th ed., Vol. iii, Part ii, Endogenous Dementias Section. Robert E. Krieger, New York.

Lambert, N., Nihira, K., and Leland, H. (1993). *AAMR Adaptive Behavior Scale-School and Community.* Pro-Ed, TX.

Lapouse, R., and Monk, M.A. (1958). An epidemiologic study of behavior characteristics of children. *American Journal of Public Health,* 48:1134–1144.

Lesniak-Karpiak, K., Mazzocco, M.M., and Ross, J.L. (2003). Behavioral assessment of social anxiety in females with Turner or fragile X syndrome. *Journal of Autism and Developmental Disorders.*33:55–67.

Lunsky, Y. (2004). Suicidality in a clinical and community sample of adults with mental retardation. *Research in Developmental Disabilities,* 25:231–243.

Mack, A.H., Feldman, J.J., and Tsuang, M.T. (2002). A case of "pfropfschizophrenia": Kraepelin's bridge between neurodegenerative and neurodevelopmental conceptions of schizophrenia. *American Journal of Psychiatry,* 159:1104–1110.

Matson, J.L. (1988). *The PIMRA manual.* International Diagnostic Systems, Inc., Orland Park, IL.

Matson, J.L., Gardner, W.J., Coe, D.A., and Sovner, R. (1990). *Diagnostic assessment for the severely handicapped (DASH) scale (User manual).* Unpublished manuscript. Louisiana State University, Baton Rouge.

Miller, M.L., Fee, V.E., and Jones, C.J. (2004). Psychometric properties of ADHD rating scales among children with mental retardation. *Research in Developmental Disabilities.* 25:477–492.

Mindham, J., and Espie, C.A. (2003). Glasgow anxiety scale for people with an intellectual disability (GAS-ID): Development and psychometric properties of a new measure for use with people with mild intellectual disability. *Journal of Intellectual Disability Research.* 47:22–30.

Minnes, P. (1998). Mental retardation: The impact upon the family. In J.A. Burack, R.M. Hodapp, and E. Zigler (eds.), *Handbook of mental retardation and development,* pp. 693–712. Cambridge University Press, New York.

Moss, S., Patel, P., Prosser, H., Goldberg, D., Simpson, N., Rowe, S., and Lucchino, R. (1993). Psychiatric morbidity in older people with moderate and severe learning disability. I: Development and reliability of the patient interview (PAS-ADD) *British Journal of Psychiatry,* 163:471–480.

National Institute of Health. (1990). *Consensus conference on treatment of destructive behaviors in persons with developmental disabilities.* U.S. Government Printing Office, Washington, DC.

NIH Workshop. Emotional and behavioral health in persons with mental retardation/ developmental disabilities: Research challenges and opportunities. November 29– December 1, 2001. Rockville, MD. (http://ord.aspensys.com/asp/workshops/search .asp)

O'Brien, G., Pearson, J., Berney, T., and Barnard, L. (2001). Measuring behaviour in developmental disability: A review of existing schedules. *Developmental Medicine and Child Neurology, 87,* 43:1–72.

Palmen, S.J., Van Engeland, H., Hof, P.R., and Schmitz, C. (2004). Neuropathological findings in autism. *Brain,* 127:2572–2583.

Patja, K., Iivanainen, M., Raitasuo, S., and Lonnqvist, J. (2001). Suicide mortality in mental retardation: A 35-year follow-up study. *Acta Psychiatrica Scandanavia,* 103: 307–311.

Powell, R. (2003). Psychometric properties of the Beck Depression Inventory and the Zung Self-Rating Depression Scale in adults with mental retardation. *Mental Retardation,* 41:88–95.

Reid, A. (1982). *The psychiatry of mental handicap.* Blackwell Scientific, Boston.

Reiss, S. (1988). *Test Manual for the Reiss Screen for Maladaptive Behavior.* International Diagnostic Systems, Orland Park, IL.

Reiss, S., and Benson, B.A. (1985). Psychosocial correlates of depression in mentally retarded adults: I. Minimal social support and stigmatization. *American Journal of Mental Deficiency,* 89:331–337.

Reiss, S., and Valenti-Hein, D. (1990). *Reiss Scales for Children's Dual Diagnosis: Test Manual.* International Diagnostic Systems, Orland Park, IL.

Rivinius, T. (1988). Alcohol use disorder in mentally retarded persons. *Psychiatric Aspects of Mental Retardation Reviews.* 7:19–26.

Robbins, L., Helzer, J.E., Croughan, J., and Ratcliff, K.S. (1981). National Institute of Mental Health Diagnostic Interview Schedule: Its history, characteristics, and validity. *Archives of General Psychiatry,* 38:381–389.

Rojahn, J. (1994). Epidemiology and topographic taxonomy of self-injurious behavior. In T. Thompson and B.B. Gray (eds.), *Destructive behavior in developmental disabilities: Diagnosis and treatment,* pp. 49–67. Sage, Thousand Oaks, CA.

Royal College of Psychiatrists. (2001). *The Diagnostic Criteria for Psychiatric Disorders for Use with Adults with Learning Disabilities/Mental Retardation'* Occasional Paper 48, pp. 1–128. Gaskell Press, London.

Rutter, M., and Graham, P. (1968). The reliability and validity of the psychiatric assessment of the child: Interview with the child. *British Journal of Psychiatry,* 11:563–579.

Sanderson, T.L., Doody, G.A., Best, J., Owens, D.G., and Johnstone, E.C. (2001). Correlations between clinical and historical variables, and cerebral structural variables in people with mild intellectual disability and schizophrenia. *Journal of Intellectual Disability Research,* 45:89–98.

Scheerenberger, R.C. (1983). *A history of mental retardation.* Paul H. Books Publishing, Baltimore, MD.

Schroeder, S.R., Oster-Granite, M.L., and Thompson, T. (2002). *Self-injurious behavior: Gene-brain-behavior relationships.* American Psychological Association, Washington, DC.

Schumann, C.M., Hamstra, J., Goodlin-Jones, B.L., Lotspeich, L.J., Kwon, H., Buonocore, M.H., Lammers, C.R., Reiss. A.L., and Amaral, D.G. (2004). The amygdala is enlarged in children but not adolescents with autism: The hippocampus is enlarged at all ages. *Journal of Neuroscience.* 24:6392–6401.

Seager, M.C., and O'Brien, G. (2003). Attention deficit hyperactivity disorder: Review of ADHD in learning disability: the Diagnostic Criteria for Psychiatric Disorders for Use with Adults with Learning Disabilities/Mental Retardation [DC-LD] criteria for diagnosis. *Journal of Intellectual Disability Research.* 47:26–31.

Siperstein, G.N., Leffert, J.S., and Wenz-Gross, M. (1997). The quality of friendships between children with and without learning problems. *American Journal of Mental Retardation,* 102:111–125.

Solnit, A., and Stark, M. (1961). Mourning and the birth of a defective infant. *Psychoanalytic Study of the Child,* 16:523–537.

Sovner, R. (1986). Limiting factors in the use of DSM-III criteria with mentally ill/mentally retarded persons. *Psychopharmocology Bulletin,* 22:1055–1059.

Sparrow, S.S., and Carter, A.S. (1992). Mental retardation: Current issues related to assessment. In I. Rapin and S.I. Segalowitz (vol. eds.), *Handbook of neuropsychology: Vol. 6, Child neuropsychology,* pp. 439–452. Elsevier Science Publishers, New York.

Sturmey, P. (1999). Classification: Concepts, progress and future. In N. Bouras (ed.), *Psychiatric and behavioural disorders in developmental disabilities and mental retardation,* pp. 3–17. Cambridge University Press, Cambridge, UK

Szymanski, L., and King, B.H. (1999). Practice parameters for the assessment and treatment of children, adolescents, and adults with mental retardation and comorbid mental disorders. American Academy of Child and Adolescent Psychiatry Working Group on Quality Issues. *Journal of the American Academy of Child and Adolescent Psychiatry,* 38:5S–31S.

Tsiouris, J.A., Mann, R., Patti, P.J., and Sturmey, P. (2003). Challenging behaviours should not be considered as depressive equivalents in individuals with intellectual disability. *Journal of Intellectual Disabilities Research,* 47:14–21.

Turner, T.H. (1989). Schizophrenia and mental handicap: An historical review, with implications for further research. *Psychological Medicine,* 19:301–314.

Vanstraelen, M., and Tyrer, S.P. (1999). Rapid cycling bipolar affective disorder in people with intellectual disability: A systematic review. *Journal of Intellectual Disability Research,* 43:349–359.

Verhoeven, W.M., Tuinier, S., van den Berg, Y.W., Coppus, A.M., Fekkes, D., Pepplinkhuizen, L., and Thijssen, J.H. (1999). Stress and self-injurious behavior; hormonal and serotonergic parameters in mentally retarded subjects. *Pharmacopsychiatry,* 32: 13–20.

Weisz, J.R. (1990). Cultural-familial mental retardation: A developmental perspective on cognitive performance and "helpless" behavior. In R.M. Hodapp, J.A. Burack, and E. Zigler (eds.), *Issues in the developmental approach to mental retardation,* pp. 137–168. Cambridge University Press, New York.

Westermeyer J., Phaobtong T., and Neider, J. (1988). Substance use and abuse among mentally retarded persons: A comparison of patients and a survey population. *American Journal of Drug and Alcohol Abuse,* 14:109–123.

Wills, K.E. (1993). Neuropsychological functioning in children with spina bifida and/or hydrocephalus. *Journal of Child Clinical Psychology,* 22:247–267.

Wing, L., and Gould, I. (1979). Severe impairments of social interaction and associated abnormalities in children: Epidemiology and classification. *Journal of Autism and Developmental Disorders,* 9:11–30.

World Health Organization. (1992). *The ICD-10 classification of mental and behavioral disorders: Clinical descriptions and diagnostic guidelines.* Author, Geneva, Switzerland.

Zammit, S., Allebeck, P., David, A.S., Dalman, C., Hemmingsson, T., Lundberg, I., and Lewis G. (2004). A longitudinal study of premorbid IQ Score and risk of developing schizophrenia, bipolar disorder, severe depression, and other nonaffective psychoses. *Archives of General Psychiatry,* 61:354–360.

Zigler, E., and Bennett-Gates, D. (1999). *Personality-motivation in individuals with mental retardation.* Cambridge University Press, New York.

7

Genetics, Behavior, and Behavioral Phenotypes

Geneticists and specialists working with individuals with intellectual disability now recognize that genetic syndromes may have characteristic physical phenotypes and behavioral features that may be linked to a specific genetic syndrome. These patterns of behavior are referred to as behavioral phenotypes. This chapter utilizes a developmental perspective to provide a definition and characterization of behavioral phenotypes in neurodevelopmental disorders and to discuss etiology, methodologies to understand underlying mechanisms, and the natural history of the disorder. Neurogenetic disorders with behavioral phenotypes include (1) Down syndrome, (2) Velocardiofacial syndrome, (3) Smith-Magenis syndrome, (4) Turner syndrome, (5) Rett's disorder, (6) Lesch-Nyhan syndrome, (7) Prader-Willi and Angelman syndromes, (8) fragile X syndrome, and (9) Williams syndrome. Each of these neurogenetic disorders involves a different genetic mechanism and provides a portal to understand neurodevelopment. A disorder that is environmentally induced, fetal alcohol syndrome, is also discussed and it, too, may provide a key to understanding aspects of the developing brain (Ikonomidou et al., 2000).

HISTORICAL BACKGROUND

The first description of behavior associated with an intellectual disability syndrome was by Down (1887). In describing the syndrome that bears his name, Down observed that "They have considerable powers of imitation, even bordering on being mimics. Their humorousness and a lively sense of the ridiculous often color their mimicry." Later, he added: "Several patients who have been under my care have been wont to convert their pillow cases into surplices (vestments) and to imitate, in tone and gesture, the clergymen or chaplain which they have recently heard." He also commented on personality traits, saying that "Another feature is their great obstinacy—they can only be guided by consummate tact." Although these stereotypes were not confirmed in subsequent studies (Gath and Gumley, 1986; Gunn, Berry, and Andrews, 1981), the prospect of linking behavior and genetics was introduced in this first description of a neurogenetic disorder. Subsequent early clinical descriptions, such as that of tuberous sclerosis complex by Critchley and Earl (1932), identified peculiar, and severe, behavioral problems in children and adult with that condition. Yet, despite the early recognition of syndrome-specific behavioral and psychiatric features, neurogenetic disorders were not empirically investigated for behavioral deficits until the end of the twentieth century when new conceptual and methodological procedures were introduced (Flint, 1998).

With the establishment of active and refined cognitive-based approaches and a better understanding of the interpretation of genetic findings, there is an expansion of research on behavioral phenotypes. There are several reasons for this (O'Brien, 1992). First, there are research findings that have been reliably reported with various syndromes. Second, there are continued reports from family members as large family organizations have developed in the United States and other countries that describe characteristic behavioral patterns and interpersonal responses in their children. Parent groups will report similar behavior problems and difficulties in management when they meet. The interest in parent groups in improving the life of their children has led to additional hypotheses and more refined observations on behavioral characteristics. Third, new techniques in genetics provide new insights into the extent and mechanisms of the human genome as the basis of behavior. Advances in other aspects of neuroscience, including neurophysiology, neuroanatomy, and neuroimaging, provide additional means of designating brain mechanisms that may be involved. With the establishment of these new methods of evaluation and the identification of rating scales to measure behavioral phenotypes, there is now an increased focus on behavioral phenotypes in developmental neuropsychiatry. Finally, comprehensive study of children with different developmental disabilities may increase our appreciation for the relative contribution of genetic variables in the pathogenesis of specific affective and behavioral disorders.

Nyhan (1972) introduced the term "behavioral phenotype" to describe outwardly observable behavior so characteristic of children with genetic disorders that its presence suggests the underlying genetic condition. In speaking of compulsive self-injury in Lesch-Nyhan disease, a disorder that he initially described, Nyhan (1976) noted:

> We feel that these children have a pattern of unusual behavior that is unique to them. Stereotypical patterns of behavior occurring in syndromic fashion in sizable numbers of individuals provide the possibility that there is a concrete explanation that is discoverable. In these children, there are so many anatomical abnormalities, from changes in hair and bones to dermatoglyphics, that it is a reasonable hypothesis that their behaviors are determined by an abnormal neuroanatomy that would be discoverable, possibly neurophysiologically, ultimately anatomically . . .

these children all seem self-programmed. These stereotypical patterns of unusual behavior could reflect the presence of structural deficits in the central nervous system. (p. 235)

Such observations have led to greater emphasis on assessment of behavior, and the recognition of behavioral phenotypes in some disorders has led to closer scrutiny of known neurodevelopmental conditions. Initially, the focus was on documenting the patterns of behavior because the study of brain and behavior requires the identification of well-defined syndromes for investigation. Now that developments in the neurosciences provide a means to understand the biological bases of such behavioral patterns, the focus has shifted to understanding the neurobiological mechanisms underlying characteristic behavioral patterns, including cognitive processes and social interactions. Such patterns are reported in a number of syndromes arising from genetic or chromosomal abnormalities. Thus, molecular analysis of the underlying genetic disorder has been initiated in several syndromes with the hope of revealing the biological basis of the behavioral phenotype. However, due to the rarity of many of these syndromes, and the complexity of their genetic basis, establishing the validity of the association between syndrome and behavioral phenotype is difficult. Nevertheless, Flint (1996, 1999) points out that evidence from animal studies with relevance to human behavioral phenotypes shows that the pathway from genotype to phenotype may be accessible following careful delineation of each of the features of the behavioral phenotypes. However, in regard to the study of cognition, he suggests (Flint, 1996, 1999) that we require a greater integration of different levels of understanding of cognition in order to exploit the genetic discoveries; "a rapprochement between molecular and systems neuroscience."

DEFINITION AND CHARACTERIZATION

The study of behavioral phenotypes emphasizes the discovery, among individuals with known chromosomal, genetic or neurodevelopmental disorders, of those mental and behavioral features causally related to the underlying condition. Examples are the characteristic self-mutilation of fingers and lips in Lesch-Nyhan disease, the hyperphagia and compulsive behaviors in Prader-Willi syndrome, gaze aversion in fragile X syndrome, the superficial sociability, hyperlalia, and language disorder in Williams syndrome. When present the behavior suggests the syndrome. As Nyhan has suggested (1995) these are "syndromes of behavior." Still, despite their behavioral presentations not all individuals with the disorder may show the classic behavioral features, but the probability is greater that they will. The essential issue is that the behavior suggests the diagnosis.

Efforts to define what is meant by a behavioral phenotype are continuing. Harris (1987, 1998a) proposed that behavioral phenotypes are stereotypical patterns of behavior that are reliably identified in groups of individuals with known neurodevelopmental disorders and are "not learned." They may be the conse-quence of neurodevelopmental abnormalities that are potentially discoverable. This approach to definition is a descriptive approach that takes as its starting point observations of the behavior itself rather than beginning with a discrete and genetically identifiable condition, such as Down syndrome. Using this approach, researchers identified Rett syndrome (The Rett Syndrome Diagnostic Criteria Work Shop, 1988), with its characteristic hand and hand-to-mouth stereotypies, as a disorder with a behavioral phenotype many years before the genetic etiology was recognized. Moreover, the descriptive approach does not discount acquired disorders, such as fetal alcohol syndrome, as having behavioral phenotypes. The impact of alcohol on cellular signaling and its consequences of cell death, ab-normal midline brain development, behavioral problems, and learning disabilities are now well known (Harris, 1998a; Ikonomidou et al., 2000).

Flint and Yule (1994) define behavioral phenotype as follows: "The behav-ioral phenotype is a characteristic pattern of motor, cognitive, linguistic, and social abnormalities that is consistently associated with a biological disorder" (p. 666). This does not mean that the behavior is present in all instances but that the probability of its occurrence is increased. In the future, more may be learned about brain mechanisms by comparing those with behavioral involve-ment with others with the same syndrome but without the behavioral features.

In understanding behavioral phenotypes, Skuse (2000) suggests that the fol-lowing points be considered: (1) The behavioral descriptions, like other physical features of neurodevelopmental disorders, have increased probability of occur-ring and do not occur in all cases; they may not be fully expressed in all affected individuals. (2) The genetic background of the individual may affect the phe-notypic expression. (3) Environmental factors may modify expression. (4) The behavioral presentation may be modified by the extent of intellectual disability associated with the disorder. (5) Mouse models, where there may be species-specific factors, may be variable such that mutant mouse models do not replicate the behavioral features found in humans. One must consider the genetic back-ground, strain differences, and differences in the rodent physiology when study-ing mouse models. In Lesch-Nyhan disease, the HPRT deficient mouse has a uricase enzyme that breaks down uric acid. Therefore, it is not a model for the hyperuricemic metabolic disorder, but it still may be a useful model to study dopamine deficiency in the brain. Thus, aspects of a disorder may be modeled in transgenic mice or in other species that may not demonstrate the full behav-ioral phenotype.

Although some (Skuse, 2000) have sought to limit the study of behavioral phenotypes to known genetic disorders, knowledge of the genetic disorder is only the first step. Links from gene to behavior are complicated in that one gene may lead to the encoding of many, perhaps 10 or more, different proteins; the number of genes and type of mutation determine complexity. For example, in Lesch-Nyhan disease, the disorder of purine metabolism clearly leads to the overproduction of uric acid and renal stones, but the pathway to the associated movement disorder and self-injury is not direct and may be mediated through effects on the arborization of dopamine neurons (Harris, 1998b). Moreover, there are variants of Lesch-Nyhan disease with different degrees of enzyme deficit, ranging up to 20%, that have clinical effects.

Pathways from genes to cognition and complex behavior require an understanding of the way genes are controlled and direct the epigenetic program. The term *epigenetics* was introduced by D.H. Waddington (1939) to describe these processes. It was derived from the eighteenth century dispute between the preformationists (who believed sperm and fertilized egg contained a preformed organism, homunculus, with all its major features present in miniature) and the epigenesists. The epigenesists believed that there were no preformed structures but that during development the embryo took on a progressively more complex form. Thus, the term epigenesis refers to the processes by which the genotype gives rise to the phenotype. If such processes are aberrant, we might speak of "the inheritance of epigenetic defects" (Holliday, 1987) in addition to genetic ones. Holliday (2002) proposes that epigenetic might be defined as nuclear inheritance that is not based on differences in DNA sequence. Lederberg (2001) suggests that for the sake of clarity the term "genetic" refers to nucleic information that is dynamically regulated by epinucleic information for development to proceed. Methylation is epinucleic and the failure of DNA methylation in fragile X syndrome is an example of a deficit in this type of epigenesis. Genetic transmission though the germline may involve imprinting or other epigenetic processes. He emphasizes that epinucleic is one aspect of epigenesis and that there are other developmental processes in keeping with Waddington's definition that do depend on sequenced base changes such as cellular senescence following shorting of the telomere at the tip of a chromosome. There is also the possibility of cytoplasmic inheritance and the role of mitochondria in inheritance. Thus, epigenesis is an important consideration where behavioral phenotypes are considered.

PREVALENCE OF BEHAVIORAL PHENOTPES

With increasing attention to neurogenetic disorders, the number of identifiable behavioral phenotypes is increasing. Although standardized rating scales and personality profiles have been developed to measure behavioral phenotypes (Ikonomidou et al., 2000; O'Brien, 1991), profiles pertinent to the specific disorder are still needed. Careful observations of behavior are necessary when considering intervention for neurogenetic disorders. Besides behavioral phenotypes, isolated special abilities that occur in genetically based syndromes also require assessment. These include special abilities in calculation and in music (Hill, 1978). Special abilities may potentially be related to the proposed modular organization of the brain. Some intellectually disabled persons with autistic disorder demonstrated such skills and have been referred to as savants.

PSYCHOPATHOLOGY AND BEHAVIORAL PHENOTYPES

Cognitive and behavioral features that are not specific features limited to one particular behavioral phenotype may be found in several neurogenetic syndromes.

These include attention problems, hyperactivity, impulsivity, self-injury, aggression, autistic-like behavior, and perseverative behaviors. These cognitive and behavioral findings indicate vulnerability of the developing brain to genetic, epigenetic, or environmental perturbation. Because these behaviors occur across many syndromes, they lack specificity and may not qualify as specific behavioral phenotypes. Still, these behavioral features should be included in the description of the disorders. For example, the relationship between aggression and antisocial behavior has been suggested in monoamine oxidase A (MAOA) deficiency. MAOA is an enzyme that oxidizes serotonin and norepinephrine.

Brunner et al. (1993) described an association between abnormal behavior and MAOA deficiency in several males from a single, large Dutch kindred. The affected males differed from unaffected males in that they tested in the borderline range of intelligence and demonstrated increased impulsive behavior, that is, aggressive behavior, abnormal sexual behavior, and arson. Yet, a specific psychiatric diagnosis was not made in four affected males who were examined by psychiatrists. Because MAOA deficiency leads to increased 5-hydroxytryptamine (5-HT) levels, the aggressive behavior in these individuals may be an exception to studies linking low 5-HT with impulsive aggression. Brunner suggests that even if a possible association between MAOA deficiency and abnormal behavior is confirmed in other kindreds, the hypothesis that MAOA constitutes an aggression gene is not supported. He noted that genes are essentially simple and code for proteins, while behavior is complex; thus, a direct causal relationship between a single gene and a specific behavior is highly unlikely. In MAOA deficiency, complexity is shown by the variability in the behavioral phenotype and by the highly complex consequences of MAOA deficiency on neurotransmitter function. Thus, the full pathway from gene to complex behavior must be considered; the concept of a gene that directly encodes behavior is overly simplistic (Brunner et al., 1993). In an attempt to understand the mechanism for the aggression, behavior was studied in MAOA-deficient mice. Mice deficient in MAOA exhibited enhanced aggression in the resident-intruder test (Cases et al., 1995) and had elevated norepinephrine and serotonin levels in the frontal cortex, hippocampus, and cerebellum. In addition, MAOA deficiency resulted in a selective effect on emotional learning (fear conditioning), yet maternal behavior and eye blink conditioning were not affected (Kim et al., 1997). Thus, chronic elevations of monoamines, due to a deletion of the gene encoding MAOA, may lead to selective alterations in emotional behavior in a mouse model. Therefore, much may be learned by considering pathways leading to behavior in neurogenetic syndromes; mouse models provide one approach. It is the "downstream" consequences of the genetic abnormality on brain chemistry, brain circuits, and brain structure that result in the abnormal behavior. Because those downstream systems may be affected by environmental and interpersonal interventions, the expression of a genetic disorder can be modified by targeted interventions.

BEHAVIORAL PHENOTYPES OF NEURODEVELOPMENTAL DISORDERS

The sections that follow discuss various syndromes where behavioral phenotypes have been identified. Characteristic behaviors will be highlighted, findings on etiology discussed, and potential neurochemical and neuroanatomical abnormalities highlighted. Behavioral and pharmacologic therapies have had limited success in many of these conditions, so better characterization of the individual condition is essential to establish treatment. Genetic studies, neuroanatomical studies, brain imaging studies, and continuing investigations of neurotransmitter systems, endocrine rhythms, and sleep studies may provide information that will be helpful in the future in treatment. Fetal alcohol syndrome is discussed in the section that follows this one.

Down Syndrome

Down syndrome was the first intellectual disability syndrome described and is the most common genetic form of intellectual disability. Because of its frequency, the general public is most aware of Down syndrome, and for many, it is the prototypical form of intellectual disability. The first description of a child with Down syndrome is found in the writings of Esquirol (1845). However, Down (1887) provided the first description of the syndrome that is now called Down syndrome. Advances in cytogenetics, resulting in improved techniques for the examination of human chromosomes, led to the recognition of the chromosomal basis of Down syndrome. The underlying genetic abnormality (trisomy 21) was identified in 1959. It was the first syndrome where a chromosomal anomaly was demonstrated as the basis for characteristic physical features.

Epidemiology

Approximately 7,000 infants are born in the United States each year with Down syndrome. The frequency of Down syndrome is one in 800 live births, in all races and economic groups. Down syndrome accounts for approximately one-third of children in special education.

Down syndrome is not attributable to any behavioral activity of the parents or environmental factors. The probability that another child with Down syndrome will be born in a subsequent pregnancy is approximately 1%, regardless of maternal age. However, a number of risk factors have been investigated, including geographic location, race ethnicity, season of birth, socioeconomic status, maternal smoking or infection, and environmental hazards such as fluoride and ionizing radiation. None of these has been found to affect the incidence of Down syndrome in a consistent manner. The life expectancy of adults with Down syndrome is variable; however, some individuals live into their 70s. Early deaths are associated with associated congenital anomalies, particularly malformations of the heart. Life expectancy has been enhanced by surgical procedures and the availability of antibiotic treatment for infections.

Genetics

The risk of having a child with Down syndrome increases with maternal age. The risk for trisomy 21 or chromosome 21 nondysjunction is increased such that the incidence is 1:1,400 for maternal age 20–24 but rises to 1:900 at age 30, 1:100 at age 40, and 1:25 among women 45 and older (Thompson, McInnes, and Willard, 2001). Moreover, if the parent is a carrier for a structural chromosomal translocation, the recurrence risk is higher. The sequencing of the chromosome 21 in the human genome, in principle, allows the identification of every gene on the chromosome (Hattori et al., 2000). In most cases, approximately 92% of the time, Down syndrome is caused by the presence of an extra chromosome 21 in all cells (trisomy 21). In approximately 2%–4% of cases, Down syndrome is due to mosaic trisomy 21. This situation is similar to simple trisomy 21, but, in this instance, the extra chromosome 21 is present in some, but not all, cells of the individual. Finally, approximately 3%–4% of individuals with Down syndrome have cells containing 46 chromosomes and translocation trisomy 21.

Prenatal Screening and Diagnosis

In the United States, prenatal screening is available by a blood test, followed by prenatal cytogenic diagnosis if indicated (Roizen and Patterson, 2003). The screening blood test measures the levels of three markers for Down syndrome: maternal serum alpha feto-protein (MSAFP), chorionic gonadotropin (hCG), and unconjugated estriol (uE3). While these measurements are not a definitive test for Down syndrome, a lower MSAFP value, a lower uE3 level, and an elevated hCG level, on average, suggests an increased likelihood of a Down syndrome fetus, and additional diagnostic testing may be carried out. When carried out in the first trimester, this test has a 69% detection rate and a 5% false positive rate (Yaron and Mashiach, 2001).

Prenatal diagnostic procedures include amniocentesis (fourteenth to eighteenth week of pregnancy, chorionic villus sampling (between 9 and 11 weeks of pregnancy), and percutaneous umbilical blood sampling (between 18 and 22 weeks). Such testing has made it possible to identify Down syndrome by chromosome analysis in gestation so that elective termination of pregnancy is possible. Chorionic villus sampling carries a 1%–2% risk of miscarriage. This risk is higher with percutaneous umbilical blood sampling. Advances in maternal serum screening and second-trimester ultrasonography have resulted in more judicious use of amniocentesis and chorionic villus sampling.

Preimplantation diagnosis or blastomere analysis before implantation is available. These tests allow clinicians to detect chromosome abnormalities before an embryo is implanted during in vitro fertilization. This technique is primarily used for couples who have suffered repeated terminations of pregnancy, couples with low fertility, couples who are at risk of passing on X-linked disorders, or those at risk for single gene disorder.

Physical Features

Down syndrome is usually diagnosed at birth. Postnatal diagnosis is generally made based on physical appearance and confirmed by chromosome analysis. The characteristic features are upturned outward slanting eyes, epicanthal folds, wide nasal bridge, brush field spots in the eyes, a large posterior fontanelle, a low hair line, a single transverse palmer crease, a large cleft between the first and second toes, and relatively short upper arms.

Infants with Down syndrome are hypotonic although this is less apparent as the individual grows older. The majority have short stature. Fifteen percent are hypothyroid by the time they reach adolescence, and approximately 50% have structural heart lesions of varying degrees. Approximately 7% have congenital upper intestinal obstructions, and 1% has a diagnosis of leukemia. In addition, hearing impairment occurs in 60%–80% along with visual problems and delayed bone maturation.

Personality and Behavioral Phenotype

Individuals with Down syndrome are generally described as placid and good-tempered. However, hyperactivity, aggression, and impulsivity may be present (Clark and Wilson, 2003). Autistic features are very rare in Down syndrome but have been described. Ghaziuddin (2000) found that in those rare cases when autistic disorder was diagnosed, autism spectrum disorder in family members was significantly more common. Down originally proposed that those in his care had considerable powers of imitation (even bordering on being mimics). He wrote that they are humorous and have a lively sense of the ridiculous, which often colors their mimicry. The finding of increased imitation ability has been reported as a trait independent of intelligence in a German study (Huffner and Redlin, 1976). These authors compared individuals with Down syndrome with both intellectually disabled and typically developing persons matched for age.

Behaviorally, Down syndrome is associated with increased sociability and decrease in problem behaviors like self-injury or aggression, relative to the developmental disabilities. Each of the differences just noted hold for both chronological age controls and mental development controls without Down syndrome (Dykens, Hodapp, and Evans, 1994). Although temperament has been described as characteristic for Down syndrome, no consistent personality type is identified. When evaluating temperament, those with Down syndrome may differ from unaffected individuals along several dimensions. As children with Down syndrome develop, the ability to respond to the environment is affected by the interaction of cognitive ability and their environmental experience. Thus, temperament is affected by the developmental course of brain maturation and experience. Temperament involves the organization of reactive capacities, emotionality, cognitive, and self-regulatory abilities. There may be differences in teachers' and parents' reports owing to the varying contexts of their observations. Those with Down syndrome may be less reactive to stimulation and possess higher thresholds to respond. As a consequence of these patterns of reactivity, they can be described as passive and less reactive. In addition, the timing of shifts and changes in temperament with age may vary because of differences in neurological maturation.

Cognitive Profile

The highest developmental scores are recorded during the early years of life, particularly during infancy, with a progressive slowing in development as the child grows older (Dykens, Hodapp, and Evans, 1994); the cognitive phenotype becomes clearer across the life span (Chapman and Hesketh, 2000). Those with Down syndrome most commonly have moderate-to-severe intellectual disability.

A developmental language delay is always present and, ordinarily, expressive language is more affected than receptive language. The pragmatics of language tend to be good; however, grammatical abilities are impaired. Visual processing tends to be better than auditory processing (Pueschel et al., 1987). Thus, the cognitive behavioral phenotype in individuals with Down syndrome includes significant delay in nonverbal cognitive development accompanied by specific deficits in speech, language production, and auditory short-term memory in infancy and childhood, but fewer adaptive behavior problems than individuals with other cognitive disabilities. Language use is generally delayed. During later development, language is characterized by word comprehension being more advanced than overall cognition, and deficits in syntax are greater than limitations in vocabulary. In terms of cognitive performance, people with Down syndrome have selective deficits in verbal short-term memory and delayed recall.

Dementia in Down Syndrome

Genetic studies and neuroimaging studies have been conducted to understand the relationship between dementia and Down syndrome. Evidence of dementia emerges for up to half the individuals with Down syndrome studied after age 50 (Wisniewski and Silverman, 1998). Janicki and Dalton (2000) studied the prevalence of dementia in a statewide sample and observed that the onset occurred in the early 50s for those with Down syndrome and in the mid-60s for other groups; Alzheimer-type dementia was the most frequent diagnosis. Rates of dementia in adults with intellectual disability without Down syndrome were equivalent to that expected in the general population unless predisposing risk factors for dementia are also present. Moreover, there is a clear discrepancy between the presumed presence of Alzheimer's neuropathology and the clinical findings of dementia of the Alzheimer's type among older people with Down syndrome. Thus, neuropathological changes are more commonly seen before behavioral manifestations and may be misleading (Devenny et al., 1996).

This high risk for dementia in adults with Down's syndrome has been linked to triplication and overexpression of the gene for amyloid precursor protein (APP) (Schupf and Sergievsky, 2002). However, there is wide variation in the age of onset; additional risk factors may account for these differences. Studies of factors that influence formation of beta-amyloid (Abeta) were reviewed, such as atypical karyotypes, susceptibility genotypes, gender and estrogen deficiency, and individual differences in Abeta peptide levels. Because various alleles of the apolipoprotein E genotype have been associated with risk for dementia, these alleles have been studied in Down syndrome. It has been proposed that the E_2 allele may be protective against the onset of dementia, while the E_4 homozygote may be associated with increased risk. Others have suggested that the E_2 allele may be associated with a more aggressive course of the disease. When studied in 100 individuals with Down syndrome and 346 intellectually disabled individuals without Down syndrome, similar genotypes have been documented (Prasher et al., 1997). However, Schupf and Sergievsky (2002) found that apolipoprotein E_4 allele, estrogen deficiency, and high levels of Abeta1-42 peptide are associated with earlier onset of dementia. Atypical karyotypes and the apolipoprotein E_2 allele were associated with reduced mortality and reduced risk of dementia. They conclude that factors that influence Abeta levels, rather than the overexpression of APP alone, may help researchers understand the differences in age of onset of dementia in Down's syndrome.

Women with Down syndrome experience early onset of both menopause and Alzheimer's disease (Schupf et al., 2003). Information from cognitive assessments, medical record review, neurological evaluation, and caregiver interviews was used to establish ages for onset of menopause and dementia in a community-based sample of 163 postmenopausal women with Down syndrome, 40 years–60 years of age. Women with early onset of menopause (46 years of age or younger) were found to have earlier onset and increased risk of Alzheimer's disease compared with women with onset of menopause after 46 years. Demented women had higher mean serum sex hormone binding globulin levels than nondemented women, but similar levels of total estradiol, suggesting that bioavailable estradiol, rather than total estradiol, is associated with dementia. These findings support the view that reductions in estrogens after menopause may contribute to the cascade of pathological processes leading to Alzheimer's disease in women with Down syndrome and suggest that estrogen replacement therapy be considered in women with Down syndrome and early menopause.

Neuroimaging in Down Syndrome

Neuroimaging studies involving volumetric MRI, single photon emission computed tomography (SPECT) scans, and positron emission tomography (PET) scans have been conducted in Down syndrome. These studies have been carried out to investigate brain structure and function. Such studies may elucidate neurodevelopment and potentially be used to monitor brain changes with aging. Individuals with Down syndrome ranging in age from early childhood to young adulthood have been shown to have smaller overall brain volumes involving both cerebral gray and white matter, disproportionately smaller cerebellar volumes and proportionately larger subcortical gray and parietal white matter volumes than control groups. There is relative preservation of parietal lobe gray and temporal lobe white matter (Pinter et al., 2001). Hippocampal volume reduction is seen in both children and adults with Down syndrome and is more likely due to early developmental differences rather than neurodegenerative changes. Amygdala volumes did not differ between Down syndrome and a control groups. Subcortical structures (basal ganglia) are preserved; this is reflected in larger adjusted subcortical gray matter volumes in the Down syndrome group (Pinter et al., 2001).

The cerebellar hypoplasia evident in Down syndrome might be linked to hypotonia and motor coordination difficulties, as well as articulatory speech disturbances, commonly found in most children with Down syndrome. Syntactic difficulties found in individuals with Down syndrome also may be due to cerebellar hypoplasia and dysfunction. The frontal lobes are small (but not proportionally so) and might be implicated in the cognitive deficits of Down syndrome such as inattention and perseveration. The preservation of the basal ganglia structures in children with Down syndrome despite significantly smaller overall cerebral volumes suggests a temporal dissociation in the development of cortical compared to subcortical regions. Embryologically, neither brain volume differences nor neuropathologic abnormalities are apparent in fetal Down syndrome brains until the third trimester. By this time, the majority of basal ganglia development is completed. However, dendritic arborization, synaptogenesis, and laminar organization are ongoing in the cerebral cortex in the third trimester.

Using an interactive anatomical segmentation technique and volume-of-interest measurements of MRI, nondemented Down syndrome adults (mean age = 41.1 years, 15 female) had significantly reduced hippocampus, entorhinal cortex, and corpus callosum sizes with increasing age. Comparable decrease of corpus callosum and hippocampal size with age in nondemented subjects with Down syndrome suggests that neocortical neuronal alterations accompany allocortical (hippocampal complex/olfactory cortex) changes in the predementia phase of Down syndrome (Teipel et al., 2004).

SPECT scanning has documented bilateral reduction in uptake in the temporoparietal region, the pattern that is suggestive of dementia. However, it may be of limited use in diagnosing dementia (Jones et al., 1997) in Down syndrome because blood flow changes are not necessarily associated with clinical finding of dementia. Twenty-six adults with Down syndrome, aged 16–55, underwent HMPAO SPECT evaluations. The findings were normal in 18 of the 26 adults, 5 showed nonspecific abnormalities, and 3 had bilateral reduction in uptake in the temporoparietal region, the pattern that is suggestive of dementia. However, only 1 of the 5 with dementia had an abnormal SPECT scan and a diagnosis of dementia suggestive of the Alzheimer's type. There was no association between dementia ratings and the SPECT scan abnormalities. Other investigators (Deb et al., 1992) carried out SPECT scans with 99mTc-exametazime in 20 adult cases of Down syndrome diagnosed with dementia using a structured psychiatric and physical examination along with a caregiver interview and case notes. Four individuals were clinically demented and all showed regional cerebral blood flow (rCBF) changes commonly found in patients with Alzheimer's disease, namely, bilateral temporoparietal deficits. These changes were also observed in approximately half of the patients without clinical evidence of dementia, but in none of the healthy controls. Across the group of patients, temporoparietal rCBF deficits were associated with evidence of deterioration, but not with advancing age. Thus, careful assessment of dementia and appropriate diagnostic criteria may be critical in the use of the SPECT scan in the assessment of dementia. The value of using SPECT to monitor cognitive decline is not yet established.

Positron emission tomography (PET) with 18-fluorodeoxyglucose was undertaken at rest with eyes covered and ears plugged and during audiovisual stimulation in eight younger (mean age 35 years) and eight older (mean age 50 years) healthy individuals with Down syndrome, none of whom had dementia. Intellectual functioning and compliance was similar in the two groups. No differences were found in the resting state, yet during audiovisual stimulation, the older group had lower rates of glucose metabolism in the inferior, superior, and medial parietal neocortical areas and in the temporal, visual, and sensorimotor regions, as well as lower overall global cerebral glucose metabolism (Pietrini et al., 1997). This study suggested that abnormal brain metabolism of the Alzheimer's disease pattern may be demonstrated before the appearance of clinical dementia in a high-risk group, using PET imaging. Continuing follow-up is necessary to confirm these findings. Thus, a stress test paradigm can identify metabolic abnormalities in preclinical stages of Alzheimer's disease, even though cerebral metabolism is normal at rest.

Treatment

The American Academy of Pediatrics (2001) and the Down Syndrome Medical Interest Group (Cohen, 1999) have developed guidelines for medical management that are found at www.denison.edu/collaborations/dsq/health99.html. These guidelines are regularly updated and include detail recommendations for all aspects of care (e.g., cardiac, hematologic, ENT, gastrointestinal, endocrine, dental, etc.) and include neonatal, infancy, childhood, adolescence, and adult age periods. The 1999 update recommended additional thyroid screening at 6 months of age, hearing evaluations at birth and every 6 months thereafter until 3 years, eye evaluations by 6 months of age and yearly, celiac disease screening between 2 and 3 years of age, and radiographic screening for atlantoaxial instability once between 3 and 5 years and then as needed, such as for participation in Special Olympics. Additional guidelines for adolescent management (Roizen, 2002) and adult management (Smith, 2001) are available. Roizen and Patterson (2003) provide advice on disorders to prevent, disorders to monitor, disorders that require vigilance, and behavioral and psychiatric disorders throughout the life span.

Velocardiofacial Syndrome (22q11.2 deletion)

Velocardiofacial syndrome (VCFS) was first described in 1981 by Robert Shprintzen and colleagues. Subsequently, it was shown to be linked to the long arm of chromosome 22 and is now referred to as a 22q11.2 deletion syndrome. The 22q11.2 deletion syndrome includes the phenotypes that were previously referred to as DiGeorge syndrome (DGS) and velocardiofacial syndrome or Shprintzen syndrome. The clinical descriptions of DiGeorge syndrome and velocardiofacial syndrome resulted from the age of ascertainment of the original syndromes. The majority of individuals with DiGeorge syndrome were identified during the neonatal period and noted to have major congenital heart defects, hypocalcemia, and immunodeficiency; those individuals with velocardiofacial syndrome were more often diagnosed in cleft palate clinics or craniofacial centers around the time they reached school age and speech and learning difficulties became evident. Other disorders, such as Pierre-Rubin syndrome, and other rarer syndromes, are also caused by a seemingly identical microdeletion in this region. Identification of the gene(s) that are affected by the deletion will be required before it is known whether the same or different genes contribute to the expression of these disorders. Together with velocardiofacial syndrome, they are collectively referred to as the 22q11 deletion syndromes (22qDS).

Prevalence

Velocardiofacial syndrome has an estimated prevalence of 1:3,000, making it the second most common genetic syndrome after Down syndrome. Given the variable expression of the 22q11.2 deletion, the incidence is probably much higher than previously estimated. The earliest reports on velocardiofacial syndrome patients involved young children. By school age, it became apparent that they demonstrated behavioral problems. They were often shy and socially withdrawn, with blunted affect, impulsive, disinhibited, and prone to temper tantrums. Psychotic and affective symptoms sometimes emerged in adolescence or early adulthood.

Genetics

The 22q11.2 deletion syndrome is inherited as an autosomal dominant trait. Approximately 93% of those affected have a spontaneous or de novo microdeletion in chromosome band 22q11.2 (Pike and Super, 1997), and approximately 7% have inherited the 22q11.2 deletion from a parent. Overall, offspring of individuals with the deletion at 22q11.2 have a 50% chance of inheriting the 22q11.2 deletion. Similar to other syndromes caused by a microdeletion, the molecular diagnosis of 22qDS is usually made by fluorescence in situ hybridization (FISH). In FISH, a fluorescently labeled sequence of a few thousand nucleotides is developed in the laboratory. This sequence is used as a probe; this probe will bind to the complementary sequence of bases on chromosome 22. Because there are two copies of each chromosome, two hybridization signals are found on the FISH examination in the normal individual. In those cases in which a deletion is present, fluorescence will be demonstrated on only one chromosome. Ninety-five percent of 22qDS can be detected with this technique. The rest may not be detected because they are caused by unique deletions or unbalanced translocations. When a 22q11.2 deletion is suspected, it is recommended that routine cytogenetic analysis be performed at the time of FISH testing because a small percentage (<1%) of individuals with clinical findings of the 22q11.2 deletion syndrome have chromosomal rearrangements involving 22q11.2, such as translocation between chromosome 22 and another chromosome.

The gene or genes that result in 22q11.2 are not known; however, the disorder does not seem to be a contiguous gene deletion syndrome like Williams syndrome, which is caused by a microdeletion on chromosome 7, and the mutations of several of approximately 16 genes involved are thought to explain the varied symptoms. The phenotype of 22q11.2 is highly variable with no clear-cut correlation between severity of the phenotype and the extent of the deletion. However, deletion might cause a disruption in the expression of a transcription factor or other protein involved in the expression of genes outside the 22qD region. The absence of such proteins might be responsible for the pathophysiology of the disorder.

One gene implicated in possible psychopathology is located within the 22qD region; it is the gene encoding for catechol-O-methyltransferase (COMT), an enzyme that degrades dopamine. Several polymorphisms exist within the gene, and at least one of these is associated with lower biochemical activity of COMT. Candidate genes in velocardiofacial syndrome include those involved in the early growth and development of the brain, such as genes that regulate the migration of neurons.

Genes encoding migratory factors that are expressed in the brain might explain the cytoarchitectural abnormalities in the brain. Such genes in the 22qD region include the goosecoid-like (GSCL) gene, which encodes for a homeobox protein; ARVCF, which is involved in the formation of adherence junctions between cells; the clathrin heavy chain-like gene, which recycles the presynaptic membrane of vesicles after release of neurotransmitters; and UFD1L, which is involved in the degradation of proteins. However, point mutations have not been detected in any of these genes.

Prenatal Diagnosis

Prenatal testing is available for both those fetuses determined to be at 50% risk by family history and for fetuses not known by family history to be at increased risk for deletion 22q11.2 but who have congenital heart disease and/or cleft palate found on ultrasound examination. Fewer than 5% of individuals with clinical symptoms of the 22q11.2 deletion syndrome have normal routine cytogenetic studies and negative FISH testing. They may have variant deletions that may be detectable with extensive additional testing.

Physical Features

The diagnosis is suspected in individuals with a range of presentations that may include combinations of the following: congenital heart disease (particularly conotruncal malformations), abnormalities of the palate, especially velopharyngeal insufficiency (VPI), hypocalcemia, immune deficiency, learning difficulties, and in some instances, characteristic facial features. The typical physical presentation in children with velocardiofacial syndrome is a narrow face, narrow palpebral fissures, a prominent tubular nose and a bulbous nasal tip, small open mouth, recessed jaw, short stature, and slender hands and digits (Shprintzen et al., 1981). Less frequent features include short stature, microcephaly, intellectual disability, minor ear anomalies, and inguinal hernia.

The presence of cleft palate and velopharyngeal insufficiency often results in feeding difficulties. Hypocalcemia, immune deficiency, and cardiac malformations are present in a majority; hypotonia is found in approximately half of the patients (Shprintzen et al., 1981; Vantrappen et al., 1999; Wang et al., 2000). Congenital heart disease is present in 74% of patients with 22qDS. The most common are tetralogy of Fallot, interrupted aortic arch, and ventricular septal defect. The prevalence of the deletion among cardiac patients is highest for those with interrupted aortic arch and tetralogy of Fallot. Palatal abnormalities are present in 83% of patients and range from velopharyngeal incompetence to cleft lip and palate. Hypocalcemia and T-cell immunodeficiency are caused by hypoplastic parathyroid and thymus glands, respectively. Seizures occur in approximately 20%; most are secondary to hypocalcemia. Approximately half of children with velocardiofacial syndrome are hypotonic. Most affected individuals have delays in gross motor development, such as crawling and walking independently, as well as fine motor development.

How might these physical features be accounted for? It is known that embryonic neural crest cells are highly migratory cells that give rise to the mesenchyme in the third and fourth pharyngeal arches. These arches differentiate into specific organs and structures of the head, neck, and aortic arch. The cardiac anomalies, cleft palate, facial dysmorphism, and maldevelopment of the thymus and parathyroid gland found in 22qDS might be the result of an embryonic defect in the migration of neural crest cells.

Behavioral Phenotype

The social deficits are the most striking features of velocardiofacial syndrome. These children are generally withdrawn and have poor social interaction skills (Heineman-de Boer et al., 1999). There is minimum spontaneous facial expression, and speech is nasal with a monotonous voice tone. Blunt and inappropriate affect are frequently present (Golding-Kushner, Weller, and Shprintzen, 1985). They are often shy and socially withdrawn, with blunted affect, but are also impulsive, disinhibited, and prone to temper tantrums.

There is a high frequency of psychiatric disorder in individuals with velocardiofacial syndrome. Psychotic and affective symptoms may emerge in adolescence or early adulthood. Approximately one-quarter of velocardiofacial syndrome patients develop psychotic symptoms, and a diagnosis of schizophrenia may be made in adolescence. Overall, the prevalence of schizophrenia in velocardiofacial syndrome patients is 25 times that of the general population prevalence. Moreover, both schizophrenic and nonschizophrenic velocardiofacial syndrome patients scored higher on a scale for schizotypal personality disorder. The psychosis associated with velocardiofacial syndrome has a chronic course with poor response to neuroleptic treatment (Gothelf et al., 1999).

Schizoaffective disorder and bipolar spectrum disorders (cyclothymia, dysthymia, and major depression) may be diagnosed. Paranoid schizophrenia is reported to occur in up to 30% of adults with velocardiofacial syndrome (Wang et al., 2000). Pulver et al. (1994) found psychotic illnesses among relatives of individuals with velocardiofacial syndrome. Moreover, schizophrenic patients have been found to have an increased rate of velocardiofacial syndrome. One team detected 22qD in 2 of 100 adult schizophrenic patients, a rate approximately 200 times greater than in the general population. A 22qD prevalence of 20% in a sample of persons with schizophrenia with at least one prominent physical manifestation of velocardiofacial syndrome, such as cardiac anomaly, cleft palate, or the typical facies, was found in one study and the likelihood of the diagnosis was higher in those with at least two physical manifestations of velocardiofacial syndrome. The Child Psychiatry Branch of the NIMH reported a 6% rate of 22qD in a cohort of 47 patients with very early-onset schizophrenia.

Similar to schizophrenia, patients with velocardiofacial syndrome show aberrant early development marked by psychomotor delays; coordination deficits; specific deficits in cognition, language, learning and attention; and social withdrawal. These features strongly suggest a disruption in normal central nervous system development. Mice with deletions for a subset of the genes that are deleted in clinical cases show deficits in sensorimotor gating and learning and memory. Sensorimotor gating deficits have been linked to schizophrenia and schizotypal personality disorder. Genetic studies in mice may aid the identification of genes that modulate these behaviors (Paylor et al., 2001).

Cognitive Profile

Intelligence is usually in the normal range, although mild intellectual disability may occur. Language and motor developmental delay and persistent coordination deficits are common. Verbal IQ is usually higher than the performance IQ (Wang et al., 2000). Learning disabilities are present. The most common form of learning disability is poor arithmetic skills, with better reading and spelling achievement (Wang et al., 2000). The relative strength in language abilities is contrasted with a delay in early language development. Speech disorder is secondary to the cleft palate. Distractibility, attention deficits, and abstract thinking problems are also characteristic features (Shprintzen et al., 1981).

Intelligence has been studied in affected preschool children, adolescents, and adults. The average total IQ score in these studies fell in the borderline intelligence range of 71 to 78. From 25% to 40% of patients were mildly intellectually disabled. Moderate to severe intellectual disability was rarely demonstrated. The performance IQ score was consistently and significantly lower (by approximately 10 points) than the verbal IQ. Information, comprehension, and coding subsets were relatively strengths, but visuospatial perception and problem-solving were weaknesses. The language skills were both delayed and impaired in all velocardiofacial syndrome subjects, with the impairment being more pronounced in the expressive than the receptive language domain. Although developmental language disorders are regarded as precursors of later disabilities in reading, the latter remained intact in velocardiofacial syndrome. However, most subjects with velocardiofacial syndrome require special education. Overall, the verbal–performance IQ split and the reading–mathematics splits are compatible with a nonverbal learning disability (Swillen et al., 1999).

Neuroimaging

High-resolution magnetic resonance imaging (MRI) scans have been used to provide quantitative measures of specified brain tissues and regions in velocardiofacial syndrome. Fifteen children and adolescents with velocardiofacial syndrome were matched by age and gender with 15 unaffected subjects (Eliez et al., 2000). Total brain volume was approximately 11% smaller in the children with velocardiofacial syndrome. Gray matter volume was reduced but to a lesser extent (7.5%) than white matter volume (16.3%). Brain region variation was found in the frontal lobe tissue, which tended to be enlarged relative to the overall reduction in total brain volume. There was a lack of normal symmetry of the parietal lobe. The authors attribute this loss of symmetry to the significant reduction of gray matter in the left parietal lobe. These brain findings may be related to the language and learning deficits associated with the syndrome. Nonspecific findings of enlarged lateral ventricles and decreased gray matter volume found in MRI studies of velocardiofacial syndrome patients, with and without schizophrenia, are similar to findings in some MRI studies of schizophrenia.

Treatment

Depending on the age and presenting problems of the individual with the 22q11.2 deletion syndrome, a multidisciplinary evaluation involving health care providers from the following specialties is often necessary: medical genetics, plastic surgery, speech pathology, otolaryngology, audiology, dentistry, cardiology, immunology, child development, child psychology, neurology, and general pediatrics. Some individuals also require evaluation by health care providers specializing in feeding disorders, endocrinology, rheumatology, gastroenterology, neurosurgery, general surgery, orthopedics, urology, hematology, psychiatry, and ophthalmology. Treatment entails surgery to correct the physical defects, and medication, therapy, and special education to assist with the cognitive, psychiatric, and neurological effects.

In the neonatal period, health care providers are encouraged to do the following: (1) Measure serum calcium concentration. Low serum calcium concentration warrants calcium supplementation and, when possible, referral to an endocrinologist. (2) Measure absolute lymphocyte count. A low absolute lymphocyte count necessitates evaluation of T and B cell subsets and referral to an immunologist. Infants with lymphocyte abnormalities should not be immunized with live vaccines (i.e., oral polio and MMR), and their immune status should be re-evaluated before receiving live vaccines during childhood. In addition, antibody studies to assess results of immunizations are warranted. (3) Perform a renal ultrasound examination owing to the approximately 37% incidence of structural renal abnormalities. (4) Obtain a chest x-ray to evaluate for thoracic vertebral anomalies. (5) Perform a baseline cardiac evaluation for all individuals diagnosed with the 22q11.2 deletion syndrome. (6) Obtain cervical spine flexion/extension films from all individuals over the age of five years. In childhood, children with growth failure should be evaluated by an endocrinologist for possible growth hormone deficiency. (7) Encourage early educational intervention and speech therapy beginning at age 1 because of the high incidence of speech and language delay. (8) Assess speech and language to aid in diagnosis of a palatal abnormality or velopharyngeal insufficiency. Referral to a craniofacial team for management is recommended. (9) Consider magnetic resonance angiography for individuals who are candidates for pharyngeal surgery to identify ectopic internal carotid arteries that may pose a risk for surgery. (10) Address feeding difficulties through strategies such as including modification of spoon placement when eating, treating gastroesophageal reflux with acid blockade, prokinetic agents, and postural therapy, and prescribing medication to treat gastrointestinal dysmotility and to facilitate bowel evacuation (Dinulos and Graf, 1998).

Smith-Magenis Syndrome

Smith-Magenis syndrome (SMS) involves multiple congenital anomalies and intellectual disability. The first detailed description was written by Ann Smith and Ellen Magenis (Smith et al., 1986). Smith-Magenis syndrome results from the interstitial deletion of chromosome 17p11.2 and is a contiguous gene deletion syndrome. Contiguous gene syndromes are chromosomal rearrangements in which the phenotype is believed to result from an altered copy number of physically linked dosage-sensitive genes. How the genes involved result in pathogenesis is unclear. It occurs sporadically and its recurrence risk is low.

Prevalence

The prevalence is estimated to be 1:25,000 births, but this probably represents an underestimate. The facial abnormalities may be subtle in infancy, so the physical features of the syndrome may not be recognized. The majority of cases have been identified as a result of improved cytogenetic techniques. The syndrome has been identified worldwide, in all ethnic groups.

Genetics

Smith-Magenis syndrome is inherited as an autosomal dominant disorder. Virtually all cases of Smith-Magenis syndrome occur de novo. It is a contiguous gene deletion syndrome with a common deletion interval spanning approximately 4 Mb in approximately 75% of cases. The Smith-Magenis syndrome critical region maps to 17p11.2 and spans less than 1.0 Mb; this critical region contains approximately 20 genes expressed in multiple tissues. Interestingly, a new dominant mutation in the *RAI1* (retinoic acid induced 1) gene has been identified in individuals who demonstrate the major developmental and behavioral features of the Smith-Magenis syndrome phenotype but do not have a 17p11.2 deletion (Slager et al., 2003). These three cases have dominant frameshift mutations, leading to truncation in the RAI1 protein. *RAI1* mutation may be responsible for the neurobehavioral, craniofacial, and otolaryngological features of the syndrome, but not for the short stature commonly seen in Smith-

Magenis syndrome patients with chromosome deletion, implying the role of other genes in the 17p11.2 region. There are no statistically significant differences between the incidence of these abnormalities in patients with the common deletion and the incidence in patients with smaller or larger sized deletions.

The diagnosis of Smith-Magenis syndrome is confirmed either by detection of an interstitial deletion of the short arm of chromosome 17, band 11.2 (del17p11.2), by G-banded cytogenetic analysis, and/or by fluorescence in situ hydridization (FISH). Although, provided the resolution is adequate, a visible interstitial deletion of chromosome 17p11.2 can be detected in all patients with the common deletion by a routine G-banded analysis, the deletion may be missed without careful inspection. Molecular cytogenetic analysis by FISH using a DNA probe specific for the Smith-Magenis syndrome critical region is required in cases of submicroscopic deletions and/or to resolve questionable cases.

Prenatal Testing

Because Smith-Magenis syndrome usually occurs as the result of a de novo deletion of 17p11.2, essentially all individuals with Smith-Magenis syndrome represent a single occurrence in a family. In the rare instance of a complex familial chromosomal rearrangement, prenatal testing is available for pregnancies at risk using a combination of routine cytogenetic studies and FISH on fetal cells that are obtained by chorionic villus sampling (CVS) at from 10 weeks to 12 weeks of gestation or amniocentesis at 16–18 weeks of gestation.

Physical Features

Smith-Magenis syndrome is characterized by distinctive facial features, developmental delay, cognitive impairment, and behavioral abnormalities. Facial features of children with Smith-Magenis syndrome include a broad, square-shaped face, brachycephaly, synophrys, midface hypoplasia with a broad nasal bridge, prominent forehead, upslanting palpebral fissures, deep-set eyes, epicanthal folds, and micrognathia in infancy changing to relative prognathia with age (Greenberg et al., 1991). The shape of the mouth is characteristic, with a fleshy upper lip with a tinted appearance. The facial features are subtle in infancy, and the diagnosis may not be made until early childhood. Cardiac defects and renal anomalies, as well as short stature and failure to thrive, hypotonia, and ocular abnormalities, along with hoarse voice and hearing loss, are characteristic (Greenberg et al., 1991). However, there is no specific pathognomonic clinical feature and no characteristic cardiovascular defect, renal anomaly, otolaryngological, or ophthalmic abnormality in Smith-Magenis syndrome. Despite the common deletion size in 75% of those affected, the only objectively defined features that are found among all affected persons are sleep disturbances, limited adaptive functioning, and intellectual disability.

Behavioral Phenotype

The behavioral phenotype, including significant sleep disturbance, stereotypies, and maladaptive and self-injurious behaviors, is most often not recognized until approximately 18 months of age or older, and it continues to change throughout early childhood into adulthood. Intellectual disability, speech delay, hyperactivity, attention deficit, decreased sensitivity to pain, and aggressive behavior are also associated.

In infancy, those affected, although sociable, are described as quiet infants. Still, infancy is often characterized by feeding difficulties, failure to thrive, hypotonia, long naps with the need to be awakened for feeding, and generalized lethargy. (Smith et al., 1998a). With increasing age, sleep disturbance, especially reductions in REM sleep, become apparent. The sleep disturbances are associated with an inverted melatonin circadian rhythm and remain a problem throughout life. Prominent sleep problems, including difficulties falling asleep, shortened sleep cycles, frequent and prolonged nocturnal awakenings, excessive daytime sleepiness, daytime napping, snoring, and bed-wetting, are seen in 65%–100%. Medication to facilitate sleep was used by 59% of persons with Smith-Magenis syndrome in one study (Smith, Dykens, and Greenberg, 1998b).

Childhood and adulthood are characterized by behavior problems including inattention, hyperactivity, impulsivity, temper tantrums linked to changes in routine, aggression, and toileting problems. A characteristic form of the behavioral phenotype is self-mutilatory behavior that occurs in 70% of individuals. The topography of the self-injury involves wrist biting, head banging, skin picking, pulling out finger nails and toe nails (onychotillomania), and insertion of foreign bodies into ears or other body orifices (polyembolokoilamania) (Smith, Dykens, and Greenberg, 1998a). Because of the severity of the self-mutilation, parents have been inappropriately reported to social services programs for suspicion of child abuse. In addition to these behavioral characteristics, individuals with Smith-Magenis syndrome show a pattern of behavior referred to as the "self-hug," which is a spasmodic pattern of squeezing the upper body. Two types have been described: (1) self-hugging and spasmodically tensing the upper body, and (2) hand clasping at the chest level or under the chin while squeezing arms tightly against the chest and sides. Such patterned behavior appears to be an expression of excitement and is involuntary (Finucane et al., 1994). Other stereotypies include mouthing objects, teeth grinding, body rocking, and spinning or twirling objects.

Mouse Model

Smith-Magenis syndrome (deletion 17p11.2 and duplication 17p11.2p11.2) is a contiguous gene syndrome associated with a heterozygous deletion or duplication of band p11.2 of chromosome 17, respectively. One group of investigators (Walz et al., 2004) engineered chromosomes carrying a deletion/deficiency [Df(11)17] (Del mutant) or a duplication [Dp(11)17] (Dup mutant) of the syntenic region on mouse chromosome 11. Heterozygous male mice carrying the engineered deletion or the duplication were hypoactive or hyperactive, respectively. In addition, male duplication mutant mice, but not deletion mutant mice, had impaired contextual fear conditioning. Moreover, circadian rhythm studies revealed period length differences in deletion mutant mice but not duplication mutant mice. These results indicate that some of the behavioral abnormalities may be gene-dosage sensitive, whereas other behavioral abnormalities are specific to mice carrying the deletion or the duplication and can be observed in a sex preferential manner. These studies in mice suggest that gene or genes present in this defined genomic interval may be responsible for behavioral abnormalities in the mouse, as has been shown in the analogous human chromosome region.

Cognitive Profile

The largest published study (Udwin, Webber, and Hom, 2001) on cognitive abilities and attainment investigated 29 children and 21 adults with Smith-Magenis syndrome. Thirteen boys and 16 girls aged 6 years–16 years, and 9 men and 12 women aged 16 years–52 years were examined. All had mild-to-severe intellectual disability: overall, there were no differences between verbal and performance skills, but the profile of cognitive abilities varied. Adaptive behavior was limited, and the group of adults was more dependent on caregivers than expected based on the individuals' general level of intellectual functioning; none of the adults lived independently. In Smith-Magenis syndrome patients, overall intellectual disability is usually in the moderate range. This was confirmed in this study, in which 75% of the children had IQ scores below 50; however, some subjects tested in the severe range and a smaller number in the mild range. In the adult sample, 16 of 21 scored in the range of 50–69 and 5 scored under 50. This suggests that there is no decline in IQ with age, but it does not confirm continued growth in cognitive ability with age. Half of the children and three-quarters of the adults were able to read, yet for both groups, the average level of attainment in reading and spelling was the 6-year to 7-year level.

Other investigators (Dykens, Finucane, and Gayley, 1997) report that long-term memory, computer skills, and perceptual skills are areas of strength in children and adults. Short-term memory is poor. Visuomotor coordination, sequencing, and response speed are areas of weakness. Speech and language delay is common, with receptive language skills being better than expressive language skills. Affected individuals are easily distracted; however, visual reasoning is a strength, so they tend to be visual learners. They have difficulty in sequential processing, which includes processes such as counting, following multistep commands, and mathematical performance. Adults show limited independence and low levels of occupational attainment (Udwin, Webber, and Horn, 2001). This may be related to high rates of aggression, self-injury, and attentional problems.

Neuroimaging

Anatomical MRI was analyzed using optimized voxel-based morphometry in one study (Boddaert et al., 2004). This method can detect structural anomalies not apparent on visual inspection of the scans. Two comparison groups with similar mean age were studied: Group A contained 12 healthy control children and Group B contained 5 children with idiopathic intellectual disability. In addition, PET and water-labeled method were used to investigate a putative localized brain dysfunction in Smith-Magenis syndrome. A significant bilateral decrease of gray matter concentration was detected in the insula and the lenticular nucleus of Smith-Magenis syndrome children. Significant hypoperfusion was found in the same brain regions of children with Smith-Magenis syndrome. These findings of bilateral insulolenticular anomalies in Smith-Magenis syndrome are consistent with neurobehavioral symptoms of the disease.

Treatment

The treatment process begins with a comprehensive evaluation (review of systems, physical and neurological examination, sleep history, cognitive testing, speech/language examination, renal ultrasound examination, echocardiogram, spine radiographs, ophthalmologic evaluation, audiological examination, parental chromosome analysis, and psychosocial assessment) to clarify the clinical presentation and develop a treatment plan.

Anticipatory care and specific interventions are provided throughout the developmental period. Infancy and early childhood intervention programs are followed by special education programs and vocational training in later years. Therapies include speech/language, physical, and occupational therapy. Speech/language pathology services may identify and treat swallowing and feeding problems and facilitate oral sensorimotor development. Adjunctive use of sign language and total communication programs, in addition to traditional speech/language therapy, may enhance communication skills. Expressive language benefits from early use of sign language and early speech/language intervention. Both behavioral management techniques and the appropriate use of psychotropic medication for attention deficits and hyperactivity may be effective in individual cases. Special education programs should emphasize individualized instruction, structure, and routine. Treatment of the sleep disorder is problematic. Sleep logs are used to ascertain the child's baseline sleep pattern. Both behavioral management and medications have been used for the sleep disorder. Melatonin is being evaluated for treatment of the sleep disturbance. Daytime behavior tends to improve following improved night time sleep. Temporary respite care may be considered, depending on the individual needs of the family.

Turner Syndrome

Turner syndrome (TS) is the most common sex chromosome disorder causing short stature in females. It results from an X-chromosome anomaly and is associated with physical, neurological, and behavioral phenotypes; the most common are short stature and gonadal dysgenesis. Turner syndrome was first described by Otto Ulrich in 1930 and by Henry Turner in 1938. Turner described a syndrome of sexual infantilism, short stature, webbed neck, and cubitus valgus (arms turned out). Turner syndrome was recognized as a genetic syndrome in 1959 when Charles Ford and colleagues described an individual with 45 chromosomes lacking one X chromosome (Ford et al., 1959), a karyotype known as

45,X. Turner sundrome is defined by a combination of characteristic physical features and complete or part absence of one of the X chromosomes, frequently accompanied by cell-line mosaicism. This syndrome provides an opportunity to study the effect of having one rather than two copies of genes on the X chromosome that are required for normal physical development and possibly for cognitive abilities.

Prevalence

Turner syndrome is one of the most common chromosomal anomalies in females, with an estimated frequency of 1:2500–1:5000 (Connor and Loughlin, 1991) of live female births. Approximately 800 new cases are diagnosed in girls and women in the United States each year. It is more common among pregnancies that do not survive to full term (miscarriages and still births). Although occurring in approximately 3% of all women conceived, it is estimated that over 99% of affected fetuses with 45,X are spontaneously aborted. Thus, it is thought that only fetuses with the least severe manifestations of the chromosomal anomaly survive. Life expectancy is generally not affected; however, this depends on associated risks, particularly cardiovascular problems. There is a risk for hypertension in adult life.

Genetics

Turner syndrome is the consequence of an error in reproductive cell division (nondisjunction) that results in an X chromosome anomaly or alteration in some or all of the cells in a female. Most cases are not inherited but occur as random events during the formation of reproductive cells. Turner syndrome occurs when a female's cells have one normal X chromosome and the other sex chromosome is missing or altered. The missing genetic material affects development and causes the characteristic features of the condition.

Approximately half of individuals with Turner syndrome have monosomy X in which each cell in a woman's body has only one copy of the X chromosome instead of the usual two copies. Turner syndrome can also occur if one of the sex chromosomes is partially missing or rearranged rather than completely missing. Some women with Turner syndrome have a chromosomal change in only some of their cells, which is known as X-chromosome mosaicism. X-chromosome mosaicism is also not inherited. It is the result of a random error during cell division early in fetal development.

Although it is not yet known which genes on the X chromosome are responsible for most signs and symptoms of Turner syndrome, one gene called *SHOX* has been identified. The *SHOX* gene is located on the short (p) arm of chromosome X between the end (terminal) of the arm and position 22.32 and on the short (p) arm of chromosome Y at position 11.3. The *SHOX* gene provides instructions for making the SHOX protein that regulates the activity of other genes. The SHOX protein is a transcription factor and part of a larger family of transcription factors, the homeobox genes. These genes act early in embryonic development; the *SHOX* gene is essential to the development of the skeleton and plays an important role in the growth and maturation of bones in the arms and legs. Most women with Turner syndrome have only one copy of the *SHOX* gene instead of the usual two copies, thus reducing the amount of SHOX protein to half the normal value. Because this gene is important for bone development and growth, missing one copy of this gene is thought to be linked to the short stature and skeletal abnormalities (such as unusual rotation of the wrist and elbow joints) in women with Turner syndrome.

Other candidate genes for gonadal dysgenesis in Turner syndrome are under investigation.

Prenatal and Postnatal Diagnosis

Prenatal diagnosis is made by ultrasound, serum markers, or karyotype and must be confirmed by postnatal karyotype (Batch, 2002). If a peripheral blood karyotype is normal and Turner's syndrome is suspected, a karyotype on a peripheral skin biopsy may be performed. A probe for Y-chromosome centromeric material to assess the risk for the development of germ cell tumors is available. If Y chromosomal material is present, the risk for gonadoblastoma is 7%–10%.

Physical Features

Most individuals with Turner syndrome are recognized at birth because of characteristic edema on the dorsal surface of their hands and feet and loose skin folds in the nape of the neck. Low birth weight and short stature are common. In childhood, clinical features include webbing of the neck, low posterior hair lines, a small mandible, prominent ears, epicanthal folds, high arched palate, a broad chest with wide spaced nipples, cubitus valgus (increased carrying angle at the elbow), and hyperconvex fingernails. Short stature is evident with growth below the third percentile. Short stature may be detected in the early years of life, at school age, or at puberty when sexual maturation fails to occur. Associated defects include coarctation of the aorta in approximately one-sixth of those affected, isolated nonstenotic bicuspid aorta valve in approximately one-third, and hypertension. There is decreased estrogen production, resulting in absent breast development, amenorrhea, and infertility (Hall and Gilchrist, 1990).

Behavioral Phenotype

Developmentally, social, and emotional adjustment varies. Younger girls are more immature, hyperactive, and anxious, while older ones report anxiety, depression, and problems with social relationships. At the beginning of puberty, a decrease in activity level has been described (Swillen et al., 1993). A correlation has been reported between structural abnormalities of the X chromosome and the severity of behavioral problems (Rovet and Ireland, 1994). A study on phenotypic variability as a result of differences in parental origin of the X chromosome in Turner syndrome was described by Skuse, Edgar, and Morris (1999). These authors found the quality of life of those with a maternal X chromosome is poorer than that of those with a paternal X chromosome. Still, girls with Turner syndrome do have a feminine gender identity. There is no evidence they have less feminine attitudes than their normal age-matched peers (El-abd, Turk, and Hill, 1995). They are less independent than age-matched girls and less frequently live with a partner or marry (Nyborg and Nielsen, 1977).

Cognitive Profile

Intelligence is generally within the normal range (Siegel, Clopper, and Stabler, 1998). Intellectual disability is found in only 5% of girls with classic Turner syndrome presentation but in 30% of those with more rare Turner syndrome anomalies (Swillen et al., 1993). Typically, the performance IQ is lower than the verbal IQ, specifically because of weaknesses on visuospatial subtests. Poor visual motor skills have been demonstrated; however, verbal and language abilities are in the normal range. Learning disabilities, particularly in math, are common (Siegel, Clopper, and Stabler, 1998). Other areas of cognitive weakness include the ability to discriminate facial affect (McCauley et al., 1987) and affective prosody (Ross et al., 1995). These deficits may impact on social relationships, as affected individuals have difficulty in processing affective cues in social situations. A nonverbal learning disability related to right hemisphere dysfunction is associated (Ross et al., 1995; Siegel, Clopper, and Stabler, 1998). Moreover, difficulties with attention, short-term memory, and executive function, including problems with verbal fluency, planning skills, and flexibility, have been demonstrated (Rovet, 1993; Siegel, Clopper, and Stabler, 1998).

Many studies indicate that girls with Turner syndrome have a characteristic IQ profile: a verbal IQ that seems to be at a (nearly) normal level and a decreased performance IQ. This profile remains into adulthood. Visuospatial problems are mentioned most frequently and there is some evidence for a relationship to particular neuroanatomical structures, hormonal dysfunction, and genotype. Although much less research has been done on motor performance in Turner syndrome, there is clear evidence that it too is disturbed in Turner syndrome. Many authors emphasize the interaction between somatic, psychological, and social factors.

Neuroimaging

Turner syndrome has been investigated with MRI, PET, and functional MRI (Kesler et al., 2004). Volumetric MRI neuroimaging studies have been used to characterize the neuroanatomical correlates of visuospatial and executive function deficits. MRI studies have demonstrated decreased volume in the right parietal/occipital cortex and a proportional decrease in gray matter in the right posterior parietal lobe, larger left amygdala gray matter, and reduced right hippocampal volume. A study of 10-year-old monozygotic twin girls showed decreased proportions of gray matter volumes in the right frontal, left and right parietal and right occipital cortices in the affected twin (Reiss et al., 1993). Two PET studies revealed decreased glucose metabolism in the parietal and occipital lobes bilaterally. These imaging studies did not report any direct correlation between parietal morphology or function and measures of cognitive performance. However, functional MRI has been used to study the neural mechanisms underlying deficits in spatial orientation processing. Thirteen individuals with Turner syndrome and 13 age-matched controls who were typically developing completed neuropsychological assessments and participated in functional MRI scanning while they carried out easy and difficult versions of a judgment of line orientation task (Kesler et al., 2004). With increasing task difficulty, the control subjects responded by recruiting executive frontal areas, but individuals with Turner syndrome did not activate alternate brain regions in response to increased task demands. Thus, individuals with Turner syndrome show activation deficits in parietal-occipital and frontal areas during the judgment of line orientation task. The authors conclude that activation, and possibly deactivation, deficits in these areas may be responsible for the visuospatial deficits observed in women with Turner syndrome.

Treatment

Turner syndrome is a systemic disorder and requires a multisystem management approach. The evaluation includes attention to the endocrine system, cardiovascular system, renal system, audiology, gastrointestinal system, ears, eyes, skeletal system, dental system, and skin, as well as to the psychology of the patient and the family. It is important to provide to girls and women with Turner syndrome, and their families, comprehensive information about the syndrome and to advise them about the availability of Turner syndrome societies that can provide information and support.

Complete spontaneous puberty may occur in approximately 16% of patients, with pregnancy in up to 4%. The final height of untreated girls with Turner syndrome is 86%–88% of the mean adult female height. Growth hormone given alone or with oxandrolone improves final height. The major factors determining the outcome of growth hormone therapy are the dose of growth hormone used and the number of years of growth hormone therapy prior to estrogenization. The induction of puberty should be individualized, taking into account both optimizing growth and psychological issues of adolescence. Adolescents and adults with Turner syndrome must deal with a wide range of medical, fertility, and psychosocial concerns. Adults with Turner syndrome may have a reduced life expectancy, in some instances, owing to excess cardiovascular risk, but they may also have multiple co-occurring problems including hypothyroidism, deafness, osteoporosis, and the consequences of estrogen deficiency and infertility. A multidisciplinary approach to focused adult care is essential. Psychological support for persons with Turner syndrome and their families is important throughout life and should be provided by both health professionals and Turner syndrome family support groups.

Rett's Disorder

Rett's disorder is the most common cause of profound intellectual disability in girls and women. It was originally reported by Andreas Rett, who observed girls in his clinic with similar behaviors. Later, Hagberg et al. (1983) published additional cases, thus generating greater interest in the disorder.

Prevalence

Rett's disorder is a pervasive neurodevelopmental disorder, with a prevalence of 1:10,000–1:12,000 girls (Hagberg et al., 1983), and occurs in all ethnic groups. Clinical features include pervasive growth failure, communication dysfunction, and stereotypical movements. Survival into the fourth decade is common. Although Rett's disorder occurs almost exclusively in girls, female sex is not a necessary diagnostic criteria because there have been a few male cases. Developmental deviations are apparent by 15 months of age in 50% of individuals, by 18 months in 80%, and by 2 years in 100%.

Genetics

Rett's disorder is inherited as an X-linked dominant condition. Approximately 99.5% of cases are a single occurrence in a family, resulting either from a de novo mutation in the child with Rett's disorder or through inheritance of the disease-causing mutation from one parent who demonstrates somatic or germline mosaicism. Although the majority of the cases are sporadic, there are rare reports of recurrence in a single family. The diagnosis of Rett's disorder is based on clinical diagnostic criteria (The Rett Syndrome Diagnostic Work Group, 1988) established for the classic disorder and/or molecular testing of the *MECP2* gene (chromosomal locus Xq28). The mutation in Rett's disorder occurs in the *MECP2* gene that encodes an X-linked methyl-CpG-binding protein. In 50% of cases, MECP2 is thought to mediate the transcriptional silencing in the cell nucleus (Amir et al., 1999). It is proposed that by binding to methylated DNA, it represses transcription.

Mutations are identified using molecular genetic testing in approximately 80% of females with classic Rett's disorder. Such testing is available clinically. It is possible for a mother, who is a carrier, to have a favorably skewed X-chromosome inactivation that can result in her being unaffected or being minimally affected. When the mother of an affected person is found to have the *MECP2* mutation identified in her affected child, the risk to siblings of the affected child of inheriting the mutant *MECP2* allele at conception is 50%. However, if a mutation is not identified in the parent, the risk to sibs of the proband is low. Still, germline mosaicism in either parent cannot be excluded even if the disease-causing *MECP2* mutation present in the proband has not been identified in either parent. If the disease-causing *MECP2* mutation has been identified in the affected patient, molecular genetic testing is offered to both parents.

Prenatal Testing

Prenatal testing is available in pregnancies at risk if the *MECP2* mutation has been identified in a family member. However, because germline mosaicism cannot be excluded, it is best to make available prenatal diagnosis to couples who have had a child with Rett's disorder or intellectual disability owing to a *MECP2* mutation regardless, whether or not the disease-causing mutation has been identified in a parent. In regard to pregnancies in women with a known *MECP2* mutation, prenatal diagnosis for pregnancies at increased risk is possible by analysis of DNA taken from fetal cells obtained by amniocentesis between 16 weeks and 18 weeks of gestation or chorionic villus sampling (CVS) between 10 weeks and 12 weeks of gestation. However, the disease-causing allele in an affected family member must be identified before prenatal testing can be performed.

A male fetus with an *MECP2* mutation who survives will, at best, have a severe intellectual disability syndrome, but the phenotype in a female with an *MECP2* mutation is more difficult to predict, and it can range from apparently normal to severely affected. In regard to pregnancies of a couple who have a child with Rett's disorder or intellectual disability caused by an *MECP2* mutation germline mosaicism cannot be ruled out in either parent even if the disease-causing *MECP2* mutation that is present in the affected patient has not been identified in parental cells. Consequently, it is important to provide prenatal diagnosis whether or not the disease-causing mutation has been identified in a parent.

Physical Features

The main features of Rett's disorder are summarized by The Rett Syndrome Diagnostic Work Group (1988) and in the DSM-IVTR (APA, 2000). Clinical course is characterized by progressive changes with identifiable stages. The disorder is not recognized at birth, and head circumference is normal at birth. Between 5 and 48 months of age, there is a deceleration of head growth. There is a loss of previously acquired, purposeful hand movements that becomes apparent between 6 and 30 months of age and is temporarily associated with communication dysfunction and social withdrawal. Because of this withdrawal secondary to the encephalopathy and behavioral features, individuals with Rett's disorder have been placed in the DSM-IVTR category of pervasive developmental disorder.

Behavioral Phenotype

In Rett's disorder, there are stereotypical midline hand movements, such as hand wringing, hand washing, clapping, tapping, and mouthing of hands and fingers. These behaviors begin at or after the time when purposeful hand movements are lost. Gait apraxia and truncal apraxia/ataxia appear between 1 and 4 years of age. There is a severe impairment in the development of expressive and receptive language, and psychomotor retardation is characteristic. By school age, the social withdrawal is less prominent and overall development reaches a plateau. The gait is awkward and worsens, with gradual motor deterioration over time leading to placement in a wheel chair. Individuals with Rett's disorder lose functional hand use in manipulating objects. Gaze is their most important way of interacting with others in their surroundings. Affected girls remain visually attentive to objects and people and they show their preferences by eye pointing (von Tetzchner et al., 1996). They also may demonstrate their excitement by increasing their midline hand movements.

Cognitive Profile

Individuals with Rett's disorder test in the severe-to-profound range of intellectual disability throughout their lives. Cognitive and communication skills are limited, but that there is limited evidence of deterioration of these abilities with age was shown in a study of 87 individuals (age range = 2 to 44 years); this is consistent with a neurodevelopmental disorder rather than a degenerative condition (Cass et al., 2003). Therefore, intervention and support to maintain and increase motor skills, daily living skills, and cognitive and communicative functioning are appropriate. In one study, the communicative and cognitive behaviors of a group of 10 girls with Rett's disorder were compared with those of a group of girls who did not have Rett's disorder but tested in the profound range of intellectual disability (Woodyatt and Ozanne, 1997). The girls with Rett's disorder were a rather homogenous group, showing similar cognitive patterns but fewer communicative behaviors, communicative functions, and total numbers of inferred communicative acts. Their visual processing and memory did deteriorate somewhat with age, but those of the comparison group showed a slight increase. Age at onset of Rett's disorder general symptomatology and speech measures were inversely correlated with visual processing and memory. This suggests that the age at regression may have different consequences for different functions.

In a study involving 42 individuals with Rett's disorder (aged 2.5 to 42 years) (von Tetzchner et al., 1996), persistent looking was associated with lower cognitive function, suggesting that preferential looking may be useful in cognitive assessment of females with Rett's disorder. All individuals maintained a profound level of intellectual disability and a preintentional level of communication. Individual variation was found in both cognitive and social interaction skills. The study findings are consistent with an increased perception of social interactiveness by the caregivers over time. The development landmark of means-end behavior was related to a measured increase in behaviors considered to be communicative by parents. There was a relative preservation of gross motor and daily living skills at the developmental level of the age of onset of the disorder.

Neuroimaging

Extensive neuroimaging studies have been conducted in Rett's disorder. Volumetric analyses of MRI, magnetic resonance spectroscopy (MRS), diffusion tensor imaging (DTI), cerebral blood flow measurements with MRI, and positron emission tomography scans (PET) by one group of investigators has provided a comprehensive view of brain structure and neurochemistry, as well as insight into mechanisms underlying the clinical features of this disorder (Naidu et al., 2001). Volumetric analyses indicated decreased brain volume in Rett's disorder that resulted from global reductions in both gray and white matter of the brain. The frontal lobes were selectively vulnerable: there was preferential reduction of blood flow in this brain region and increased choline, and reduced n-acetyl aspartate (NAA) was demonstrated by magnetic resonance spectroscopy. Increased glucose uptake in these same regions was shown by 18-fluorodeoxyglucose PET scans. The authors hypothesize that the increased glucose uptake relates to increased glutamate cycling in synapses. This might result in neuroexcitotoxic injury to the developing brain and contribute to the seizures, behavioral disturbance, and respiratory irregularities commonly seen in clinical phases 1 and 2 of this disorder.

Another group of investigators (Dunn et al., 2002) carried out volumetric measurements of basal ganglia using MRI and compared the findings in 9 individuals with Rett's disorder (aged 14 years to 26 years, mental age 4 months to 15 months) with those in 9 age-matched volunteer females. Mutations in the coding regions of the *MECP2* gene were present in all nine patients. Positron emission scans with [18F]-6-fluorodopa and [11C]-raclopride were performed under light anesthesia with intravenous propofol. Magnetic resonance scans of basal ganglia detected a significant reduction in the size of the caudate heads and thalami in the individuals with Rett's disorder. Positron emission scans demonstrated that the mean uptake of fluorodopa in Rett's disorder was 13.1% lower in the caudate and 12.5% lower in the putamen than in corresponding areas of the control group, but dopamine D2 receptor binding measured with [11C]-raclopride was 9.7% higher in the caudate and 9.6% higher in the putamen. These results suggest a mild presynaptic deficit of nigrostriatal activity in Rett's disorder.

Treatment

Everyday life for a person with Rett's disorder is complicated by other characteristic clinical features of the disorder that include seizures, breath-holding spells, periodic hyperventilation, periodic apnea, dystonia, spasticity, scoliosis, and peripheral vasomotor problems. The optimal treatment for Rett's disorder is based on understanding the underlying processes and the brain mechanisms that lead to the clinical features. Interventions are multidisciplinary and current management of patients with Rett's disorder focuses on supportive and symptomatic therapy. Although no treatment has been shown to improve the neurologic outcome of patients with Rett's disorder, seizure management is essential. Video/EEG monitoring is the best way to obtain definitive information about the occurrence of seizures and the need for antiepileptic drugs. Ample fluid intake and a high fiber diet along with the use of stool softeners, as indicated, can help prevent acute intestinal crises. Gastroesophageal reflux may be decreased by treatment with antireflux agents, smaller and thickened feedings, and positioning. Occupational and physical therapy are important for maintaining function and preventing scoliosis and deformities. Interventions include physical therapy and occupational therapy for maintaining function and preventing scoliosis and deformities. Augmentative communication, swimming, and music therapy are often beneficial. Pharmacotherapy for treatment of behavioral difficulties may include the use of low doses of risperidone, or selective serotonin uptake inhibitors, for excessive agitation. Sleep disturbances have been treated with antihistamine sedatives, such as diphenylhydramine, or with melatonin.

A major aspect of the intervention is the facilitation of supportive activities for parents to carry out with their children. The phases of parent adjustments to Rett's disorder are similar to those of other disorders. Parental education is the first step and may be supplemented by educational sessions in parent groups. There may be an increased risk of mood disorder in family members. Mood disorder should be considered when developing treatment plans for the child and family. Working with parents and parent associations and using parents' support for one another is an essential aspect of the management of Rett's disorder.

Lesch-Nyhan Disease

Lesch-Nyhan disease is a rare sex-linked recessive disease caused by an inborn error of purine nucleotide metabolism. Self-injury is the major behavioral manifestation; this behavior was sufficiently characteristic that Nyhan (1972) introduced the term "behavioral phenotype." Lesch-Nyhan disease is of psychosocial and psychiatric importance because of the lifelong suffering experienced by the involved child and his family, the uniqueness of the behavioral phenotype, and the resources needed for lifelong patient supervision. Moreover, an understanding of the neurobiological basis of this disease might contribute to a better understanding of brain mechanisms involved in self-injurious and compulsive behaviors.

Prevalence

The prevalence of classic Lesch-Nyhan disease is estimated to be approximately 1:380,000. Lesch-Nyhan variants (HPRT levels above 2%) are less frequent.

Genetic/Metabolic Aspects

Lesch-Nyhan disease is inherited in an X-linked recessive manner. The father of an affected male will not have the disease and will not be a carrier of the mutant allele. The risk to siblings of a proband depends upon the carrier status of the mother. Carrier mothers have a 50% chance of transmitting the Hypoxanthine-guanine phosphoribosyltransferase (HPRT1) mutation in each pregnancy. Sons who inherit the mutation will be affected; daughters who inherit the mutation are carriers. Therefore, with each pregnancy, a female who is a carrier has a 25% chance of having an affected male, a 25% chance of having a carrier female, and a 50% chance of having an unaffected male or female.

The HPRT-encoding gene is located on the X chromosome in the q26-q27 region and is made up of nine exons and eight introns, totaling 57 kb. The HPRT gene is transcribed to produce an mRNA of 1.6 kb that contains a protein-encoding region of 654 nucleotides. Over 200 different mutations throughout the coding regions have been identified. Techniques that provide information on the three-dimensional structure of the HPRT protein make it possible to correlate structure and function of the enzyme (Eads et al., 1994). Eads et al. (1994) report the effects of single amino acid substitutions on the stability and activity of HPRT.

The gene involved in Lesch-Nyhan disease is on the X-chromosome, so the disorder occurs almost entirely in males; occurrence in females is extremely rare. The metabolic abnormality is the result of an abnormal gene product, a deficiency in the enzyme hypoxanthine-guanine phosphoribosyltransferase (HPRT). This enzyme is normally present in each cell in the body and is highest in the brain, especially in the basal ganglia. Its absence prevents the normal metabolism of hypoxanthine, resulting in excessive uric acid production and manifestations of gout without specific drug treatment (i.e., allopurinol). The full disease requires the virtual absence of the enzyme. Other syndromes with partial HPRT deficiency are associated with gout without the neurological and behavioral symptoms. Page and Nyhan (1989) have reported that HPRT levels are related to the extent of motor symptoms, the presence or absence of self-injury, and possibly the level of cognitive function. Hypoxanthine accumulates in the cerebral spinal fluid, but uric acid does not because it is not produced in the brain and does not cross the blood-brain barrier.

Prenatal Testing

Prenatal testing is available and may be utilized to inform parents about the presence of the disorder. Prenatal testing has been used for preimplantation genetic diagnosis (Ray et al., 1999).

Clinical Features

The clinical features may be categorized into five main areas: (1) overproduction of uric acid and consequences thereof, (2) movement disorder, (3) cognitive disability, (4) behavioral manifestations including self-injurious behavior, and (5) a miscellaneous category including growth retardation and anemia.

Though Lesch-Nyhan disease is often regarded as a single disorder, there is a marked phenotypic variability among patients with HPRT deficiency. A subgroup of HPRT-deficient patients displays a partial syndrome. This condition, characterized by hyperuricemia but virtually without neurobehavioral features, is called HPRT-related hyperuricemia. In addition, intermediate clinical presentations have been identified, showing hyperuricemia and definite neurological abnormalities but lacking the behavioral symptoms including self-injurious behavior. These patients are referred to as Lesch-Nyhan variants.

Behavioral Phenotype

Self-injurious behavior usually is expressed as self-biting; however, other patterns of self-injurious behavior may emerge with time. It is not uncommon for self-injury to progress to deliberate self-harm (Anderson and Ernst, 1994; Harris, 1998b). Characteristically, the fingers, mouth, and buccal mucosa are mutilated. The biting pattern is often asymmetrical so that the patient may mutilate the left or right side of the body and become anxious if he perceives this side of the body is threatened. Other associated maladaptive behaviors include head or limb banging, eye poking, pulling fingernails, and psychogenic vomiting (Anderson and Ernst, 1994).

Self-mutilation in Lesch-Nyhan disease is conceptualized as a compulsive behavior that the child tries to control but generally is unable to resist. With increasing age, the affected child becomes more adept at finding ways to control his self-injury. He may enlist the help of others to protect him against these impulses or may learn to self-restrain. A language pattern that consists of repeated ambivalent statements with anxiety and coprolalia (vulgar speech) is characteristic. Moreover, the patient may be compulsively aggressive and inflict injury to others through pinching, grabbing, or verbal forms of aggression. Frequently, he will apologize for this behavior immediately afterward and say that the behavior was out of his control.

Cognitive Profile

The mean IQ for persons with Lesch-Nyhan disease is in the mild-to-moderate range of intellectual disability. Those with partial HPRT deficiency test in the low-normal IQ range. Fifteen patients with LND, 9 variants, and 13 normal adolescents and adults were compared on cognitive tests (Shretlen et al., 2001). Testing revealed qualitatively similar cognitive deficits in both patient groups. The variants produced scores that were intermediate between those of patients with LND and normal participants on nearly every cognitive measure.

Etiology/Neuroimaging Studies

The etiology of the neurological and behavioral symptoms is not clearly established. Early neuroimaging studies including computed tomography (CT) and magnetic resonance imaging (MRI) showed no obvious structural changes in the brain; however, mild diffuse atrophy was noted in several patients. Quantitative MRI demonstrated smaller total brain volumes in Lesch-Nyhan disease patients than in age-matched controls (Harris et al., 1998). In this study, the basal ganglia were disproportionately affected, averaging 66% of controls, thus demonstrating that there are structural brain changes in Lesch-Nyhan disease.

Abnormalities in dopamine function have been demonstrated (Lloyd et al., 1981) in three autopsied cases. The behavior is not caused by hyperuricemia or excess hypoxanthine since partial variants with hyperuricemia (HPRT levels >2.0%) do not self-injure and infants treated for hyperuricemia from birth do develop self-injury. To address the issue of dysfunction of dopamine systems in vivo, dopamine axon integrity was measured in six patients using positron emission tomography (PET) (Wong et al., 1996). This study showed a reduction of binding of the dopamine transporter ligand WIN 35,428 by 68% and 42% in the putamen and caudate, respectively. Another PET-study that included 11 patients showed reduced accumulation of the levodopa analogue [18F]-fluorodopa into fibers in the putamen and caudate by 69% and 61%, respectively (Ernst et al., 1996). These results provide important correlative evidence for dysfunction of nigrostriatal dopaminergic pathways in vivo.

To further clarify the relationship between presynaptic dopamine transporter binding in the striatum and self-injurious behavior, Harris et al. (1999) studied 7 Lesch-Nyhan variant patients (HPRT levels 1.8%–20.0%) and 2 cases with HPRT levels <1.5%, all 9 without self-injurious behavior (age range = 12 years–37 years). The extent of motor findings was documented on quantitated neurological examination. Two patients with HPRT levels <1.5% and two patients with HPRT levels of 1.8% and 2.5% and with severe movement disorder were not different in WIN 35,428 dopamine transporter binding in PET imaging from the previously described classical Lesch-Nyhan patients who do self-injure. The study of variant cases with motor symptoms but without self-injurious behavior suggests that reductions in dopamine receptor density are not a sufficient explanation of the self-injury. However, these authors found that HPRT level and the extent of motor deficit was correlated with dopamine transporter binding in the caudate and putamen in the nine cases. Dopamine transporter binding was significantly correlated with HPRT levels in whole cells. Moreover, when the movement disorder was rated on a standardized dystonia rating scale, putamen dopamine transporter density was significantly correlated with symptom severity. These findings suggest that dopamine reduction is linked to the extent of the movement disorder but may not be a sufficient explanation for self-injurious behavior and that other neurotransmitters need to be examined.

Future investigation will need to take into account the existence of a variety of mutations in the HPRT gene structure. Why partial HPRT deficiency does not lead to behavioral symptoms remains unclear; perhaps trophic factors are active with minute amounts of the enzyme.

Treatment

A multimodal approach to treatment focuses on the following:

1. *Medical management.* Allopurinol reduces the risk of hyperuricemia-associated urological and joint complications by reducing serum uric acid levels and by inhibiting the conversion of xanthine and hypoxanthine to uric acid. Nephrolithiasis is best prevented by allopurinol in combination with generous oral hydration.

2. *Neurological features.* Effective treatment for the neurological features of Lesch-Nyhan disease is currently not available. Because basal ganglia dopamine is markedly depleted, attempts have been made to treat dystonia by restoring dopamine. However, treatment with the dopamine precursor levodopa has not been shown to be effective. Neurosurgical interventions aimed at the extrapyramidal features in Lesch-Nyhan disease have not been beneficial. Bilateral chronic deep brain stimulation in the globus pallidus pars interna in a single 19-year-old patient improved the dystonia by 33%, and had beneficial effects on the behavioral features (Taira, Kobayshi, and Hori, 2003). His parents reported at 3-month follow-up that self-mutilating behavior had stopped. At 24-month follow-up there was no self-mutilating behavior. Pyramidal manifestations such as spasticity can be treated with baclofen or benzodiazepines. Benzodiazepines

also reduce anxiety but may exacerbate the extrapyramidal and behavioral features of the disease.

3. *Behavior and self-injury*. Stress and anxiety exacerbate self-injury so that supportive behavioral approaches are important aspects of treatment. No fully effective treatment for self-injury is available, so the use of restraints and protective equipment is critical. Because affected individuals can cooperate in their use, an active collaboration is needed so that the affected person can let the caregiver know when it is safe to remove restraints. Restraints for arms and legs should be applied to prevent self-injury such as hitting, biting fingers, and poking in the eyes. Flexible arm splints (Ball, et al., 1985) or helmets with retractable mouth barriers may provide an alternative to protective straps. Other patients find that covering their hands with gloves or socks provides enough of a deterrent to prevent self-injury. Dental devices, constructed to prevent self-biting of the lips and tongue while preserving the teeth, have showed inconsistent results, so the prevention of self-inflicted tissue damage may require tooth extraction. A properly designed wheelchair is one of the most critical supportive elements for the management of Lesch-Nyhan disease patients (Letts and Hobson, 1975). It should be individually adapted, comfortable, and fully padded without any sharp parts within reach. In addition, it should be impossible for the patient to put fingers into the wheel spokes or abrade the ankles on the sides of foot supports. A soft but firm support should stabilize the head because frequent opisthotonic spasms and extreme backward head thrusts may lead to cervical spine injury (Watts et al., 1982).

Behavior management using extinction techniques consisting of actively ignoring an unwanted behavior so that it is not positively reinforced has proven to be one of the more effective behavior modification approaches. Negative reinforcement (punishment methods) in Lesch-Nyhan disease is ineffective and may increase undesirable behavior. In most patients, a combination of ignoring inappropriate behaviors and positive reinforcement for alternative behaviors is the best approach to behavioral modification.

Pharmacotherapy for behavior management is symptomatic and focused on mood lability, aggression, and impulsive self-injury. Treatment approaches include reducing hyperuricemia by the administration of allopurinol, increasing brain serotonin levels by the administration of the serotonin precursors 5-hydroxytryptophan and tryptophan or serotonin reuptake inhibitors such as clomipramine and fluoxetine, treating mood lability by the administration of mood stabilizers such as carbamazepine and gabapentin, and reducing anxiety with benzodiazepine anxiolytics. Low doses of the atypical antipsychotic risperidone have been used to treat self-injury and aggression.

Prader-Willi Syndrome

The Prader-Willi syndrome (PWS) is one of the five most common syndromes that is diagnosed and treated by birth defects clinics. It is the most common dysmorphic form of obesity. It is of particular interest as a neuropsychiatric disorder because of the associated behavioral phenotype that involves compulsive hyperphagia, other food related behaviors, and compulsive behaviors. Prader-Willi syndrome was initially described in 1956 as a new disorder involving obesity, short stature, cryptorchidism, and intellectual disability (Prader, Labhart, and Willi, 1956).

Prevalence

The incidence of Prader-Willi syndrome is estimated to fall between 1:10,000 and 1:22,000 live births. Over 90% of cases occur sporadically. Life span is related to management of weight; with successful weight control, long-term survival is reported.

Genetics

Prader-Willi syndrome results from either paternal deletion of 15q11-q13 or maternal uniparental disomy (UPD) of chromosome 15 or imprinting center mutation. The latter involves a cluster of imprinted genes on human chromosome 15q11-q13 (the Prader-Willi syndrome/Angelman syndrome domain) and its ortholog on mouse chromosome 7c believed to be regulated by an imprinting control center. In UPD, two copies of the maternal chromosome are inherited with no paternal contribution (Nicholls, Saitoh, and Horsthemke, 1998). Without the presence of the chromosome donated by the father, the normal imprinting of the two maternally donated chromosomes leads to absence of gene expression in this interval. This results in a functional abnormality that is essentially equivalent to the structural abnormality found in a deletion in the 15q11-q13 region that is associated with the disorder. Moreover, in approximately 5% of cases, abnormalities in the mechanism of imprinting may occur when the imprinting control center itself has a mutation.

Several genes are included in the most commonly deleted region in Prader-Willi syndrome. Some are paternally imprinted and others are maternally imprinted (State and Dykens, 2000). Among those paternally imprinted are *ZNF 127, NDN, SNURF-SMRPN,* and *IPW.* Another gene, *UBE3A* (E6-AP ubiquitin lipase), is maternally imprinted. Other genes in this region that are expressed from both maternal and paternal chromosomes include three GABA receptor subunits (GABRB3, GABRA5, and GABRG3) (State and Dykens, 2000). Because similar phenotypes result from deletions and from imprinting in Prader-Willi syndrome, it is less likely that nonimprinted genes play a role in Prader-Willi syndrome or Angelman syndrome. Among these genes, a specific gene for Prader-Willi syndrome has not been established, so several of these genes may contribute to the phenotype. For example, the *SMRPN* gene is involved in protein slicing and is expressed throughout the brain; however, it is not thought that Prader-Willi syndrome is the direct outcome of this deficit. The *NCD* (necdin) gene does lead to failure to thrive in certain mouse strains, so it may be a factor; however, those mice that survive do develop into apparently normal adults. Thus, the disorder is most likely linked to the loss of more than one gene in this region. On the other hand, the mutation of a single gene, *UBE3A,* has been found in cases of Angelman syndrome (Moncla et al., 1999a).

Mouse Model

A mouse model deficient for necdin has been suggested for Prader-Willi syndrome (Muscatelli et al., 2000). Viable necdin mutants demonstrate a reduction in both oxytocin-producing neurons and luteinizing hormone–releasing, hormone–producing neurons in hypothalamus. Necdin-deficient mice display increased skin scraping activity in the open field test and improved spatial learning and memory in the Morris water maze. The features may be analogous to skin picking and improved spatial memory that are characteristics of the Prader-Willi syndrome phenotype. Necdin may be involved in at least a subset of the clinical manifestations of Prader-Willi syndrome.

Prenatal Diagnosis

Prenatal diagnosis of Prader-Willi syndrome is indicated for chromosomal parental translocation involving chromosome 15 and for decreased fetal movements during the third trimester of gestation. The prenatal diagnosis of Prader-Willi syndrome during the first trimester may utilize chorionic villus sampling (CVS), amniocentesis, fetal ultrasound, and molecular analysis.

Physical Features

Prader-Willi syndrome is a neurodevelopmental disorder characterized by obesity, short stature, cryptorchidism, intellectual disability, hyperphagia, learning disability, short stature, hypogonadism, hypotonia, small hands and feet, and dysmorphic facies. There is an increased prevalence of daytime sleepiness, scoliosis, and other orthopedic abnormalities. Because of the obesity, heart failure and diabetes may occur as complications.

Some of the features, such as neonatal hypotonia and feeding problems in infancy, may lead to diagnosis of the syndrome in the first few years of life. Other features, such as excessive eating, are useful for diagnosis during early childhood. Hypogonadism is most useful in diagnosis during and after adolescence. Based on the sensitivities of the published criteria, testing all newborns/infants with otherwise unexplained hypotonia with poor suck is suggested. For children between 2 years and 6 years of age, hypotonia, a history of poor suck, and global developmental delay are sufficient criteria to prompt testing. Between 6 and 12 years of age, testing those with hypotonia (or history of hypotonia with poor suck), global developmental delay, and excessive eating with central obesity is suggested. At age 13 and older, testing patients with cognitive impairment, excessive eating with central obesity, hypogonadotropic hypogonadism, and/or behavior problems, such as temper tantrums and obsessive-compulsive preoccupations, is recommended.

Behavioral Phenotype

The behavioral phenotype includes unusual food-related behavior (compulsive food seeking, hoarding, and gorging), skin picking, irritability, anger, low frustration tolerance, and stubbornness. Standardized methods of assessment have documented increased rates of depression, anxiety, and compulsive behavior. Up to 50% of children and adults with Prader-Willi syndrome demonstrate behavioral disorders.

Compulsive eating is the most disabling of these behavioral manifestations, and it leads to obesity and the complications of severe obesity, such as respiratory impairment and diabetes. The hyperphagia, which has been consistently found, has received the most systematic behavioral evaluation. Holm and Pipes (1976) evaluated food-related behavior in the Prader-Willi syndrome. They found that behavioral problems were most commonly related to food and included food stealing, foraging for food, gorging, and indiscriminate eating with little food selectivity. No special circumstances that resulted in food stealing or gorging were identified. When not carefully supervised, patients may steal food and, in some instances, eat unpalatable food, although this can be avoided with appropriate supervision.

Besides the food-related compulsions, nonfood related compulsive behaviors, emotional lability with temper tantrums, stubbornness, negativism, skin picking, and scratching have been examined. A questionnaire survey involving 369 cases identified compulsive and impulsive aggressive behavior (Stein, Keating, and Zar, 1993). These authors used the Overt Aggression Scale, the Yale-Brown Obsessive-Compulsive Disorder Scale, a clinical global rating, and DSM-III-R (APA, 1987) criteria to diagnose self-stimulation and self-injury, compulsive behavior, and obsessive behaviors. They found that skin picking was the most common form of self-injury, being observed in 19.6% of this sample. Other types of self-injury with lower frequency were nose picking, nail biting, lip biting, and hair pulling. The second behavioral problem area was compulsive behavior; food hoarding was the most severe manifestation and occurred in 17.7%. Other compulsive behaviors included counting, symmetrical arrangements of objects, and checking and hand washing, but these were less common. Obsessive thinking was far less characteristic, with only 1.4% rated in the severe range on an item dealing with concerns about contamination. State and colleagues review the evidence in regard to compulsive behaviors in Prader-Willi syndrome (State et al., 1999) and the relationship to obsessive compulsive disorder. Behavioral problems identified in the preschool years persisted throughout the school years and continue into adolescence and adulthood.

Cognitive Profile

The extent of cognitive impairment is variable in Prader-Willi syndrome. Some individuals test in the normal range of intelligence, but most test in the mild-to-moderate range of intellectual disability. Others may test in the severe range of intellectual disability. Individuals with Prader-Willi syndrome may have greater learning disabilities and cognitive deficits than would be expected for their IQ level. Learning disabilities in arithmetic and writing, as well as reading problems, are reported. Performance on executive function, memory, and visuospatial tasks has ranged from 2.1 to 7.0 standard deviations below the expected means. Behavioral problems, including attention-deficit hyperactivity disorder (ADHD), may also be associated and affect the overall management.

Etiology

The genetic abnormality in Prader-Willi syndrome leads to hypothalamic dysfunction that results in aspects of the clinical phenotype, for example, regulation of feeding, delay in sexual development, sleep disorder, and abnormality of thermoregulation. In support of hypothalamic dysfunction, Swaab, Purba, and Hofman (1995), in a postmortem study, found reduction in oxytocin cells in certain regions of the hypothalamus. However, other brain regions and neuropeptides may be involved in Prader-Willi syndrome. Because of the loci of GABA subunits in the area around the 15q11-13 region, GABA has been measured in Prader-Willi syndrome, and abnormalities have been reported in plasma levels in some subjects.

To further clarify the mechanism leading to the behavioral phenotype, differences between deletion and maternal uniparental disomy have been assessed (Roof et al., 2000). Similar studies have been completed in Angelman syndrome (Moncla et al., 1999b). Differences in intellectual functioning in individuals with Prader-Willi syndrome with a paternal 15q11-q13 deletion rather than maternal uniparental disomy (UPD) of chromosome 15 were evaluated using measures of intelligence and academic achievement in 38 individuals with Prader-Willi syndrome (24 with deletion and 14 with UPD). The subjects with UPD had significantly higher verbal IQ scores than those with deletion ($p < 0.01$). The magnitude of the difference in verbal IQ was 9.1 points (69.9 versus 60.8 for UPD and deletion Prader-Willi syndrome subjects, respectively). Only 17% of subjects with the 15q11-q13 deletion had a verbal IQ > or = 70, while 50% of those with UPD had a verbal IQ > or = 70. Performance IQ scores did not differ between the two Prader-Willi syndrome genetic subtype groups. This report documents the difference between the verbal and performance IQ score patterns of Prader-Willi syndrome subjects with the deletion and Prader-Willi syndrome patients with the UPD subtype.

Neuroimaging Studies

Magnetic resonance imaging techniques allow the developing brain to be visualized in sufficient detail to perform "in vivo neuropathology" in Prader-Willi and Angelman syndromes. These two syndromes are of particular interest regarding neuroimaging because, although they are both caused by deletions in the same region of chromosome 15, persons with Angelman syndrome are far more severely affected and are nonverbal. The cortical morphology in six children with Angelman and four with Prader-Willi syndrome were compared (Leonard et al., 1993). When these authors studied the length of the banks of the Sylvian fissure in both syndromes, they found that, in Angelman syndrome, a significantly larger proportion (75%) had anomalous fissures than did those with Prader-Willi syndrome (12%). Such deviant cortical growth might result from abnormal timing in the expression and recognition of macromolecules involved in axonal guidance, target recognition, and pruning. The misrouting of long projection axons might be related to the Sylvian fissure anomalies and the language disorder in Angelman syndrome. Others have demonstrated abnormal cortical development, using 3-D MRI in Prader-Willi syndrome (Yoshii, Krishnamoorthy, and Grant, 2002). A preliminary fMRI study (Shapira et al., 2005) documented delay in activation of the hypothamamus and other brain regions linked to satiety (insula, ventromedial prefrontal cortex, and nucleus accumbens) following a glucose meal.

Treatment

A comprehensive treatment program includes medical management, family intervention, and behavioral treatment. To reduce obesity, close supervision is needed to prevent access to food. Interventions emphasize a low calorie diet, ensuring adequate calcium intake, periodic weigh-ins, and regular exercise (with a goal of at least 30 minutes/day). Medications have not been effective in curbing the drive for food. Obesity, poor growth, and hypotonia in children with Prader-Willi syndrome are accompanied by abnormal body composition resembling a growth hormone–deficient state. Hypothalamic dysfunction in Prader-Willi syndrome suggests partial growth hormone deficiency; this has led to FDA approval for growth hormone for short stature from Prader-Willi syndrome. Growth hormone treatment leads to increase in lean body mass and may prevent massive obesity. Initially used in adults, growth hormone trials are now being conducted beginning in infancy. Growth hormone significantly increased lean body mass and decreased body fat in one group of 25 infants with an average age of 15.5 months. Age-equivalent motor scores improved four months in the treated group. Studies of four years' duration have demonstrated growth hormone–induced alterations in body composition (decreased body fat and increased lean body mass) and increased linear growth in children with Prader-Willi syndrome (Wilson et al., 2003). Many of these children appear to have growth hormone deficiency, although this should be interpreted in the context of the patients' body mass index because short, nonobese children with Prader-Willi syndrome may not have biochemical evidence of growth hormone deficiency. Higher doses may be necessary to sustain improvements in body composition. In children, the dose of growth hormone to sustain effects is 1 mg/m^2 or higher. Still, despite improved body composition and physical functioning, abnormalities in these areas remain after 4 years of growth hormone therapy. Thus far, growth hormone therapy has not increased the risk of diabetes mellitus in these children; however, it is a concern. Diabetic ketoacidosis is a rare complication of growth hormone therapy, so screening for carbohydrate intolerance before and during growth hormone treatment in patients with Prader-Willi syndrome is recommended. Although sleep is expected to improve with changes in body composition, sleep apnea and pulmonary complications are risks and should be carefully monitored while growth hormone is given (Vleit et al., 2004). Growth hormone treatment does not change ghrelin, leptin, or neuropeptide Y. Ghrelin and other compounds continue to be studied in regard to obesity.

Prader-Willi syndrome symptoms are typically exacerbated over time, and consequently, parents need continuous support throughout childhood and adolescence. Greater attention should be paid to idiosyncrasies in cognitive functioning and to clinical markers of neuropsychiatric problems. Dykens and Shah (2003) suggest the following behavioral management and intervention techniques for individuals with Prader-Willi syndrome in order to provide clear, consistent limits and daily routines across living settings: (1) Offer extra help with transitions and getting individuals "unstuck" from compulsions (e.g., give ample warning, use special cues, and use behavioral programming). (2) Base the school curriculum on the profile of the student's strengths and weaknesses. (3) Increase the frequency of adapted physical education. (4) Provide speech-language therapy to improve articulation and pragmatic skills. (5) Consider occupational therapy for hypotonia and developing daily living skills. (6) Consider social skills training for help with rudimentary skills, such as perspective taking. (7) Provide close supervision around food across multiple living settings (school cafeteria, playground, at work, at home, and in the community). (8) Implement a low-calorie diet (approximately 1200 calories daily, ensuring adequate calcium intake). (9) Have periodic weigh-ins. (10) Ensure participation in regular exercise or sustained physical activity (up to 30 minutes daily). (11) Use environmental modifications as needed (e.g., locks on cabinets and refrigerator). (12) Encourage appropriate decision making and independence in nonfood areas of living. (13) Consider growth hormone treatment for hypotonia, increasing height and muscle mass.

Pharmacotherapy for the eating disorder, maladaptive behaviors, self-injurious behaviors, and psychosis is reviewed by Dykens and Shah (2003). Stimulant medications and other anorectic medications have not proven effective for the eating disorder. Topiramate may have some effect on suppressing eating behavior. Selective serotonin reuptake inhibitors (SSRIs) have been effective in reducing skin-picking behavior, compulsions, and depression in some individuals with Prader-Willi syndrome. Mood stabilizers have been utilized for mood lability and intermittent explosive disorder. Atypical antipsychotics have been effective for psychotic symptoms and severe aggression. Controlled medication trials are needed to determine overall risks and benefits.

Angelman Syndrome

Angelman syndrome is a rare intellectual disability syndrome that is associated with a characteristic physical and behavioral phenotype. Interest in Angelman syndrome has grown with the recognition that it involves a deficiency in the same region on chromosome 15 as Prader-Willi syndrome, an example of genomic imprinting (Hall, 1990). Angelman syndrome demonstrates that the parental origin of genetic material may have a major effect on the clinical expression of a defect.

Prevalence

The prevalence of Angelman syndrome is 1:12,000–1:20,000 persons.

Genetics

The deletion occurs at the same site on chromosome 15 as is seen in Prader-Willi syndrome. Despite deletions of the same chromosome region, these are distinct clinical phenotypes. Minor similarities, such as fair hair and blue eyes, occur in both syndromes, but the major clinical features do not overlap. In Angelman syndrome, the deletion always arises on the chromosome 15 that is inherited from the mother, whereas in Prader-Willi syndrome the same deletion is inherited from the father. The two disorders, Angelman syndrome and Prader-Willi syndrome, provide a human model for genomic imprinting (Hall, 1990), a phenomenon where genetic information is expressed differently depending on the parental chromosome inherited.

Angelman syndrome may arise from several genetic mechanisms. Most reported cases are sporadic, but familial inheritance has been reported. Angelman syndrome is caused by the loss of maternally imprinted contribution in the 15q11.2-q13 (AS/PWS) region that can occur by one of at least five different known genetic mechanisms. Analysis of parent-specific DNA methylation imprints in the 15q11.2-q13 chromosome region detects approximately 78% of patients with Angelman syndrome, including those with a deletion, uniparental disomy, or an imprinting defect; fewer than 1% of patients have a cytogenetically visible chromosome rearrangement (i.e., translocation or inversion). *UBE3A* sequence analysis detects mutations in approximately 11% of patients. Accordingly, molecular genetic testing identifies alteration in approximately 90% of patients. Fewer than 1% of patients with Angelman syndrome have a cytogenetically visible chromosome rearrangement (i.e., translocation or inversion) of one number 15 chromosome involving 15q11.2-q13 that can be detected. At the present time, it is presumed that the cardinal features of Angelman syndrome are due to deficient expression or function of the maternally inherited *UBE3A* allele.

Moncla et al. (1999a) describe the phenotypic expression in 14 Angelman syndrome cases involving eight *UBE3A* mutations. These were made up of 11 familial cases from five families and three sporadic cases. Some subtle differences from the typical phenotype of Angelman syndrome were noted. Consistent features were psychomotor delay, a happy disposition, a hyperexcitable personality, EEG abnormalities, and intellectual disability with severe speech impairment. The other main features of Angelman syndrome were ataxia, epilepsy, and microcephaly; these were either milder or absent in various combinations among these cases. Moreover, myoclonus of cortical origin was commonly observed with severe myoclonic seizures. The majority of these cases were overweight. This study showed that ataxia, myoclonus, EEG abnormalities, speech impairment, characteristic behavioral phenotype, and abnormal head circumference are attributable to a deficiency in the maternally inherited *UBE3A* allele.

Prenatal Detection

Prenatal detection of all the known molecular genetic abnormalities in the 15q11.2-q13 region that give rise to Angelman syndrome is possible through

DNA and/or chromosomal/FISH analysis of fetal cells collected by chorionic villus sampling at approximately 10 weeks–12 weeks of gestation or amniocentesis at 16 weeks–18 weeks of gestation. Prenatal testing should be undertaken only after the genetic mechanism in the index case has been established and the couple has been counseled regarding the risk to their unborn child.

Physical Features

Dysmorphic facial features are characteristic and become apparent during the second year of life (Clayton-Smith, 1992). The mouth is typically wide and smiling, with a thin upper lip, pointed chin, and prominent tongue with wide-spaced teeth. The head circumference is usually below the 50th percentile; however, approximately a quarter of cases are microcephalic. Approximately half of those affected have fair hair and skin, and most have blue eyes. Approximately two-thirds demonstrate alternating strabismus.

Feeding problems are common in the neonatal period, with difficulty in breast feeding, poor weight gain, and gastroesophageal reflux. Parents frequently describe tremulousness and jerky movements with handling during the first several months of life. Motor milestones are delayed, and truncal hypotonia may be apparent. Independent walking generally is not achieved until between three years and four years of age, although some children may walk during their second year. A minority does not ambulate and may have associated scoliosis or cerebral palsy. The gait of a child with Angelman syndrome is ataxic, with a wide base and stiff legs. Because they maintain a characteristic posture with arms upheld and flexed and laugh frequently, the designation "happy puppet syndrome" has been used (Bower and Jeavons, 1967; Clayton-Smith, 1992). However, the appropriate characterization is "Angelman syndrome."

Seizure disorder occurs in approximately 80% of cases, with an onset between 18 months and 24 months. Commonly, the first convulsion is a febrile one. A variety of seizure types are noted; myoclonic jerks and drop attack are most frequent. Seizures may be difficult to control and may occur episodically. Speech development is significantly delayed, with the acquisition of perhaps three or four words of speech. Because of the speech disturbance, sign language may be used for communication.

Behavioral Phenotype

Children with Angelman syndrome appear happy and sociable. They laugh frequently and often inappropriately. Although the laughter is not uncontrollable, it occurs unexpectedly and with minimal stimulation. In addition to laughter, hand flapping may occur with excitement. There is no associated EEG change with the laughter. The happy, sociable appearance in a severely intellectually disabled child provides clues to a diagnosis of Angelman syndrome in young children before dysmorphic facial features are apparent. Sleep disturbances are also characteristic, with frequent nighttime waking.

Cognitive Profile

Overall, cognitive level is in the severe-to-profound range of intellectual disability; however, it may be difficult to obtain accurate psychological testing because of the child's difficulties in speech and coordination. Comprehension abilities are significantly better than their expressive speech.

Neuroimaging

Neuroimaging studies show an apparently structurally normal brain with MRI or CT; however, mild cortical atrophy or dysmyelination may be observed. Angelman and Prader-Willi syndromes were compared using MRI measuring the length of the banks of the Sylvian fissure in a gapless series of thin sagittal images. Children with Angelman syndrome had a significantly larger proportion (75%) of anomalous Sylvian fissures than the children with Prader-Willi syndrome (12%) (Leonard et al., 1993).

Treatment

Treatment begins with the recognition of the syndrome. Hyperactivity, seizures, and severe intellectual disability with absent speech are usually the major management concerns. Family counseling is initiated to assist with the associated clinical symptoms. Parental chromosome study may be used to rule out one of the rare familial forms. Adaptation to the child's intellectual disability and clarification of the expected behavior disorder is crucial. Behavioral modification is used in treating undesirable behaviors that are socially disruptive or self-injurious. Most children with Angelman syndrome do not receive drug therapy for hyperactivity, although some may benefit from the use of stimulant medications. Management of seizure disorder may be difficult and require multiple anticonvulsant drug trials. Sleep disturbances are common and may respond to a combination of pharmacotherapy and behavior management (Summers et al., 1992).

Fragile X Syndrome

Fragile X syndrome is the most common known cause of inherited intellectual disability and may also result in learning disabilities and social deficits in those who do not test in the intellectual disability range. After the identification of the fragile X mental retardation-1 (*FMR1*) gene, the cytogenetic marker (a fragile site at Xq27.3) was replaced by molecular diagnosis. Recognition of this gene has broadened our understanding of the spectrum of the fragile X syndrome.

Prevalence

Prevalence studies using molecular genetic testing of *FMR1* have estimated a prevalence of 1 in 2,200 schoolchildren in an English study. A Canadian study found 1 in 259 women with a premutation of 55 repeats or larger. The premutation was identified in 1in 755 males in Quebec, Canada. A population-based prevalence study of affected African-American males found a higher estimate than reported for Caucasians. The prevalence of fragile X syndrome in females is thought to be approximately one-half the male prevalence. The frequency of the premutation and mutation may be variable in different populations because of founder effects (Hagerman, 1999a).

Genetics

The fragile X syndrome was one of the first examples of a class of disorders caused by a dynamic mutation: the progressive expansion of the polymorphic (CGG) trinucleotide repeats located in the promoter region of the *FMR1* gene in the X chromosome at Xq27.3. Thus, it is caused by massive expansion of CGG triplet repeats located in the 5'-untranslated region of the fragile X mental retardation-1 (*FMR1*) gene. In the normal population, the CGG repeat varies from 6 to 54 units. Affected subjects have expanded CGG repeats (>200) in the first exon of the *FMR1* gene (the full mutation). Phenotypically normal carriers of the fragile X syndrome have a repeat in the 43–200 range (the premutation). There are two additional disorders that result in a fragile site at Xq27.3. These are FRAXE, which is associated with a milder form of intellectual disability, and FRAXF, which is not consistently associated with intellectual disability. Both of these mutations also have CGG repeat expansions and are distal to the *FMR1* site. The transcriptional silencing of the *FMR2* gene has been implicated in FRAXE intellectual disability. Individuals with FRAXE have learning deficits, including speech delay and reading and writing problems.

The cloning of the *FMR1* gene allowed the characterization of its protein product FMRP. The full mutation is linked to a process of methylation involving the addition of methyl groups along the DNA helix. In patients with fragile X syndrome, the expanded CGG triplet repeats are hypermethylated; this results in the expression of the *FMR1* gene being repressed. The process of methylation silences gene transcription, and a fully methylated full mutation results in no FMR1 protein being produced. The result of the absence of FMR1 protein is fragile X syndrome. The encoded FMR1 protein is a ribosome-associated, RNA-binding protein that is thought to play a role in translational regulation of selective messenger RNA transcripts. This protein is thought to be involved in protein translation and found associated with polyribosomes and the rough endoplasmic reticulum.

The diagnosis of fragile X syndrome rests on the detection of an alteration in the *FMR1* gene. More than 99% of affected individuals have a full mutation in the *FMR1* gene caused by an increased number of CGG trinucleotide repeats (>200 typically) accompanied by aberrant methylation of the *FMR1* gene. Both increased trinucleotide repeats and methylation changes in *FMR1* can be detected by molecular genetic testing. Such testing is clinically available.

Mouse and Drosophila Models

The physiological function of the FMR1 protein has been studied in both mouse and drosophila models. In the mouse, a loss-of-function mouse model demonstrates slightly enlarged testes, a subtle behavioral phenotype, and discrete anomalies of dendrite spines that are similar to those observed in brains of persons with fragile X syndrome (Kooy, 2003). Studies in drosophila (fruit fly) show that FXMR plays a major role in synaptogenesis and axonal arborization. This might underlie the observed deficits in flight ability and circadian behavior of FXR mutant flies (Bakker and Oostra, 2003).

Prenatal Diagnosis

Prenatal testing is conducted through molecular genetic testing of DNA from cells obtained by chorionic villus sampling (CVS) or amniocentesis. Prenatal testing for fetuses at increased risk for *FMR1* full mutations can be performed using DNA extracted from cells obtained by amniocentesis at 16 weeks–18 weeks of gestation or CVS at approximately 10 weeks–12 weeks of gestation. For pregnancies evaluated by CVS, follow-up amniocentesis or testing using the polymerase chain reaction (PCR) may be necessary to determine the size of the *FMR1* alleles in a methylation-independent manner. Prenatal testing should be undertaken after carrier status has been confirmed and the couple has been counseled regarding the risk of recurrence. All mothers of a child with an *FMR1* gene full mutation (expansion >200 CGG trinucleotide repeats) are carriers of an *FMR1* gene expansion. Molecular genetic testing and recurrence risk counseling should be provided. The optimal time for determination of genetic risk, clarification of carrier status, and discussion of availability of prenatal testing is before pregnancy. The increased risk for premature ovarian failure (i.e., menopause before age 40) in female premutation carriers should be taken into account when providing genetic counseling.

Premutation genetic diagnosis for fragile X is feasible for a number of couples. A premutation genetic diagnosis should include a determination of the premutation or mutation carrier status, the maternal or paternal origin of the premutation, and an estimation of the ovarian reserve of the patient. Fragile X premutation carriers should be advised not to postpone reproduction if they plan to have children.

Etiology

The FMR1 protein is expressed most abundantly in neurons and testes with the localization primarily in the cytoplasm. High concentrations of *FMR1* mRNA have been found at the synapse in rat brains, especially in areas involved in synaptogenesis in the hippocampus, cerebral cortex, and cerebellum. Hinton et al. (1991) found thin and immature dendritic branches with small synapses in neuroanatomical studies of the neocortex in three males with fragile X syndrome. The expression of the FMR2 protein also has been characterized. To characterize the expression of the fragile X mental retardation 2 (FMR2) protein, polyclonal antibodies were raised against two regions of the human FMR2 protein and used in immunofluorescence experiments on cryosections of mouse brain. The FMR2 protein is localized in neurons of the neocortex, Purkinje cells of the cerebellum, and the granule cell layer of the hippocampus. FMR2 staining is shown to colocalize with the nuclear stain 4,6-diamidino-2-phenylindole (DAPI), confirming that FMR2 is a nuclear protein. The localization of FMR1 and FMR2 protein to the mammalian hippocampus and other brain structures involved with cognitive function is consistent with the learning deficits seen in fragile X individuals.

Physical Features

Characteristics of fragile X syndrome are present at birth. It is characterized by intellectual disability, behavioral characteristics, and physical findings such as an elongated face with large protruding ears, a protruding jaw, hyperextensible joints, and enlarged testes in postpubescent males (Hagerman, 1999b). People with fragile X also have poor motor coordination and an increased incidence of epilepsy. Common peripheral symptoms are heightened sensitivity to tactile irritation and loose bowel movements.

Behavioral Phenotype

There is a substantial degree of heterogeneity in the physical, cognitive, and behavioral phenotype. The behavioral phenotype has been the subject of considerable study and includes intellectual disability and learning disabilities, language impairment, hand flapping, gaze aversion, perseveration, and neuropsychiatric disturbance, principally attention deficit hyperactivity disorder and pervasive developmental disorder-like symptoms. The patients are more interested in social interactions than those with autistic disorder; the avoidance of social contact may be secondary to hyperarousal or increased sensitivity to stimuli associated with social situations. The behavioral phenotype may be more helpful than the physical phenotype in diagnosis because most prepubertal patients do not have macroorchidism or the characteristic long face.

Attentional difficulty and concentration problems are commonly associated, and hyperactivity may be a presenting symptom in non–intellectually disabled boys with fragile X syndrome. Behavioral features include increased social avoidance, anxiety, and hyperactivity (Hatton et al., 1999). Self-injury, most commonly hand biting and scratching, may be elicited by excitement and frustration. Fragile X females may be unaffected, although abnormalities in social interaction, thought process, and affect regulation have been reported in carriers. Both schizotypal features and depression have also been found in carriers. These differences are primarily evidenced by individuals who show the full gene mutation.

The majority of the girls with the full mutation exhibit shyness and social anxiety. In women with the full mutation, the social anxiety is associated with social awkwardness and schizotypal features. Anxiety disorders, avoidance disorder, and mood disorder symptoms are common (Hagerman, 1999b).

Gaze Aversion. Gaze aversion is a striking feature of affected males with fragile X syndrome. There is consistency in gaze aversion over repeated trials in the same individual; nearly all fragile X males over the age of eight or nine avert gaze on greeting another person. Their unusual greeting is characterized by both head and gaze aversion along with an appropriate recognition of the social partner (Wolff et al., 1989). This greeting response is qualitatively different from gaze aversion that is described in individuals with autistic disorder. Those with Down syndrome and nonspecific intellectual disability do not show this behavioral pattern on greeting. The idiosyncratic gaze behavior in fragile X syndrome may disrupt social interactions. Despite their apparent social anxiety and aversion to eye contact, males with fragile X syndrome are otherwise socially responsive and can be affectionate.

Speech and Language. Speech and language in fragile X syndrome is generally delayed even though the IQ may be in the normal range. Deficits in both receptive and expressive language include dysfluency, production of incomplete sentences, echolalia, palilalia (reiteration of the speaker's own words and phrases in a perseverative manner), verbal perseveration, and poor fluency in conversation. Compulsive utterances and shifts in speech pitch are common and auditory processing and memory deficits are present.

Cognitive Profile

The extent of intellectual disability is correlated with the number of trinucleotide repeats and ranges from severe intellectual disability to low-average intelligence. Cognitive and language features of fragile X syndrome include deficits consistent with the level of intellectual disability but with more pronounced deficits in visual–spatial skills, attention, and executive functioning (Mazzocco, 2000). These include intellectual disability in the moderate-to-severe range, developmental delay, attention deficit and hyperactivity, anxiety with mood lability, and obsessive-compulsive and autistic-like behaviors.

Neuroimaging

Autopsy studies indicate that although the brain is grossly normal, dendritic spines are longer and immature in appearance. Neuroimaging studies have shown selective changes in brain size of fragile X patients, including a reduction in the posterior cerebellar vermis, an age-dependent increase in hippocampal volume, and an enlarged caudate nucleus and thalamus. Magnetic resonance imaging studies demonstrate a reduction in temporal lobe volume (primarily gray matter) and relative preservation/enlargement of parietal white matter volume in fragile X males (Kates et al., 2002). Diffusion tensor imaging has been used to investigate whether white matter tract integrity and connectivity are altered in fragile X syndrome. Results from these studies in fragile X females suggest a relative involvement of white matter in frontostriatal pathways, as well as in parietal sensory-motor tracts. Such observations indicate that FMRP absence may also affect axons and not just dendrites and postsynaptic neurons.

Functional magnetic resonance imaging has been employed to explore the activated brain areas during either arithmetic processing or a cognitive interference task in fragile X females (Tamm et al., 2002). Some brain areas were more extensively activated (for example, the anterior prefrontal cortex), while others failed to show the expected activation (for example, the association areas of the parietal lobe) compared with normal controls.

Treatment

Although at this time there is no specific cure for fragile X syndrome, a number of recent advances are hopeful. These include a neuropharmacological approach acting on either critical receptors or aimed at reactivating the silenced *FMR1* gene (Antar et al., 2004; Rattazzi, LaFauci, and Brown, 2004). Autopsy studies demonstrate that although the brain is grossly normal in fragile X syndrome, dendritic spines are longer and immature in appearance. Fragile X syndrome is caused by the absence of the mRNA-binding protein, fragile X mental retardation protein (FMRP), which may play a role in activity-regulated localization and translation of mRNA in dendrites and at synapses. A key aspect of the effects of the absence of fragile X protein in the brain may be unregulated synaptic protein synthesis. Metabotropic glutamate receptor (mGluR) activation, in particular mGluR5 activation, was found to be necessary for localization of FMRP into dendrites (Antar et al., 2004). This suggests that regulation of FMRP trafficking in dendrites and synapses occurs in response to specific glutamatergic signals. If so, mGluR5 antagonists might provide a potential treatment for the neurological and psychiatric symptoms of fragile X expressed in adults. Thus, it might be possible to overcome the loss of FMRP by dampening the protein synthesis triggered by activation of these signals. The other approach is gene therapy. In the fragile X syndrome, the approach most likely to have a chance of being effective should consist of a small, diffusible vector derived from the adeno-associated virus, carrying an *FMR1* cDNA comprising the 5' promoter region and the 3' untranslated region of the gene, delivered to the entire brain (Rattazzi, LaFauci, and Brown, 2004).

Current supportive therapy consists of the use of behavioral techniques to assist in behavior management and social learning, and educational intervention with an individualized education plan aimed specifically at the known problems in learning. Parents and teachers of children with fragile X syndrome have recognized the need for individual attention, small class size, and the avoidance of sudden change. Pharmacological management of behavioral issues that significantly affect social interaction may be helpful. However, no specific pharmacological treatment has been shown to be uniquely beneficial; therapy must be individualized and closely monitored. Stimulants appear to be quite useful for management of distractibility, hyperactivity, and impulsive behavior; antidepressants help with anxiety, obsessive-compulsive behaviors, and mood dysregulation; and atypical antipsychotics can reduce aggression. These medications are used for support and help minimize dysfunctional behaviors and maximize functioning. As more is learned about the neural functions of FMRP, medications in the future might be targeted to specific synaptic mechanisms that are dysfunctional in the brain and thus focus directly on the cognitive deficit. Detailed treatment recommendations are found in Hagerman (1999b).

Williams (Williams-Beuren) Syndrome

Williams and colleagues described a syndrome with supravalvular aortic stenosis, a specific heart defect, intellectual disability, and unusual facial appearance (Williams, Barratt-Boyes and Lowe, 1961). Williams syndrome is a specific neurodevelopmental disorder associated with a characteristic physical, linguistic, and behavioral phenotype, which provides a unique opportunity to study personality development, linguistic functioning, and visuospatial development in a well-defined population of children with known cognitive deficits.

Prevalence

The prevalence of Williams syndrome (WMS) was initially estimated to occur in approximately 1:20,000 live births. However, a population study in 30,037 Norwegian children found a prevalence of 1:7,500 live births (Stromme, Bjornstad, and Ramstad, 2002).

Genetics

Williams syndrome is caused by a chromosomal deletion at 7q11.23. In Williams syndrome (WMS), a deletion of 1.5 Mb on one copy of chromosome 7 results in specific physical, cognitive, and behavioral features. It is a contiguous gene deletion disorder that results from hemizygous deletion of at least 15 genes. This chromosomal region is highly repetitive, and the deletion arises from recombination between misaligned repeat sequences flanking the Williams syndrome region. The deletion breakpoints cluster within the repeats, so that most patients with Williams syndrome have similar, although not identical, deletions of 1.5 Mb. The first deleted gene identified in the critical region was that for elastin (*ELN*). Studies of patients having deletions or point mutations confined to this gene show that hemizygosity for *ELN* causes supravalvular aortic stenosis (SVAS) but not the other typical features of Williams syndrome.

Several other genes that are deleted in most patients with Williams syndrome have now been identified. These include *LIMK1*, which codes for a protein tyrosine kinase expressed in the developing brain and has been implicated in the visuospatial cognition defect. *GTF2I* (general transcription factor II, I) encodes transcription factor TFII-I and BAP-135, a B cell protein. Deletion mapping of "SVAS plus" families has suggested that deletion of this gene may impact IQ (Morris et al., 2003). Other genes in this region include that for syntaxin 1A (*STX1A*), which encodes a component of the synaptic apparatus; *RFC2*, which codes for a subunit of the replication factor C complex involved in DNA replication; and *FZD3*, which is homologous to the drosophila tissue-polarity gene, "frizzled" (Korenberg et al., 2000).

Prenatal Testing

Due to the theoretical risk for germline mosaicism, prenatal testing may be offered to couples in which neither member has Williams syndrome, but who have had a child with Williams syndrome. FISH testing may be used to detect the microdeletion of the Williams syndrome critical region in fetal cells. These cells are procured by chorionic villus sampling at approximately 10 weeks–12 weeks of gestation or by amniocentesis at 16 weeks–18 weeks of gestation. Most cases are the only case in the family.

Physical Features

The syndrome is characterized by congenital facial and cardiovascular anomalies (supravalvular aortic stenosis and peripheral pulmonary stenosis), failure to thrive, and intellectual disability that may be accompanied by transient idiopathic infantile hypercalcemia (Williams, Barratt-Boyes, and Lowe, 1961). The cluster of unusual facial features is one of the most characteristic aspects of Williams syndrome. The typical facial features include a broad forehead, medial eyebrow flare, depressed nasal bridge, stellate pattern in the iris, widely spaced teeth, and full lips. Their full prominent cheeks, wide mouth, short turned-up nose, and flat nasal bridge have often been described as distinctive elfin-like faces. (Although some use the term "elfin" face, the term "Williams syndrome face" is preferable [Greenberg, 1990]). Others features are digestive disorders in infancy, apparent auditory sensitivity, mild microcephaly, and renal problems.

Behavioral Phenotype

Williams syndrome patients often have an overly friendly, engaging personality that is characterized by excessive sociability with strangers, excessive empathy, attention problems, and anxiety (Jones, Bellugi, and Lai, 2000). Individuals with Williams syndrome show an unusual positive response in their social judgments of unfamiliar individuals. In intellectually disabled persons with Williams syndrome, linguistic abilities, especially expressive language ability, may be better than expected for cognitive level (Bellugi et al., 2000). Behavior problems in Williams syndrome include perseveration, anxiety, attention deficit disorder, and sleep difficulties.

Cognitive Profile

Intellectual disability, usually in the mild range, occurs in 75% of individuals. Adaptive behavior is less than expected for IQ in adults and affects independent living in the community. The cognitive profile consisting of strengths in auditory rote memory and language, but deficits in visuospatial constructive cognition. Thus, children with Williams syndrome tend to score higher on verbal subtests than on tests measuring visuospatial construction. Academically, there is a wide range of achievement, so individuals with Williams syndrome may demonstrate reading ability up to the high school level. However, there are significant difficulties with writing, drawing, and math.

Howlin, Davies, and Udwin (1998) investigated cognitive, linguistic, and academic assessments in a representative sample of 62 adults with Williams syndrome (average age of the group = 26 years; mean full scale IQ = 61). Less difference was found between verbal and performance IQ, and between receptive and expressive language skills, in the adults than was found in children. Still, subtest scores documented an almost identical cognitive profile to that found in children. Reading, spelling, arithmetic, and social adaptation remained at a low level, with functioning around a 6-year to 8-year age equivalent. The consistency in intellectual abilities found in studies of both adults and children with Williams syndrome supports the notion of a syndrome-specific pattern of cognitive, linguistic, and adaptive functioning.

Williams syndrome is an example of why it is important to apply a developmental approach to neurogenetic disorders. Karmiloff-Smith et al. (1997) have proposed that in Williams syndrome, language follows a different path to normal acquisition and may turn out to be more like second language learning. Bellugi et al. (2000) propose that the distinguishing cognitive feature of Williams syndrome is the dissociation between language and face processing (relative strengths) and spatial cognition (profound impairment). However, other authors emphasize that there is both delay and deviance in face processing in Williams syndrome and stress the importance of building developmental trajectories for each specific task.

Finally, Tager-Flusberg, Boshart, and Baron-Cohen (1998) tested the hypothesis that the Williams syndrome phenotype involves sparing abilities involved in the domain of understanding other minds (mentalizing or theory of mind). They compared a group of intellectually disabled adults with Williams syndrome to an age-, IQ-, and language-matched group of adults with Prader-Willi syndrome, and a group of age-matched normal adults, on a task that tests mentalizing ability. The task involved identifying the correct labels to match photographs of complex mental state expression focused on the eye region of the face. The adults with Williams syndrome performed significantly better than the adults with Prader-Willi syndrome on this task, and approximately half the group performed in the same range as the normal adults. Such findings provide support for the proposal that mentalizing is a distinct cognitive domain. The authors propose that this sparing of cognitive capacity may be related to the relative sparing of limbic-cerebellar neural substance in Williams syndrome, which is linked to corticofrontal regions that are involved in understanding complex mental states.

Linking Genes and Cognition in Williams Syndrome

Molecular dissection of the Williams syndrome phenotype may lead to identification of genes important in human cognition and behavior. An approach to studying cognition is to carry out genetic and psychometric testing of patients who have small deletions within the Williams syndrome critical region. LIM kinase 1 (*LIMK1*) and *STX1A* are good candidate genes to investigate cognitive or behavioral aspects of Williams syndrome. The gene for *LIMK1* has been implicated (Frangiskakis et al., 1996) as a cause for the visuospatial characteristics of Williams syndrome; however, other investigators were unable to substantiate this association in three further cases (Tassabehji et al., 1999). The genes for STX1A and FZD9 have been proposed to be involved based on brain-specific gene expression in the adult (*STX1A*) and developing (*FZD9*) central nervous system, respectively. Korenberg et al. (2000) reports that deletion of these genes is not associated with significant effects on overall cognition. However, these authors do propose that genes responsible for intellectual disability and other features of the disorder are located in the region telometric to RFC2 through GTF21 at the telometric border of the deletion. Moreover, mild cognitive deficits reported in a subject with deletions of the elastin and *LIMK1* genes (Tassabehji et al., 1999) are consistent with findings that those with deletion of genes in the *WMSTF* through *LIMK1* region have mild cognitive deficits. Thus, studies of individuals with rare and atypical deletions may be informative in identifying candidate genes to understand the cognitive deficit.

Neuroimaging Studies/Event-Related Potential Studies

Williams syndrome is associated with specific neuromorphological and neurophysiological findings. There is proportional sparing of frontal, limbic, and neocerebellar structures on MRI (Reiss et al., 2000). Abnormal functional organization of the neural systems that underlie language processing is revealed through studies using event-related potentials (ERPs) (Mills et al., 2000). ERP studies suggest abnormal cerebral specialization for spared cognitive functions in Williams syndrome. The nonuniformity in the cognitive, neuromorphological, and neurophysiological domains of Williams syndrome make it a compelling model for elucidating the relationships between cognition, the brain, and, ultimately, the genes.

Another approach is to investigate anatomical changes in brain regions of Williams syndrome patients that may be the result of gene deletions. In individuals with Williams syndrome, Galaburda and Bellugi (2000) found that the overall shape of the brain is not consistently abnormal, although, in some cases, abnormal brain shape is apparent. The most consistent anatomical finding is abnormal length of the central sulcus, producing an unusual configuration of the dorsal central region. This includes the distal portion of the superior-parietal lobule and dorsal frontal gyrus. These regions may be linked to abnormal behavior in patients with Williams syndrome. Cytoarchitecture of Williams syndrome forebrain appears mostly normal, although subtle dysplastic changes are noted. Abnormal neuronal size of cortical neurons was suggested in one region and might be linked to increased subcortical connectivity. Elastin does not stain in the cerebellum, while LIM kinase does stain in cortical neurons.

Thus, in Williams syndrome the link between neuroanatomy and behavior seems to fit a dorsal-ventral dichotomy and not a frontal-caudal, left-right, or cortical-subcortical dichotomy. Galaburda and Bellugi (2000) propose that the dorsal portions of the hemispheres, the frontal and parietal-occipital regions, may be involved. They note that some language functions that are linked to ventral systems are preserved. Face recognition, also a ventral function, is preserved despite severe visuospatial dysfunction, a dorsal function. Anatomical findings also suggest possible involvement of the visually linked lateral nucleus of the amygdala. Galaburda and Bellugi speculate that this might be related to the lack of appropriate fear Williams syndrome patients have for new, unfamiliar, and perhaps threatening faces. Moreover, because this region may receive auditory projections, Williams syndrome subjects may not be sensitive to threatening voice and speech. Further work is needed at architechtronic and histologic levels to confirm sparing of ventral regions. To understand the linking of genes with neuroanatomy, it is necessary to find more genes with brain developmental effects. Of particular interest in this regard is the proposal that the region deleted in Williams syndrome may be a hotspot in mammalian brain evolution (Korenberg et al., 2000).

Treatment

Guidelines for medical management are available on the Williams Syndrome website (www.williams-syndrome.org) (Morris et al., 1999). These include guidelines for cardiac evaluation, urinary tract evaluation, calcium determinations, thyroid function testing, and eye examination. The cardiovascular system requires lifelong monitoring, since arterial stenosis may worsen. Surgical treatment of SVAS or renal artery stenosis may be required. Because hypercalcemia may occur at any age, concentration of calcium in serum and urine should be monitored every two years. Hyperopia is treated with corrective lenses. Adults should be screened for sensorineural hearing loss, hypothyroidism, and diabetes mellitus.

The developmental disability requires early intervention programs, special education programs, and vocational training for adults. Verbal strengths should be encouraged when learning spatial tasks. Speech/language, physical, and occupational therapies are recommended. Behavioral therapy and psychotropic medication may be used for management of behavior problems, especially attention deficit disorder. Hypercalcemia may contribute to irritability, vomiting, constipation, and muscle cramps. Because hypercalcemia may occur at any age, concentration of calcium in serum and urine should be monitored every two years. Hagerman outlines additional recommendations for treatment for Williams syndrome (Hagerman, 1999b).

Fetal Alcohol Syndrome (FAS) and Fetal Alcohol Spectrum Disorders (FASD)

Fetal alcohol syndrome was originally described in 1968 by Lemoine et al. These authors described anomalies observed in 127 children of alcoholic parents, with emphasis on the effects of alcohol on the developing fetus (Lemoine et al., 1968). Subsequently, Jones et al. (1973) outlined the pattern of malformation in the offspring of chronic alcoholic mothers and described the characteristics of the fetal alcohol syndrome in detail. It has since become apparent that prenatal alcohol exposure is associated with a more extensive range of abnormalities that include physical, cognitive, and behavioral dysfunction. Thus, the effects of alcohol on development are broad and result in a spectrum of problems, ranging from severe intellectual disability to poor adaptive living skills, impaired social understanding, and dependency on others. Fetal alcohol syndrome and fetal alcohol spectrum disorders result in preventable behavioral, cognitive, and psychosocial problems. Fetal alcohol syndrome is one of the most commonly recognized causes of intellectual disability.

Genetics

Discordance in dizygotic twins affected by alcohol exposure in utero suggests that genetic factors may lead to susceptibility to fetal alcohol syndrome. Riikonen (1994) described discordant twins exposed to heavy maternal alcohol consumption only during the second half of pregnancy. One twin showed greater susceptibility to the effects of alcohol and had prenatal growth retardation, neonatal withdrawal symptoms, delayed motor milestones, and poorer cognitive function in the first year of life, as well as central and cortical brain atrophy on neuroimaging studies. The other twin was normal at the 17-month follow-up. Streissguth and Dehaene (1993) reported prenatal alcohol exposure in 5 pairs of monozygotic twins and 11 pairs of dizygotic twins. The concordance rate of monozygotic twins was 5/5 and 7/11 for dizygotic twins. In two dizygotic pairs, one twin had fetal alcohol syndrome and the other had alcohol-related effects. In the two other dizygotic pairs, one twin had no diagnosis, and one had alcohol-related effects. IQ scores were similar in the monozygotic twin pairs and dissimilar in the discordant dizygotic pairs. Despite similar levels of alcohol exposure, differences in susceptibility in discordant twins indicate that genes may modulate the influence of alcohol. Understanding how alcohol affects gene regulation is critical to understanding the mechanisms underlying fetal alcohol syndrome.

Genetic variability is one factor that may influence the deleterious effects of alcohol during gestation; allelic differences in alcohol dehydrogenase in mother and fetus may be one element that leads to variability in the phenotype. The alcohol dehydrogenase enzyme affects maternal blood levels of alcohol, and thus, may be higher in some individuals than in others. The level of alcohol in the body results in effects on developing fetal tissues. Heavy maternal alcohol use results in the full fetal alcohol syndrome in less than 40% of those who are exposed during pregnancy. Therefore, other factors that influence the developmental outcome, in addition to alcohol, must be considered. These include genetic factors, smoking, physical illness and infection, nutrition, trauma, the use of other drugs, stress, parity, age of the mother, and having given birth to a child with fetal alcohol syndrome. Alcohol is both directly and indirectly neurotoxic and causes a disturbance in normal brain architecture. Fetal alcohol exposure results in growth retardation in mice and rats. The distinctive facial features of fetal alcohol syndrome have been documented in monkeys and in mice.

Ethanol-induced cell death leads to hypoplasia of the basal ganglia and various frontosubcortical nuclei involved in cognitive function and mood regulation. These effects may result in memory deficits, perseverative behaviors, and mood disorders in children with fetal alcohol spectrum disorders.

Prevalence

Fetal alcohol syndrome is a common and preventable cause of intellectual disability, with a worldwide incidence of approximately 5.2:10,000 live births (Abel, 1998). The CDC (2002) estimates 0.3 to 1.5 per 1,000 live-born infants. Rates in selected subgroups—for instance, Native Americans—approach 30: 10,000 live births. The rates of occurrence of both fetal alcohol syndrome and alcohol-related neurodevelopmental disorder in a Seattle study was 9.1:1,000 cases or approximately one child for every 100 live births (Sampson et al., 1997). Mills et al. (1984) prospectively studied 31,000 pregnancies to establish the amount of alcohol that a pregnant woman may safely consume. One or more drinks per day increased the risk of infant growth retardation. One drink is defined as 1.5 oz of distilled spirits, 5 oz. of wine, or 12 oz. of beer. Despite its frequency, the syndrome may go unrecognized because physicians may not systematically inquire about alcohol use (Donovan, 1991).

Clinical Features

Over 80% of children with fetal alcohol syndrome show prenatal and postnatal growth deficiency, microcephaly, infantile irritability, mild-to-moderate intellectual disability, and a characteristic facial appearance (Clarren and Smith, 1978; Jones, 1986; Jones et al., 1973). Approximately half are poorly coordinated, hypotonic, and have attention deficits. An additional 20% to 50% have other birth defects including eye and ear anomalies and cardiac anomalies. Those children who are exposed to alcohol in utero who do not show growth retardation, congenital anomalies, or intellectual disability may demonstrate more subtle changes. These more subtle abnormalities are referred to as "fetal alcohol spectrum disorders" and include cognitive, behavioral, and psychosocial problems.

The three general criteria used to make the diagnosis of fetal alcohol syndrome include the following: (1) prenatal and postnatal growth retardation, (2) dysmorphic facial features (flat philtrum and flat midface, thin upper lip, and small palpebral fissures), and (3) evidence of central nervous system dysfunction (behavioral, neurological, and/or cognitive disabilities) in children born of mothers who abuse alcohol (American Academy of Pediatrics Committee on Substance Abuse and Committee on Children with Disabilities, 2000).

Behavioral Phenotype

The behavioral phenotype is characterized by subnormal intellectual functioning, particularly in arithmetic, and difficulty understanding cause and effect and generalizing from one situation to another. Inattention, poor concentration, impaired

judgment, memory deficits, and problems in abstract reasoning are also characteristic. Behavioral problems related to impulsivity and hyperactivity include
oppositional and conduct disorders. The behavioral phenotype includes cognitive, behavioral, and psychosocial problems that may persist throughout the life
span (American Academy of Pediatrics Committee on Substance Abuse, 2000).
The extent of these problems is indicative of the impact of alcohol as a teratogen
that affects brain development. Neurodevelopmental problems interact with psychosocial risks linked to the mother's alcohol problems and result in chronic
neuropsychiatric disorders (Streissguth and O'Malley, 2000). Cognitive deficits
include problems with abstract and cause and effect reasoning, difficulties in
generalizing from one situation to another and specific mathematics problems
consistent with social-emotional learning disability. Of particular concern are
difficulties making the "moral connection" between one's actions and their consequences and effects on others. Such deficits in social understanding may lead
to antisocial behavior without antisocial intent. Conduct problems, such as lying,
stealing, stubbornness, and oppositional behavior are common, relatively distinct, and qualitatively and quantitatively different from behavior in other intellectual disability syndromes. Affected individuals have poor attention and concentration, memory deficits, and impaired judgment. They may present with
hyperactivity and impulsiveness but with a different neurocognitive and behavioral profile than children with a primary diagnosis of attention deficit/hyper-
activity disorder.

Fetal alcohol syndrome is not only a childhood disorder; the cognitive and
behavioral effects and psychosocial problems may persist through adolescence
into adulthood in both fetal alcohol syndrome and spectrum disorders. After
puberty, the faces of patients with fetal alcohol syndrome or those who had fetal
alcohol effects are not as distinctive. These individuals generally remained short
and microcephalic but achieve a weight close to the mean for chronological age.
Streissguth et al. (1991) found in a follow-up study that the average IQ was 68,
although the range of IQ scores widely varied. IQ was stable on retesting. Average academic functioning was at the second- to fourth-grade levels, although
arithmetic deficits were most characteristic. Maladaptive behaviors included
poor judgment, distractibility, difficulty perceiving social cues, and problems in
modulating mood. The family environment continued to be unstable. None of
the subjects in the study had age-appropriate socialization and communication
skills.

Clinical descriptions of patients with fetal alcohol syndrome and fetal alcohol
effects suggest major problems with adaptive behavior. Five operationally defined adverse outcomes and 18 associated risk/protective factors were examined
using a Life History Interview with knowledgeable informants of 415 patients
with fetal alcohol syndrome or fetal alcohol effects (median age = 14 years,
range 6–51 years; median IQ = 86, range = 29–126). Eighty percent of these
patients were not raised by their biological mothers. For adolescents and adults,
the life span prevalence was 61% for disrupted school experiences, 60% for
trouble with the law, 50% for confinement (in detention, jail, prison, or a psychiatric or alcohol/drug inpatient setting), 49% for inappropriate sexual behav-

iors on repeated occasions, and 35% for alcohol/drug problems. The odds of escaping these adverse life outcomes are increased 2- to 4-fold by receiving the diagnosis of fetal alcohol syndrome or fetal alcohol effects at an earlier age and by being reared in good stable environments.

Cognitive Effects

Executive function also is impaired in individuals with prenatal alcohol exposure whether or not they test in the intellectually disabled range. Mattson et al. (1999) found that executive function was impaired in individuals with and without fetal alcohol syndrome and intellectual disability on several domains of executive functioning. These include planning ability, cognitive flexibility, selective inhibition, concept formation, and reasoning. Thus, Mattson et al. (1999) classified children with heavy prenatal alcohol exposure and nonexposed controls, using four measures of attentional functioning: the Freedom from Distractibility index from the Wechsler Intelligence Scale for Children-Third Edition (WISC-III), the Attention Problems scale from the Child Behavior Checklist (CBCL), and omission and commission error scores from the Test of Variables of Attention (TOVA). Data from two groups of children—children with heavy prenatal alcohol exposure and nonexposed controls—were analyzed. Children in the alcohol-exposed group included children both with and without fetal alcohol syndrome. Groups were matched on age, sex, ethnicity, and social class. Data were analyzed using backward logistic regression. The final model included the Freedom from Distractibility index from the WISC-III and the Attention Problems scale from the CBCL. The TOVA variables were not retained in the final model. Classification accuracy was 91.7% overall. Specifically, 93.3% of the alcohol-exposed children and 90% of the control children were accurately classified. These data indicate that children with heavy prenatal alcohol exposure can be distinguished from nonexposed controls with a high degree of accuracy using two commonly used measures of attention.

Neuroimaging

Six boys and 5 girls with a mean age of 8.6 years (range = 3–13 years) with fetal alcohol syndrome were studied by MRI and single photon emission computed tomography (SPECT) to discern specific areas of vulnerability (Riikonen et al., 1999). Morphological anomalies shown in 6 of 11 patients by MRI were found both cortically and subcortically: cortical atrophy ($N = 2$), dilated ventricle ($N = 1$), corpus callosum hypoplasia ($N = 1$), cerebellar atrophy ($N = 2$), and one of the latter with Arnold-Chiari malformation ($N = 1$). Delayed myelination of the white matter was seen in two patients. Volumetric studies of the hippocampus showed morphological left-right asymmetry in five of eight patients. However, SPECT showed mild hypoperfusion of the left hemisphere in all 10 subjects. The negative left-right index was located especially in the left parietooccipital region, that is, in the brain areas implicated in arithmetical and logical-grammatical functions, which are known to be affected in fetal alcohol syndrome. Normal left-right dominance was also lacking in the frontal area, which is the brain area affected in attention-deficit-hyperactivity disorder (ADHD). Diverse morphological and functional abnormalities were more frequent than has been believed even in less impaired children with fetal alochol syndrome.

Bookstein et al. (2002) combined neuroanatomical measures with neurocognitive and neuromotor measures in to determine the consequences of alcohol exposure on brain. Midline curves of the corpus callosum were carefully digitized in three dimensions from MR scans of 15 adult males diagnosed with fetal alochol syndrome, 15 with fetal alcohol spectrum disorder, and 15 who were not exposed to alcohol and were clinically normal. These authors identified abnormality in the shape of the corpus callosum as a consequence of gestational substance abuse. Neuropsychological ratings pertaining to attention, memory, executive function, fine and gross motor performance, and intelligence were also identified. Callosal midline shape in fetal alcohol spectrum disorder subgroups was strikingly more variable than it was in normal individuals. Excess shape variation was associated with two different profiles of behavioral deficit unrelated to full-scale IQ or to the fetal alcohol syndrome/fetal alcohol spectrum distinction within the exposed subgroup. These authors found a relatively thick callosum was associated with a pattern of deficit in executive function; a callosum that is relatively thin was associated with a deficit in motor function.

Treatment

The first approach to treatment is prevention. There is no clearly established safe dose of alcohol for pregnant women. However, mothers of children with fetal alcohol syndrome drank more alcohol and drank excessively early in gestation when contrasted with those with less severe clinical features. Alcohol use in late pregnancy is primarily associated with prematurity and infants who are small for gestational age rather than with fetal alcohol syndrome (Jones et al., 1973). One prospective study of 31,604 pregnancies found that the consumption of 1 to 2 drinks a day was associated with an increased risk of giving birth to a baby who was growth retarded (Mills et al., 1984).The Committee on Substance Abuse and the Committee on Children's Disabilities of the American Academy of Pediatrics (2000) recommends that because there is no known safe amount of alcohol consumption during pregnancy, abstinence from alcohol for women who are pregnant or who are planning a pregnancy is recommended. The committee recommends special efforts toward education about the harmful effects of alcohol, that identified children be referred for early educational services, and that federal legislation for print and broadcast alcohol advertisements read: "Drinking during pregnancy may cause mental retardation and other birth defects. Avoid alcohol during pregnancy."

The development of statewide networks of local fetal alcohol syndrome and fetal alcohol spectrum disorders diagnostic clinics is recommended. Such clinics may coordinate local community care, facilitate early diagnosis, and reduce socially disruptive behavior and school problems. A coordinated system of parent and citizen education courses and a system of ongoing in-service training for care providers is needed. Such programs should focus on strategies for improving quality of life, lengthening the duration of stay in placements out of home, providing life skills, and facilitating job training.

SUMMARY

The recognition and neurobiological investigation of behavioral phenotypes in intellectual disability syndromes is leading to new knowledge about the relationship of brain development to behavior. Studies of these neurogenetic syndromes make clear that the relationship between genes and behavior is not a simple one. Knowing the genetic abnormality is only the first step in beginning to understand the cascade of changes that occur in the brain as a result of a genetic disorder. Finally, studies of brain functioning in carriers of genetic mutations and those with partial expression of the clinical syndromes also can play an important role in understanding cognition, brain, and behavior.

KEY POINTS

1. The first full description of behavior in a genetic syndrome was by J.L.H. Down in 1887.
2. When evaluating a genetic disorder, both physical and behavioral features must be considered.
3. "Behavioral phenotype" is a term that describes outwardly observable behavior that is so characteristic of a genetic disorder that its presence suggests the underlying condition.
4. The behavioral phenotype is a characteristic pattern of motor, cognitive, linguistic, and social behavior.
5. Following characterization of the behavioral phenotype, neurobiologic features linked to it may provide a better understanding of brain development.
6. Behavioral phenotypes from various disorders may be compared for a better understanding of certain behaviors (e.g., obsessive compulsive behaviors and self-injurious behavior).
7. Routine screening for and ongoing monitoring of behavioral phenotypes is essential.
8. Parent organizations play an important role in identifying behavioral phenotypes.
9. Ongoing research on epigenesis is needed to better understand pathways from genes to cognition and complex behaviors.
10. Future interventions must consider the role of preimplantation genetic diagnosis and the application of new research to treatment (e.g., fragile X syndrome and gene reactivation therapy).

General References

Harris, J. (1998). Behavioral phenotypes. In J. Harris *Assessment, diagnosis and treatment of developmental disorders*, pp. 251–376. Oxford University Press, New York.

O'Brien, G. (ed.). (2002). *Behavioural phenotypes in clinical practice*. MacKeith Press, London. Distributed by Cambridge University Press, Cambridge.

O'Brien, G., Pearson, J., Berney, T., and Branard, L. (2001). Measuring behaviour in developmental disability: a review of existing schedules. *Developmental Medicine and Child Neurology* (suppl.), 87:1–72.

O'Brien, G. and Yule, W. (eds.). (1995). *Behavioural phenotypes*. Cambridge University Press, Cambridge.

References

Abel, E.L. (1998). Prevention of alcohol abuse-related birth effects–I. Public education efforts. *Alcohol and Alcoholism*, 33:411–416.

American Academy of Pediatrics Committee on Genetics. (2001). Health supervision for children with Down syndrome. *Pediatrics*, 107:442–449.

American Academy of Pediatrics Committee on Substance Abuse and Committee on Children with Disabilities. (2000). Fetal alcohol syndrome and alcohol-related neurodevelopmental disorders. *Pediatrics*, 106(2 pt. 1):358–361.

American Psychiatric Association. (1987). *Diagnostic and statistical manual of mental disorders*, 3rd ed., revised. Author, Washington, DC.

American Psychiatric Association. (2000). *Diagnostic and statistical manual of mental disorders*, 4th ed., text rev. Author, Washington, DC.

Amir, R.E., Van den Veyver, I.B., Wan, M., Tran, C.Q., Francke, U., and Zoghbi, H.Y. (1999). Rett syndrome is caused by mutations in X-linked *MECP2*, encoding methyl-CpG-binding protein 2. *Nature Genetics*, 23:185–188.

Anderson, L., and Ernst, M. (1994). Self-injury in Lesch-Nyhan disease. *Journal of Autism and Developmental Disorders*, 24:67–81.

Antar, L.N., Afroz, R., Dictenberg, J.B., Carroll, R.C., and Bassell G.J. (2004). Metabotropic glutamate receptor activation regulates fragile X mental retardation protein and *FMR1* mRNA localization differentially in dendrites and at synapses. *Journal of Neuroscience*, 24:2648–2655.

Bakker, C.E., and Oostra, B.A. (2003). Understanding fragile X syndrome: Insights from animal models. *Cytogenetic and Genome Research*, 100:111–123.

Ball, T.S., Datta, P.C., Rios, M., and Constantine, C. (1985). Flexible arm splints in the control of a Lesch-Nyhan victim's finger biting and a profoundly retarded client's finger sucking. *Journal of Autism and Developmetal Disorders*, 15:177–184.

Batch, J. (2002). Turner syndrome in childhood and adolescence. *Best Practices and Research. Clinical Endocrinology and Metabolism*. 16:465–482.

Bellugi, U., Lichtenberger, L., Jones, W., Lai, Z., and St. George, M. (2000). The neurocognitive profile of Williams syndrome: A complex pattern of strengths and weaknesses. *Journal of Cognitive Neuroscience*, 12:7–29.

Bishop, D.V. (1999). Perspectives: cognition. An innate basis for language? *Science*, 286: 2283–2284.

Boddaert, N., De Leersnyder, H., Bourgeois, M., Munnich, A., Brunelle, F., and Zilbovicius, M. (2004). Anatomical and functional brain imaging evidence of lenticulo-insular anomalies in Smith Magenis syndrome. *Neuroimage*, 21:1021–1025.

Bookstein, F.L., Streissguth, A.P., Sampson, P.D., Connor, P.D., and Barr, H.M. (2002). Corpus callosum shape and neuropsychological deficits in adult males with heavy fetal alcohol exposure. *Neuroimage*, 15:233–251.

Bower, B.D., and Jeavons, P.M. (1967). The "happy puppet" syndrome. *Archives of Diseases of Childhood,* 42:298–302.

Brunner, H.G., Nelen, M.R., van Zandvoort, P., Abeling, N.G., van Gennip, A.H., Wolters, E.C., Kuiper, M.A., Ropers, H.H., and van Oost, B.A. (1993). X-linked borderline mental retardation with prominent behavioral disturbance: Phenotype, genetic localization, and evidence for disturbed monoamine metabolism. *American Journal of Human Genetics,* 52:1032–1039.

Cases, O., Seif, I., Grimsby, J., Gaspar, P., Chen, K., Pournin, S., Muller, U., Aguet, M., Babinet, C., Shih, J.C., et al. (1995). Aggressive behavior and altered amounts of brain serotonin and norepinephrine in mice lacking MAOA. *Science,* 268:1763–1766.

Cass, H., Reilly, S., Owen, L., Wisbeach, A., Weekes, L., Slonims, V., Wigram, T., and Charman, T. (2003). Findings from a multidisciplinary clinical case series of females with Rett syndrome. *Developmental Medicine and Child Neurology,* 45:325–337.

CDC (2002). Fetal alcohol syndrome—Alaska, Arizona, Colorado, and New York, 1995–1997. *MMWR Morbidity and Mortality Weekly Reports,* 51:433–435.

Chapman R.S., and Hesketh, L.J. (2000). Behavioral phenotype of individuals with Down syndrome. *Mental Retardation and Developmental Disability Research Reviews,* 6: 84–95.

Clark, D., and Wilson, G.N. (2003). Behavioral assessment of children with Down syndrome using the Reiss psychopathology scale. *American Journal of Medical Genetics,* 118A:210–216.

Clarren, S.K., and Smith, D.W. (1978). The fetal alcohol syndrome. *New England Journal of Medicine,* 298:1063–1067.

Clayton-Smith, J. (1992). Angelman syndrome. *Archives of Disease in Childhood,* 67: 889–891.

Cohen, W.I. (1999). Health care guidelines for individuals with Down syndrome: 1999 revision. *Down Syndrome Quarterly,* 4:1–15. (www.denison.edu/collaborations/dsq/health99.html)

Connor, J.M., and Loughlin, S.A.R. (1991). Molecular genetic analysis in Turner syndrome. In M.B. Rande and R.G. Rosenfeld (eds.), *Turner syndrome: Growth promoting therapies,* pp. 3–8. Elsevier, Amsterdam.

Critchley, M., and Earl, C.J.C. (1932). Tuberous sclerosis and allied conditions. *Brain,* 55:311–346.

Deb, S., de Silva, P.N., Gemmell, H.G., Besson, J.A., Smith, F.W., and Ebmeier, K.P. (1992). Alzheimer's disease in adults with Down's syndrome: The relationship between regional cerebral blood flow equivalents and dementia. *Acta Psychiatrica Scandinavica,* 86:340–345.

Devenny, D.A., Silverman, W.P., Hill, A.L., Jenkins, E., Sersen, E.A., and Wisniewski, K.E. (1996). Normal ageing in adults with Down's syndrome: A longitudinal study. *Journal of Intellectual Disability Research,* 40:208–221.

Donovan, C.L. (1991). Factors predisposing, enabling, and reinforcing routine screening of patients for preventing fetal alcohol syndrome: A survey of New Jersey physicians. *Journal of Drug Education,* 21:35–42.

Down, J.L. (1887). *Mental affectations of childhood and youth.* J.A. Churchill, London.

Dunn, H.G., Stoessl, A.J., Ho, H.H., MacLeod, P.M., Poskitt, K.J., Doudet, D.J., Schulzer, M., Blackstock, D., Dobko, T., Koop, B., and de Amorim, G.V. (2002). Rett syndrome: Investigation of nine patients, including PET scan. *Canadian Journal of Neurological Science,* 29:345–357.

Dykens E., Finucane, B.M., and Gayley, C. (1997). Brief report:Cognitive and behavioral profiles in persons with Smith-Magenis syndrome. *Journal of Autism and Developmental Disorders*, 27:203–211.

Dykens, E., Hodapp, R.M., and Evans, E.W. (1994). Profiles and development of adaptive behavior in children with Down syndrome. *American Journal of Mental Retardation*, 98: 580–558.

Dykens, E., and Shah, B. (2003). Psychiatric disorders in Prader-Willi Syndrome. *CNS Drugs*, 17:167–178.

Eads, J.C., Scapin, G., Xu, Y., Grubmeyer, C., and Sacchettin, C. (1994). The crystal structure of human hypoanthine-guanine phosphoribosyltransferase with bound GMP. *Cell*, 78:325–334.

el Abd, S., Turk, J., and Hill, P. (1995). Psychological characteristics of Turner syndrome. *Journal of Child Psychology and Psychiatry*, 36:1109–1125.

Eliez, S., Schmitt, J.E., White, C.D., and Reiss, A.L. (2000). Children and adolescents with velocardiofacial syndrome: A volumetric MRI study. *American Journal of Psychiatry*. 157:409–415.

Ernst, M., Zametkin, A.J., Matochik, J.A., Pascualvaca, D., Jons, P.H., Hardy, K., Hankerson, J.G., Doudet, D.J., and Cohen, R.M. (1996). Presynaptic dopaminergic deficits in Lesch-Nyhan disease. *New England Journal of Medicine*. 334:1568–1572.

Esquirol, J.E. (1965). *Mental maladies: A treatise on insanity.* Facsimile of the English edition of 1845. Hafner, New York.

Finucane, B.M., Konar, D., Haas-Givler, B., Kurtz, M.B., and Scott, C.I., Jr. (1994). The spasmodic upper-body squeeze: A characteristic behavior in Smith-Magenis syndrome. *Developmental Medicine and Child Neurology*, 36:78–83.

Flint J. (1996). Annotation: Behavioural phenotypes: A window onto the biology of behaviour. *Journal of Child Psychology and Psychiatry*, 37:355–367.

Flint J. (1998). Behavioral phenotypes: Conceptual and methodological issues. *American Journal of Medical Genetics*, 81:235–240.

Flint J. (1999). The genetic basis of cognition. *Brain*, 122:2015–2031.

Flint J., and Yule, W. (1994). Behavioural phenotypes. In M. Rutter, E. Taylor, and L. Hersov, (eds.), *Child and adolescent psychiatry*, 3rd ed., pp. 666–687. Blackwell Scientific, Oxford.

Ford, C.E., Jones, K.W., Polani, P.E., de Almeida, J.C., and Briggs, J.H. (1959). A sex-chromosome anomaly in a case of gonadal dysgenesis (Turner syndrome). *Lancet*, 1:711–713.

Frangiskakis, J.M., Ewart, A.K., Morris, C.A., Mervis, C. B., Bertrand, J., Robinson, B. F., Klein, B. P., Ensing, G. J., Everett, L. A., Green, E. D., et al. (1996). LIM-kinase 1 hemizygosity implicated in impaired visuospatial constructive cognition. *Cell*, 86: 59–69.

Galaburda, A.M., and Bellugi, U. (2000). Multi-level analysis of cortical neuroanatomy in Williams syndrome. *Journal of Cognitive Neuroscience*, 12:74–88.

Gath, A., and Gumley, D. (1986). Behavior problems in retarded children with special reference to Down's syndrome. *British Journal of Psychiatry*, 149:156–161.

Ghaziuddin M. (2000). Autism in Down's syndrome: A family history study. *Journal of Intellectual Disability Research*, 44:562–566.

Golding-Kushner, K.J., Weller, G., and Shprintzen, R.J. (1985). Velo-cardio-facial syndrome: Language and psychological profiles. *Journal of Craniofacial Genetics and Development Biology*, 5:259–266.

Gothelf, D., Frisch, A., Munitz, H., Rockah, R., Laufer, N., Mozes, T., Hermesh, H., Weizman, A., and Frydman, M. (1999). Clinical characteristics of schizophrenia associated with velo-cardio-facial syndrome. *Schizophrenia Research*, 35:105–112.

Graf, W.D., Unis, A.S., Yates, C.M., Sulzbacher, S., Dinulos, M.B., Jack, R.M., Dugaw, K.A., Paddock, M.N., and Parson, W.W. (2001). Catecholamines in patients with 22q11.2 deletion syndrome and the low-activity COMT polymorphism. *Neurology,* 57:410–416.

Greenberg, F. (1990). Willams syndrome professional symposium. *American Journal of Medical Genetics,* 6:85–88.

Greenberg, F., Guzzetta, V., Montes de Oca-Luna, R., Magenis, E., Smith, A.C., Richter, S.F., Kondo, I., Dobyns, W.B., Patel, P.I., and Lupski, J.R. (1991). Molecular analysis of the Smith-Magenis syndrome: A possible contiguous-gene syndrome associated with del(17)(p11.2). *American Journal of Human Genetics,* 49:1207–1218.

Gross-Tsur, V., Landau, Y.E., Benarroch, F., Wertman-Elad, R., and Shalev, R.S. (2001). Cognition, attention, and behavior in Prader-Willi syndrome. *Journal of Child Neurology,* 16:288–290.

Gunn, P., Berry P., and Andrews, R.J. (1981). The temperament of Down's syndrome in infants: A research note. *Journal of Child Psychology and Psychiatry,* 22:189–194.

Hagberg, B., Aicardi, J., Dias, K., and Ramos, O. (1983). A progressive syndrome of autism, dementia, ataxia, and loss of purposeful hand use in girls: Rett's syndrome: Report of 35 cases. *Annals of Neurology,* 14:471–479.

Hagerman, R. (1999a). Clinical and molecular aspects of fragile X syndrome. In H. Tager-Flusberg (ed.), *Neurodevelopmental disorders,* pp. 27–42. MIT Press, Cambridge, MA.

Hagerman, R.J. (1999b). Neurodevelopmental disorders: Diagnosis and treatment. In J. Harris, (ed.), *Series developmental perspectives in psychiatry.* Oxford University Press, New York.

Hagerman, R.J., and Cronister, A.C. (eds.) (1996). *The fragile X syndrome: Diagnosis, treatment, and research,* 2nd ed. Johns Hopkins University Press, Baltimore.

Hall, J.G. (1990). Genomic imprinting: Review and relevance to human diseases. *American Journal of Human Genetics,* 46:103–123.

Hall, J.G., and Gilchrist, D.M. (1990). Turner syndrome and its variants. *Pediatric Clinics of North America,* 37:1421–1440.

Harris, J. (1987). Behavioral phenotypes in mental retardation syndromes. In R. Barrett and J. Matson (eds.), *Advances in developmental disorders,* Vol. 1, pp. 77–106. Jai Publishing, New York.

Harris, J. (1998a). Introduction to behavioral phenotypes. In J. Harris (ed.), *Assessment, diagnosis and treatment of developmental disorders,* pp. 245–249. Oxford University Press, New York.

Harris, J. (1998b). Lesch-Nyhan disease. In J. Harris (ed.), *Assessment, diagnosis and treatment of developmental disorders,* pp. 306–318. Oxford University Press, New York.

Harris, J., Lee, R.R., Jinnah, H.A., Wong, D.F., Yaster, M., and Bryan, R.N. (1998). Craniocerebral magnetic resonance imaging measurement and findings in Lesch-Nyhan syndrome. *Archives of Neurology,* 55:547–553.

Harris, J., Wong, D.F., Jinnah, H.A., Schretlen, D., Yokoi, F., Stephane, M., and Dogen, S. (1999). Dopamine transporter binding of WIN 35,428 correlates with HPRT level and extent of movement disorder but not with self-injurious behavior. Abstracts, *Society for Neuroscience,* 25.

Hatton, D.D., Bailey, D.B., Hargett-Beck, M.Q., Skinner, M., and Clark, R.D. (1999). Behavioral style of young boys with fragile X syndrome. *Developmental Medicine and Child Neurology,* 41:625–632.

Hattori, M., Fujiyama, A., Taylor, T.D., Watanabe, H., Yada, T., Park, H.S., Toyoda, A.,

Ishii, K., Totoki, Y., and Choi, D.K., (2000). The DNA sequence of chromosome 21. *Nature,* 405:311–319.

Heineman-de Boer, J.A., Van Haelst, M.J., Cordia-de Haan, M., and Beemer, F.A. (1999). Behavior problems and personality aspects of 40 children with velo-cardio-facial syndrome. *Genetic Counseling,* 10:89–93.

Hill, A.L. (1978). Savants: Mentally retarded individuals with special skills. *International Review of Research in Mental Retardation,* 9:277–298.

Hinton, V.J., Brown, W.T., Wisniewski, K., and Rudelli, R.D. (1991). Analysis of neocortex in three males with fragile X syndrome. *American Journal of Medical Genetics,* 41:289–294.

Holliday R. (1987). The inheritance of epigenetic defects. *Science,* 238:163–170.

Holliday R. (2002). Epigenetics comes of age in the twenty first century. *Journal of Genetics,* 81:1–4.

Holm, V.A., and Pipes, L. (1976). Food and children with the Prader-Willi syndrome. *American Journal of Diseases of Children,* 130:1063–1067.

Holm, V.A., Sulzbacher, S., and Pipes, P.L. (1981). *The Prader-Willi syndrome.* University Park Press, Baltimore.

Howlin, P., Davies, M., and Udwin, O. (1998). Cognitive functioning in adults with Williams syndrome. *Journal of Child Psychology and Psychiatry,* 39:183–189.

Huffner, U.T.E., and Redlin, W. (1976). Imitation responses in mongoloid children. *Zeitschrift fur Klinische Psychologie. Forschung und Praxis,* 5:277–286.

Ikonomidou, C., Bittigau, P., Ishimaru, M.J., Wozniak, D.F., Koch, C., Genz, K., Price, M.T., Stefovska, V., Horster, F., Tenkova, T., et al. (2000). Ethanol-induced apoptotic neurodegeneration and fetal alcohol syndrome. *Science,* 287:1056–1058.

Institute of Medicine. (1996). *Fetal alcohol syndrome, diagnosis, epidemiology, prevention and treatment,* K. Stratton, C. Howe, and F. Battaglia, (eds.), pp. 4–5, National Academy Press, Washington, DC.

Janicki, M.P., and Dalton, A.J. (2000). Prevalence of dementia and impact on intellectual disability services. *Mental Retardation,* 38:276–278.

Jin, P., and Warren, S.T. (2000). Understanding the molecular basis of fragile X syndrome. *Human Molecular Genetics,* 9:901–908.

Jones, A.M., Kennedy, N., Hanson, J., and Fenton, G.W. (1997). A study of dementia in adults with Down's syndrome using 99Tc(m)-HMPAO SPECT. *Nuclear Medicine Communications,* 18:662–667.

Jones, K.L. (1986). Fetal alcohol syndrome. *Pediatrics in Review,* 8:122–126.

Jones, K.L., Smith, D.W., Ulleland, C.N., and Streissguth, A.P. (1973). Pattern of malformation in offspring of chronic alcoholic mothers. *Lancet,* 1267–1271.

Jones, W., Bellugi, U., and Lai, Z. Hypersociability in Williams syndrome. (2000). *Journal of Cognitive Neuroscience,* 12:30–46.

Karmiloff-Smith, A., Grant, J., Berthoud, I., Davies, M., Howlin, P., and Udwin, O. (1997). Language and Williams syndrome: How intact is "intact"? *Child Development,* 68:246–262.

Kates, W.R., Folley, B.S., Lanham, D.C., Capone, G.T., and Kaufmann, W.E. (2002). Cerebral growth in fragile X syndrome: Review and comparison with Down syndrome. *Microscopy Research and Technique,* 57:159–167.

Kesler, S.R., Haberecht, M.F., Menon, V., Warsofsky, I.S., Dyer-Friedman, J., Neely, E.K., and Reiss, A.L. (2004). Functional neuroanatomy of spatial orientation processing in Turner syndrome. *Cerebral Cortex,* 14:174–180.

Kim, J.J., Shih, J.C., Chen, K., Chen, L., Bao, S., Maren, S., Anagnostaras, S.G., Fanselow, M.S., De Maeye, E., Seif, I., and Thompson, R.F. (1997). Selective enhancement of emotional, but not motor, learning in monoamine oxidase A-deficient mice. *Proceedings of the National Academy of Sciences USA.* 94:5929–5933.

Kooy, R.F. (2003). Of mice and the fragile X syndrome. *Trends in Genetics,* 19:148–154.

Korenberg, J.R., Xiao-Ning, C., Hirota, H., Lai, Z., Bellugi, U., Burian, D., Roe, B., and Matsuoka, R. (2000). Genome structure and cognitive map of Williams syndrome. *Journal of Cognitive Neuroscience,* 12:89–107.

Lederberg, J. (2001). The meaning of epigenetics. *The Scientist,* 15:6–7.

Lee, K.T., Mattson, S.N., and Riley, E.P. (2004). Classifying children with heavy prenatal alcohol exposure using measures of attention. *Journal of the International Neuropsychological Society,* 10:271–277.

Lemoine, P., Harrousseau, H., Borteryu, J.P., and Menuet, J.C. (1968). Les enfants de parents alcooliques: Anomalies observees a propos de 127 cas. [The children of alcoholic parents: Anomalies observed in 127 cases.] *Quest Medicale,* 21:476–482.

Leonard, C.M., Williams, C.A., Nicholls, R.D., Agee, O.F., Voeller, K.K., Honeyman, J.C., and Staa, E.V. (1993). Angelman and Prader-Willi syndrome: A magnetic resonance imaging study of differences in cerebral structure. *American Journal of Medical Genetics,* 46:26–33.

Letts, R.M., and Hobson, D.A. (1975). Special devices as aids in the management of child self-mutilation in the Lesch-Nyhan syndrome. *Pediatrics,* 55:852–855.

Lloyd, K.G., Hornykiewicz, O., Davidson, L., Shannak, K., Farley, I., Goldstein, M., Shibuya, M., Kelley, W.N., and Fox, I.H. (1981). Biochemical evidence of dysfunction of brain neurotransmitters in the Lesch–Nyhan syndrome. *New England Journal of Medicine,* 305:1106–1111.

Mattson, S.N., Goodman, A.M., Caine, C., Delis, D.C., and Riley, E.P. (1999). Executive functioning in children with heavy prenatal alcohol exposure. *Alcoholism Clinical and Experimental Research,* 23:1808–1815.

Mazzocco, M.M. (2000). Advances in research on the fragile X syndrome. *Mental Retardation and Developmental Disability Research Reviews,* 6:96–106.

McCauley, E., Kay, T., Ito, J., and Treder, R. (1987). The Turner syndrome: Cognitive deficits, affective discrimination, and behavior problems. *Child Development,* 58:464–473.

Miller, W.J., Skinner, J.A., Foss, G.S., and Davies, K.E. (2000). Localization of the fragile X mental retardation 2 (FMR2) protein in mammalian brain. *European Journal of Neuroscience,* 12:381–384.

Mills, D.L., Alvarez, T.D., St. George, M., Appelbaum, L.G., Bellugi, U., and Neville, H. (2000). Electrophysiological studies of face processing in Williams syndrome. *Journal of Cognitive Neuroscience,* 12:47–64.

Mills, J.L., Graubard, B.I., Harley, E.E., Rhoads, G.G. and Berends, H.W. (1984). Maternal alcohol consumption and birth weight: How much drinking in pregnancy is safe? *Journal of the American Medical Association,* 252:1875–1879.

Moncla, A., Malzac, P., Livet, M.O., Voelckel, M.A., Mancini, J., Delaroziere, J.C., Philip, N., and Mattei, J.F. (1999a). Angelman syndrome resulting from *UBE3A* mutations in 14 patients from eight families: Clinical manifestations and genetic counselling. *Journal of Medical Genetics,* 36:554–560.

Moncla, A., Malzac, P., Voelckel, M.A., Auquier, P., Girardot, L., Mattei, M.G., Philip, N., Mattei, J.F., Lalande, M., and Livet, M.O. (1999b). Phenotype-genotype correlation in 20 deletion and 20 non-deletion Angelman syndrome patients. *European Journal of Human Genetics,* 7:131–139.

Morris, C.A., Mervis, C.B., Hobart, H.H., Gregg, R.G., Bertrand, J., Ensing, G.J., Sommer, A., Moore, C.A., Hopkin, R.J., Spallone, P.A., et al. (2003). *GTF2I* hemizygosity implicated in mental retardation in Williams syndrome: Genotype-phenotype analysis of five families with deletions in the Williams syndrome region. *American Journal of Medical Genetics,* 123:45–59.

Morris, C.A., Pober, B., Wang, P., et al. (1999). *Medical guidelines for Williams syndrome.* Williams Syndrome Association (www.williams-syndrome.org).

Muscatelli, F., Abrous, D.N., Massacrier, A., Boccaccio, I., Le Moal, M., Cau, P., and Cremer, H. (2000). Disruption of the mouse Necdin gene results in hypothalamic and behavioral alterations reminiscent of the human Prader-Willi syndrome. *Human Molecular Genetics,* 9:3101–3110.

Naidu, S., Kaufmann, W.E., Abrams, M.T., Pearlson, G.D., Lanham, D.C., Fredericksen, K.A., Barker, P.B., Horska, A., Golay, X., Mori, S., et al. (2001). Neuroimaging studies in Rett syndrome. *Brain and Development,* 23:62–71.

Nicholls, R.D., Saitoh, S., and Horsthemke, B. (1998). Imprinting in Prader-Willi and Angelman syndromes. *Trends in Genetics,* 14:194–200.

Nyborg, H., and Nielsen, J. (1977). Sex chromosome abnormalities and cognitive performance: III. Field dependence, frame dependence, and failing development of perceptual stability in girls with Turner's syndrome. *Journal of Psychology,* 96:205–211.

Nyhan, W. (1972). Behavioral phenotypes in organic genetic disease. Presidential address to the Society for Pediatric Research, May 1, 1971. *Pediatric Research,* 6:1–9.

Nyham, W. (1976). Behavior in Lesch-Nyham syndrome. *Journal of Autism and Childhood Schizophrenia,* 6:235–252.

Nyhan, W. (1995). Lesch-Nyhan syndrome. In G. O'Brien and W. Yule (eds.), *Behavioural phenotypes.* Cambridge University Press, Cambridge.

O'Brien, G. (1991). *Behavioural measurement in mental handicap: A guide to existing schedules.* Society for the Study of Behavioural Phenotypes, Oxford, England.

O'Brien, G. (1992). Behavioural phenotypy in developmental psychiatry. *European Journal of Child and Adolescent Psychiatry,* 1:1–61.

Page T., and Nyhan, W.L. (1989). The spectrum of HPRT deficiency: An update. *Advances in Experimental Medicine and Biology,* 253A:129–132.

Paterson, S.J., Brown, J.H., Gsodl, M.K., Johnson, M.H., and Karmiloff-Smith, A. (1999). Cognitive modularity and genetic disorders. *Science,* 286:2355–2358.

Paylor, R., McIlwain, K.L., McAninch, R, Nellis, A., Yuva-Paylor, L.A., Baldini, A., and Lindsay, E.A. (2001). Mice deleted for the DiGeorge/velocardiofacial syndrome region show abnormal sensorimotor gating and learning and memory impairments. *Human Molecular Genetics,* 10:2645–2650.

Pietrini, P., Dani. A., Furey, M.L., Alexander, G.E., Freo, U., Grady, C.L., Mentis, M.J., Mangot, D., Simon, E.W., Horwitz, B., et al. (1997). Low glucose metabolism during brain stimulation in older Down's syndrome subjects at risk for Alzheimer's disease prior to dementia. *American Journal of Psychiatry,* 154:1063–1069.

Pike, A.C., and Super, M. (1997). Velocardiofacial syndrome. *Postgraduate Medical Journal,* 73:771–775.

Pinter, J.D., Eliez, S., Schmitt, J.E., Capone, G.T., and Reiss, A.L. (2001). Neuroanatomy of Down's syndrome: A high-resolution MRI study. *American Journal of Psychiatry,* 158:1659–1665.

Prader, A., Labhart, A., and Willi, H. (1956). Ein syndrom von adipositas, kleinwuchs, kryptorchismus und oligophrenie nach myatonieartigem zustand in neugeborenenalter. *Schineizerische Medizinische Wochenschrift,* 86:1260–1261.

Prasher, V.P., Chowdhury, T.A., Rowe, B.R., and Bain, S.C. (1997). ApoE genotype and Alzheimer's disease in adults with Down syndrome: Meta-analysis. *American Journal of Mental Retardation,* 102:103–110.

Pueschel, S.M., Gallagher, P.L., Zartler, A.S., and Pezzullo, J.C. (1987). Cognitive and learning processes in children with Down syndrome. *Research in Developmental Disabilities,* 8:21–37.

Pulver, A.E., Nestadt, G., Goldberg, R., Shprintzen, R.J., Lamacz, M., Wolyniec, P.S., Morrow, B., Karayiorgou, M., Antonarakis, S E., Housman, D., et al. (1994). Psychotic illness in patients diagnosed with velo-cardio-facial syndrome and their relatives. *Journal of Nervous and Mental Disease,* 182:476–478.

Rattazzi, M.C., LaFauci, G., and Brown, W.T. (2004). Prospects for gene therapy in the fragile X syndrome. *Mental Retardation and Developmental Disability Research Reviews,* 10:75–81.

Ray, P.F., Harper, J.C., Ao, A., Taylor, D.M., Winston, R.M., Hughes, M., and Handyside, A.H. (1999). Successful preimplantation genetic diagnosis for sex linked Lesch-Nyhan Syndrome using specific diagnosis. *Prenatal Diagnosis,* 19:1237–1241.

Reiss, A.L., Freund, L., Plotnick, L., Baumgardner, T., Green, K., Sozer, A.C., Reader, M., Boehm, C, and Denckla, M.B. (1993). The effects of X monosomy on brain development: Monozygotic twins discordant for Turner's syndrome. *Annals of Neurology,* 34:95–107.

Reiss, A.L., Eliez, S., Schmitt, E., Straus, E., Lai, Z., Jones, W., and Bellugi, U. (2000). Neuroanatomy of Williams syndrome: A high resolution MRI study. *Journal of Cognitive Neuroscience,* 12(Suppl. 1):65–73.

Riikonen, R., Salonen, I., Partanen, K., and Verho, S. (1999). Brain perfusion SPECT and MRI in foetal alcohol syndrome. *Developmental Medicine and Child Neurology,* 41:652–659.

Riikonen, R.S. (1994). Difference in susceptibility to teratogenic effects of alcohol in discordant twins exposed to alcohol during the second half of gestation. *Pediatric Neurology,* 11:332–336.

Roizen, N.J. (2002). Medical care and monitoring for the adolescent with Down syndrome. *Adolescent Medicine Sate of the Arts Reviews,* 13:345–358.

Roizen, N.J., and Patterson, D. (2003). Down's syndrome. *Lancet,* 361:1281–1289.

Roof, E., Stone, W., MacLean, W. Feurer, I.D., Thompson, T., and Butler, M.G. (2000). Intellectual characteristics of Prader-Willi syndrome: Comparison of genetic subtypes. *Journal of Intellectual Disability Research,* 44:25–30.

Ross, J.L., Stefanatos, G., Roeltgen, D., Kushner, H., and Cutler, G.B., Jr. (1995). Ullrich-Turner syndrome: Neurodevelopmental changes from childhood through adolescence. *American Journal of Medical Genetics,* 58:74–82.

Rovet, J., and Ireland, L. (1994.) Behavioral phenotype in children with Turner syndrome. *Journal of Pediatric Psychology,* 19:779–790.

Rovet, J.F. (1993). The psychoeducational characteristics of children with Turner syndrome. *Journal of Learning Disability,* 26:333–341.

Sampson, P.D., Streissguth, A.P., Bookstein, F.L., Little, R.E., Clarre, S.K., Dehaene, P., Hanson, J.W., and Graham, J.M. Jr. (1997). Incidence of fetal alcohol syndrome and prevalence of alcohol-related neurodevelopmental disorder. *Teratology,* 56: 317–326.

Schupf, N., Pang, D., Patel, B.N., Silverman, W., Schubert, R., Lai, F., Kline, J.K., Stern, Y., Ferin, M., Tycko, B., and Mayeux, R. (2003). Onset of dementia is associated with age at menopause in women with Down's syndrome. *Annals of Neurology,* 54: 433–438.

Schupf, N., and Sergievsky, G.H. (2002). Genetic and host factors for dementia in Down's syndrome. *British Journal of Psychiatry*, 180:405–410.

Seegmiller, J.E., Rosenbloom, F.M., and Kelley, W.N. (1967). Enzyme deficit associated with a sex-linked human neurological disorder and excessive purine synthesis. *Science*, 155:1682–1684.

Shapira, N.A., Lessig, M.C., He, A.G., James, G.A., Driscoll, D.J., and Lui, Y. (2005). Satiety dysfunction i Prader-Willi syndrome demonstrated by fMRI. *Journal of Neurology, Neurosurgery and Psychiatry*, 76:260–262.

Shprintzen, R.J., Goldberg, R.B., Young, D., and Wolford, L. (1981). The velo-cardio-facial syndrome: A clinical and genetic analysis. *Pediatrics*, 67:167–172.

Shretlen, D., Harris, J., Park, K.S., Jinnah, H.A., and del Pozo, N.O. (2001). Neurocognitive functioning in Lesch-Nyhan disease and partial hypoxanthine-guanine phosphoribosyltransferase deficiency. *Journal of the International Neuropsychological Society*, 7:805–812.

Siegel, P.T., Clopper, R., and Stabler, B. (1998). The psychological consequences of Turner syndrome and review of the National Cooperative Growth Study psychological substudy. *Pediatrics*, 102:488–491.

Simeon, D., Stein, D.J., Gross, S., Islam, N., Schmeidler, J., and Hollander, E. (1997). A double-blind trial of fluoxetine in pathologic skin picking. *Journal of Clinical Psychiatry*, 58:341–347.

Skuse, D., Elgar, K., and Morris, E. (1999). Quality of life in Turner syndrome is related to chromosomal constitution: Implications for genetic counselling and management. *Acta Paediatrica*, 88:110–113.

Skuse, D.H. (2000). Behavioural phenotypes: What do they teach us? *Archives of Disease in Childhood*, 82:222–225.

Slager, R.E., Newton, T.L., Vlangos, C.N., Finucane, B., and Elsea, S.H. (2003). Mutations in *RAI1* associated with Smith-Magenis syndrome. *Nature Genetics*, 33:466–468.

Smith, A.C. (2001). Health care management of adults with Down syndrome. *American Family Physician*, 64:1031–1040.

Smith, A.C., Dykens, E, and Greenberg, F. (1998a). Behavioral phenotype of Smith-Magenis syndrome (del 17p11.2). *American Journal of Medical Genetics*, 81:179–185.

Smith, A.C., Dykens, E, and Greenberg, F. (1998b). Sleep disturbance in Smith-Magenis syndrome (del 17 p11.2). *American Journal of Medical Genetics*, 81:186–191.

Smith, A.C., McGavran, L., Robinson, J., Waldstein, G., Macfarlane, J., Zonona, J., Reiss, J., Lahr, M., Allen, L., and Magenis, E. (1986). Interstitial deletion of (17)(p11.2p11.2) in nine patients. *American Journal of Medical Genetics*, 24:393–414.

State, M.W., and Dykens, E.M. (2000). Genetics of childhood disorders: XV. Prader-Willi syndrome: genes, brain, and behavior. *Journal of the American Academy of Child and Adolescent Psychiatry*, 39:797–800.

State, M.W., and Dykens, E.M., Rosner, B., Martin, A., and King, B.H. (1999). Obsessive-compulsive symptoms in Prader-Willi and "Prader-Willi-like" patients. *Journal of the American Academy of Child and Adolescent Psychiatry*, 38:329–334.

Stein, D.J., Keating, J., and Zar, H. (1993). Compulsive and impulsive symptoms in Prader-Willi syndrome. *Abstracts in New Research (NR33)*. Annual Meeting of the American Psychiatric Association. San Francisco, CA, May.

Streissguth, A.P., Aase, J.M., Clarren, S.K., Randels, S.P., Ladue, R.A. and Smith, D.F.

(1991). Fetal alcohol syndrome in adolescents and adults. *Journal of the American Medical Association,* 265:1961–1967.

Streissguth, A.P., Bookstein, F.L., Barr, H.M., Sampson, P.D., O'Malley, K., Young J.K. (2004) Risk factors for adverse life outcomes in fetal alcohol syndrome and fetal alcohol effects. *Journal of Developmental and Behavioral Pediatrics,* 25:228–238.

Streissguth, A.P., and O'Malley, K. (2000). "Neuropsychiatric implications and long-term consequences of fetal alcohol spectrum disorders." *Seminars in Clinical Neuropsychiatry* 5:177–190.

Stromme, P., Bjornstad, P.G., and Ramstad, K. (2002). Prevalence estimation of Williams syndrome. *Journal of Child Neurology,* 17:269–271.

Summers, J.S., Lynch, P.S., Harris, J.C., Burke, J.C., Allison, D.B., and Sandler, L. (1992). A combined behavioral/pharmacological treatment of sleep-wake schedule disorder in Angelman syndrome. *Journal of Developmental and Behavioral Pediatrics,* 13:284–287.

Swaab, D.F., Purba, J.S., and Hofman, M.A. (1995). Alterations in the hypothalamic paraventricular nucleus and its oxytocin neurons (putative satiety cells) in Prader-Willi syndrome: A study of five cases. *Journal of Clinical Endocrinology and Metabolism,* 80:573–579.

Swillen, A., Fryns, J.P., Kleczkowska, A., Massa, G., Vanderschueren-Lodeweyck, M., and Van den Berghe, H. (1993). Intelligence, behaviour and psychosocial development in Turner syndrome. A cross-sectional study of 50 pre-adolescent and adolescent girls (4–20 years). *Genetic Counseling,* 4:7–18.

Swillen, A., Vandeputte, L., Cracco, J., Maes, B., Ghesquiere, P., Devriendt, K., and Fryns, J.P. (1999). Neuropsychological, learning and psychosocial profile of primary school aged children with the velo-cardio-facial syndrome (22q 11 deletion): evidence for a nonverbal learning disability? Neuropsychology, development, and cognition. Section C, *Child Neuropsychology,* 5:230–241.

Tager-Flusberg, H., Boshart, J., and Baron-Cohen, S. (1998). Reading the windows to the soul: Evidence of domain-specific sparing in Williams syndrome. *Journal of Cognitive Neuroscience,* 10:631–639.

Taira, T., Kobayashi, T., and Hori, T. (2003). Disappearance of self-mutilating behavior in a patient with Lesch-Nyhan syndrome after bilateral chronic stimulation of the globus pallidus internus. Case report. *Journal of Neurosurgery,* 98:414–416.

Tamm, L., Menon, V., Johnston, C.K, Hessl, D.R., and Reiss, A.L. (2002). fMRI study of cognitive interference processing in females with fragile X syndrome. *Journal of Cognitive Neuroscience,* 14:160–171.

Tassabehji, M., Metcalfe, K., Karmiloff-Smith, A., Carette, M.J., Grant, J., Dennis, N., Reardon, W., Splitt, M., Read, A. P., and Donnai, D. (1999). Williams Syndrome: Use of chromosomal microdeletions as a tool to dissect cognitive and physical phenotypes. *American Journal of Human Geneticst,* 64:118–125.

The Rett Syndrome Diagnostic Criteria Work Group. (1988). Diagnostic criteria for Rett syndrome. *Annals of Neurology,* 23:425–428.

Thompson, M.G., McInnes, R.R., and Willard, H.F. (2001). *Genetics in medicine,* 5th ed., p. 215. W.B. Saunders, Philadelphia.

Teipel, S.J., Alexander, G.E., Schapiro, M.B., Moller, H.J., Rapoport, S.I., and Hampel, H. (2004). Age-related cortical grey matter reductions in non-demented Down's syndrome adults determined by MRI with voxel-based morphometry. *Brain,* 127: 811–824.

Tower, C. (1989). *Understanding child abuse and neglect.* Allyn and Bacon, Boston, MA.

Turner, H H. (1938). A syndrome of infantilism, congenital webbed neck, and cubitus valgus. *Endocrinology,* 23:566–574.

Udwin, O., Webber, C., and Horn, I. (2001). Abilities and attainment in Smith-Magenis syndrome. *Developmental Medicine and Child Neurology,* 43:823–828.

Ullrich, O. (1930). *Z. Kinderheilk,* 49:271–276.

Valenti-Hein, D., and Schwartz, L. (1995). *The sexual abuse interview for those with developmental disabilities.* James Stanfield Company, Santa Barbara, CA.

Vantrappen, G., Devriendt, K., Swillen, A., Rommel, N., Vogels, A., Eyskens, B., Gewillig, M., Feenstra, L., and Fryns, J.P. (1999). Presenting symptoms and clinical features in 130 patients with the velo-cardio-facial syndrome. The Leuven experience. *Genetic Counseling,* 10:3–9.

Vliet, G.V., Deal, C.L., Crock, P.A., Robitaille, Y., and Oligny L.L. (2004). Sudden death in growth hormone-treated children with Prader-Willi syndrome. *Journal of Pediatrics.* 144:129–131.

von Tetzchner, S., Jacobsen, K.H., Smith, L., Skjeldal, O H., Heiberg, A., and Fagan, J.F. (1996). Vision, cognition and developmental characteristics of girls and women with Rett syndrome. *Developmental Medicine and Child Neurology,* 38:212–225.

Waddington, C.H. (1939). *An introduction to modern genetics.* Allen and Unwin, London.

Walz, K., Spencer, C., Kaasik, K., Lee, C.C., Lupski, J.R., and Paylor, R. (2004). Behavioral characterization of mouse models for Smith-Magenis syndrome and dup(17)(p11.2p11.2). *Human Molecular Genetics,* 13:367–378.

Wang, P.P., Woodin, M.F., Kreps-Falk, R., and Moss, E.M. (2000). Research on behavioral phenotypes: Velocardiofacial syndrome (deletion 22q11.2). *Developmental Medicine and Child Neurology,* 42:422–427.

Watts, R.W., Spellacy, E., Gibbs, D.A., Allsop, J., McKeran, R.O., and Slavin, G.E. (1982). Clinical, post-mortem, biochemical and therapeutic observations on the Lesch-Nyhan syndrome with particular reference to the neurological manifestations. *Quarterly Journal of Medicine,* 51:43–78.

Whitman, B., Carrel, A., Bekx, T., Weber, C., Allen, D., and Myers, S. (2004). Growth hormone improves body composition and motor development in infants with Prader-Willi syndrome after six months. *Journal of Pediatric Endocrinology and Metabolism.* 17:591–600.

Williams, J.C.P., Barratt-Boyes, B.G., and Lowe, J.B. (1961). Supravalvular aortic stenosis. *Circulation,* 24:1311–1318.

Wilson, T.A., Rose, S.R., Cohen, P., Rogol, A.D., Backeljauw, P., Brown, R., Hardin, D.S., Kemp, S.F., Lawson, M., Radovick, S., Rosenthal, S.M., Silverman, L., and Speiser, P. (2003). Update of guidelines for the use of growth hormone in children: The Lawson Wilkins Pediatric Endocrinology Society Drug and Therapeutics Committee. *Journal of Pediatrics,* 143:415–421.

Wisniewski, H.M., and Silverman, W. (1998). Aging and dementia of the Alzheimer type in persons with mental retardation. *Advances in Experimental Medicine and Biology,* 446:223–225.

Wolff, P.H., Gardner, J., Paccia, J., and Lappen, J. (1989). The greeting behavior of fragile X males. *American Journal of Mental Retardation,* 93:406–411.

Wong, D.F., Harris, J.C., Naidu, S., Yokoi, F., Marenco, S., Dannals, R.F., Ravert, H.T., Yaster, M., Evans, A., Rousset, O., et al. (1996). Dopamine transporters are markedly reduced in Lesch Nyhan disease in vivo. *Proceedings of the National Academy of Sciences USA,* 93:5539–5543.

Woodyatt, G., and Ozanne, A. (1997). Rett syndrome (RS) and profound intellectual disability: cognitive and communicative similarities and differences. *European Child and Adolescent Psychiatry*, 6:31–32.

Yaron, Y., and Mashiach, R. (2001). First trimester biochemical screening for Down syndrome. *Clinical Perinatology,* 28:321–331.

Yoshii, A., Krishnamoorthy, K.S., and Grant, P.E. (2002). Abnormal cortical development shown by 3D MRI in Prader-Willi syndrome. *Neurology,* 59:644–645.

8

A Life Span Developmental Approach

Intellectual disability is a neurodevelopmental disorder that continues throughout the life span of the affected person. It is essential to understand how persons with intellectual disability progress throughout their life span from infancy to old age. The maturation of the brain, their environmental experiences, and the mastery of developmental challenges and tasks must all be considered. A focus on brain development is in keeping with neuroscience research indicating that progressive brain maturation is accompanied by successive synaptic reorganization as one moves from one developmental stage to the next. Anatomical Magnetic Resonance Imaging Studies are playing a major role in understanding the developmental trajectories of normal brain development (Durston et al., 2001; Giedd et al., 1999). Understanding the developmental trajectories of normal brain development is crucial to the interpretation of brain development in neurodevelopmental disabilities. During normal development, white matter volume increases with age, and although gray matter volumes increase during childhood, they decrease before adulthood. These changes in the brain are accompanied by changes in cognitive processing; for example, executive functioning shows a progressive emergence from the preschool years (Espy et al., 1999) into the adolescent years. Working memory and inhibitory processes may be measured during the preschool years. By adolescence, abstract reasoning, anticipatory planning, and mental judgment have emerged and may be measured. Cognitive abilities in adolescence are qualitatively different from those of young children as a result of the reorganization of the prefrontal cortex during maturation. How genetic background and environment interact in producing these changes is the object of ongoing study, yet investigators are beginning to understand how physiological processes of synaptic development, circuits, and neuronal network formation relate to processes of cognitive development (Fossella et al., 2003).

The development of persons with intellectual disability is now being evaluated systematically, and developmental trajectories are being established for known neurogenetic syndromes. These studies are making up for a surprising lack of application of a developmental perspective to persons with intellectual disability. Developmental theorists have, for the most part, monitored and measured development in normally intelligent persons in establishing developmental landmarks. Now similar approaches are being applied to establish the developmental trajectory of many neurogenetic syndromes and other etiologies of intellectual disability, such as fetal alcohol spectrum disorder as discussed in chapter 7.

This chapter introduces a developmental perspective and then proceeds to discuss transitions from one developmental stage to the next. Specific patterns of intellectual and cognitive development, in particular neurogenetic syndromes, are described along with personality development and aging.

A DEVELOPMENTAL PERSPECTIVE

A developmental perspective on intellectual disability is a dynamic one and focuses on how the person engages other people and meets environmental challenges. This dynamic approach to intelligence emphasizes fluid intelligence, which refers to those general inferential and reasoning abilities (Demetriou et al., 2002; Gustafson and Undheim, 1996) that underlie thinking and problem solving. Fluid intelligence is closely associated with general intelligence (Demetriou et al., 2002; Gustafson and Undheim, 1996) and strongly associated with working memory, executive functioning, and cognitive processing efficiency. Intelligence tests measure crystallized intelligence, knowledge that is already possessed. Considering fluid intelligence as it relates to processing efficiency and working memory in intellectual disability suggests a re-evaluation of the stage model of intellectual disability proposed by Barbel Inhelder, who, in her book, *Diagnosis of Reasoning in the Retarded* (1968), did propose a developmental approach to intellectual disability. She suggested that a failure of progression along Piaget's conceptual developmental stages corresponded to profound (sensorimotor stage), severe (early preoperational stage), moderate (late preoperational stage), and mild (concrete operational stage) levels of intellectual disability.

While Inhelder's intellectually disabled subjects were in the moderate or mild range of intellectual disability, Mary Woodward (1959a, 1959b, 1979) studied severely and profoundly intellectually disabled persons, using Piaget's approach, and reached the same conclusions as Inhelder with this group in regard to cognitive progression. She emphasized the importance of studying the process of intellectual development, as well as measuring developmental acquisitions on standardized tests. Her emphasis was on understanding developmental processes rather than primarily placing the emphasis on the age of knowledge acquisition. In doing so, like Inhelder, she concluded that the reasoning process follows a sequence of stages that represent thresholds of cognitive problem solving and understanding. Thus, she concluded that persons with intellectual disability follow similar stages but tend to stop early, failing to progress in their conceptual development.

Recently, Piagetian tests of categorization, seriation, and conservation of discrete quantities have been linked to academic achievement. Pasnak, Willson-Quayle, and Whitten (1998), conducted one such study in which the students also completed psychometric tests. The authors found correlations of 0.66 with IQ and of 0.77 with mental age. This study suggests the value of combining tests of reasoning with standardized psychometric tests in evaluating academic achievement.

A developmental approach shows promise in unraveling the dynamics of development by analyzing the failure to progress from one cognitive developmental stage to the next. A functional, developmentally focused approach may transcend the long-standing developmental delay (similarity to younger children) and difference (less cognitive efficiency or speed of information processing at a given chronological age) debate (Paour, 2001). It may shift the focus to consideration of cognitive efficiency (speed of information processing), working memory, and controlled attention to task mastery (Demetriou et al., 2002).

Inhelder wrote that ". . . the retardate who has reached the elementary forms of operatory organization is capable of remaining at this level for years. It is as though he lacked the interest, the curiosity, and the general activity, which in the normal child leads the subject to ask new questions and find the solutions, both of which lead him to superior levels" (Inhelder, 1968, p. 291). She found that within a conceptual stage, answers to questions were like those of younger children of the same mental age, yet there was also lower efficacy in their cognitive effort at problem solving. What is the basis of this failure of conceptual progression and reduced cognitive efficiency?

Demetriou et al. (2002) have reframed Inhelder's earlier proposals in their studies of the development of mental processing by combining information processing models, differential psychology, and neo-Piagetian developmental theory. Like Inhelder, they emphasize the importance of cognitive efficacy in problem solving. They extend the developmental approach and provide a modern framework by discussing the emergence and maturation of working memory, executive functioning, and thinking. They note that all aspects of processing efficiency, working memory, and problem solving systematically improve with age. Processing efficiency indicated by speed of processing is critical to memory development, but memory also involves executive and storage processes in addition to processing efficiency. This model allows us to move beyond the debate about whether development occurs in stages (developmental discontinuity) or is continuous and to consider how and when development occurs in stages, as growth proceeds, and how and when it shows continuous patterns (Fisher and Dawson, 2002). Thus, the question of how individual learning and social support shape development can be investigated with new tools to understand how an individual masters new challenges in life. Advances in the neurosciences regarding dendritic spine architecture, the processes of synaptic development and synaptic plasticity brain circuits, neuronal connectivity, interneuron development, and neuronal network formation may also allow the failure of cognitive progression to be better understood.

The developmental perspective contributes to resolving "the dual nature" of proposals about intellectual disability. The traditional view has focused on what is referred to as the developmental delay and the developmental difference hypotheses. The emphasis was on intellectual disability with or without known brain damage. Those individuals without known brain damage were referred to as "familial" intellectual disability and thought to be similar to non–intellectually disabled individuals in the developmental sequences they follow, although progressing at a slower rate based on their ability level. Those who were delayed were thought to be similar to younger children of the same mental age. Those with symptomatic brain dysfunction were proposed to have atypical development and thus to be different in their development, showing less cognitive efficacy at a given mental age and, because of their brain dysfunction, to have cognitive defects in areas such as memory and attention.

Developmental Delay or Failure of Cognitive Progression

The use of the term "developmental delay" can be misleading and sometimes confuses family members of persons with intellectual disability. It does not mean the person is delayed in development in the sense that they will eventually "catch up" as they grow older. Instead, the person, once properly diagnosed, will continue to be intellectually disabled throughout his or her life span. Perhaps it would be better to speak of a failure of cognitive progression and seek the contributory causes or conditions leading to it and provide individuals with appropriate positive personal supports and focused education. This would help them reach their potential, keeping in mind that the individual will continue to adapt and develop within the constraints of his or her intellectual and cognitive abilities.

Similar Sequences in Development and Alternative Developmental Pathways

Developmentalists currently propose an expanded developmental approach and postulate that development theory is applicable both to "familial" intellectual disability without demonstrable brain damage and to symptomatic brain dysfunction. Evidence suggests that despite brain dysfunction, there are universal sequences in development in several chromosomal disorder syndromes (Hodapp, Burack, and Zigler, 1990). Studies of developmental sequences carried out in intellectual disability syndromes with different etiologies are helping to clarify the degree that developmental processes might be altered in intellectual disability, particularly in specific syndromes. By acknowledging the many causes (heterogeneity) of intellectual disability and associated cognitive and behavioral features for each of them, the developmental questions can be addressed more directly than is the case if people with intellectual disability are considered to be one homogeneous group. Differences in development may be studied among the various etiologic groups, such as Down syndrome, fragile X syndrome,

Lesch-Nyhan disease, Rett's disorder, Williams syndrome, and Prader-Willi syndrome. Moreover, subgroups may also be investigated within syndromes, such as Down syndrome, where there are several genetic causes—for example, trisomy (3 copies of chromosome) 21, translocation (chromosomal transfer), mosaic (a mixture of chromosome pattern) groups, and Prader-Willi syndrome—where different genetic mechanisms, uniparental disomy (one parent's chromosome segment is copied twice) of chromosome 15 and gene deletion (crucial genes are missing) at chromosome 15, may result in this syndrome. Animal models of both fragile X syndrome and Rett's disorder are of importance in understanding postsynaptic organization of brain systems.

Developmental Trajectory

Besides these broad developmental sequences, the developmental rate or trajectory over the life span must also be considered in intellectual disability syndromes to understand fully the importance of maturational changes in neurological structures that are involved in specific syndromes. Thus, in Down syndrome, the importance of developmental rate is demonstrated in studies that show a gradual decline in IQ from infancy into early childhood. During the first two years of life, infants with Down syndrome fall further and further behind peers who are not intellectually disabled. This apparent slowing in development may be due to problems in moving qualitatively from one developmental stage transition to another in the preschool years and primary school years and in the kinds of IQ tests used for infants. Some of these differences may be attributed to infant intelligence tests having relatively greater motor than cognitive components. In Down syndrome, problems in transition from one developmental stage to the next become evident to the family when the school-aged child seems to have lost developmental momentum and younger peers or siblings move beyond them in mastering developmental tasks.

In contrast, in fragile X syndrome and Lesch-Nyhan disease, change in IQ test scores and intellectual progression becomes more apparent in early adolescence, during the transition from middle childhood to adolescence. Mental age tends to plateau at adolescence in these syndromes, and for some, a decline in IQ test scores in the adolescent years may be demonstrated. Test items requiring abstract reasoning on IQ tests used for testing in the adolescent years may be more difficult to master. This is consistent with the idea that brain mechanisms involved in developing abstract reasoning may require synaptic reorganization processes that accompany brain development in adolescence.

Neuroimaging and the Maturation of the Brain

Neuroimaging methods may be used in the future to monitor brain development in various syndromes now that normative neuroimaging data is available. Brain imaging studies document dynamic changes in brain anatomy and development throughout the adolescent years. White matter increases in an essentially linear pattern, with minor differences in slope in the frontal, parietal, temporal, and occipital (Giedd, 2004). Cortical gray matter is shown to follow an inverted Ushaped developmental course, with greater regional variation than white matter. For example, frontal gray matter volume peaks at approximately 11 years of age in girls and 12.1 years of age in boys. However, temporal gray matter volume peaks at approximately 16.7 years of age in girls and 16.2 years of age in boys. The dorsal lateral prefrontal cortex, a major brain region for impulse control, is among the last brain regions to mature; this region does not reach adult dimensions until the early twenties. The relationships between anatomical changes and behavioral changes and the underlying processes that influence brain development are now beginning to be established in various neurodevelopmental disorders.

Normative information on brain development has been utilized to study maturational changes in the amygdala and hippocampus in children with the diagnosis of autistic disorder with and without intellectual disability. Children with autistic disorder, both with and without intellectual disability, had a larger right hippocampal volume than typically developing control individuals. The amygdala in typically developing children increases substantially in volume from 7.5 years to 18.5 years of age; however, the amygdala in children with autistic disorder was initially larger but did not undergo the age-related increase in size observed in typically developing children. Thus, there may be an abnormality in early amygdala development over time in autistic disorder and an abnormal pattern of hippocampal development that persists through adolescence (Schumann et al., 2004). These findings are consistent with neuroanatomical studies that show increased cell packing density and smaller neuronal size in the hippocampus and amygdala in autopsies of individuals with a diagnosis of autistic disorder (Palmen et al., 2004). They are consistent with clinical observation of changes in disturbances of affective contact and emotional development in autistic disorder with age.

Environmental Interface

It is not only maturation in brain development but also the environmental interface that is essential for development, although it is unclear which aspects of the environment are most important and at which times in development they are most crucial. Because experience can shape the brain, this should lead to adoption of intervention models that highlight greater parent- or teacher-child interactions and a focus on structured language stimulation and early parent-child dialogues. These interactions structure both linguistic and nonlinguistic environments to facilitate development. The development of social communication is particularly important. Most studies emphasize mother-child relationships, but the role of the father in language facilitation is also critical. Environmental outcomes that must be monitored include not only intelligence but also the emergence of social competence and the management of emotions, especially help in stabilizing mood. Children with Down syndrome, fragile X syndrome, autistic disorder, and those with multiple disabilities do differ from one another in their natural histories, in their reactions to others and in the behaviors of caregivers toward them. Therefore, the type of early intervention must consider the natural history of the particular disorder.

Individual Mastery Motivation

Development not only in maturation of the brain and psychosocial experience but also in individual motivation is critical. This is referred to as mastery or effective motivation. Personal success in completing a task is intrinsically rewarding and motivating. Task mastery is a critical component for every developing person. When tasks are tailored to the ability level of the person, taking into account intelligence and cognitive skills, then motivation is enhanced. When psychologists test children with intellectual disability, they note that personal effort and pleasure diminish as the task becomes more difficult. When less complex tasks are reintroduced, motivation increases. For example, studies in young children with Down syndrome have found that they can be just as persistent and goal-directed as typically developing children of the same mental age (Gilmore, Cuskelly, and Hayes, 2003).

LIFE TRANSITIONS

The transition from school completion to adult life can be particularly difficult if the young person moves from a carefully monitored individualized program with peers of the same age to an adult program with individuals of all ages and many different diagnoses. This transition can be distressing. For example, the young woman, Tina (described in chapter 3), who had done well in her school program, completed her formal education at age 22 and, subsequently entered a workshop but had a difficult transition from school to adult life. She was referred for diagnosis and treatment. At age 24, she became socially withdrawn, had lost interest in all her usual activities and was not eating; she lost 20 pounds following entry into an adult sheltered workshop program. Her physician had read that Down syndrome is associated with Alzheimer's disease and, assuming this was her diagnosis, Tina and her family were referred for Alzheimer's disease counseling, despite her youth.

She did not have Alzheimer's disease, but she did have a diagnosis of major depression, a treatable illness, and subsequently responded well to supportive therapy and to antidepressant medication. Within 8 weeks, she was back in her program, eating and engaged in her preferred activities. But how did she become depressed? Although there is vulnerability to separation anxiety and depression in Down syndrome, what happened during Tina's transition from school to workshop in our system of care for persons with developmental disabilities deserves consideration.

Before she reached age 21, Tina was in an excellent school program. After age 21, she left her protective school environment and transitioned to a community sheltered workshop program where she was exposed for the first time to people of all ages, with many different types of behavioral difficulties; she was not prepared. This exposure was very stressful and a precipitant to depression in a vulnerable person. When persons with intellectual disability are transitioned to a new setting, continuity and positive personal supports for life transitions are particularly important. An emphasis on self-determination and personal task mastery in school programs is essential to transition into adult life.

With treatment for her depression and positive supports at her workshop, Tina has continued to do well. However, she subsequently developed hearing problems and was diagnosed with otosclerosis, a problem associated with aging in Down syndrome. With a hearing aid, she is again making progress. An understanding of the natural history of Down syndrome regarding physical, emotional, and behavioral risk factors is essential to ongoing care. Tina's situation illustrates the importance of a comprehensive physical and mental health assessment by caregivers who are knowledgeable about the specific disorder.

DEVELOPMENTAL MODELS

The expected developmental sequence and the developmental pathway or trajectory associated with the intellectual disability syndrome must be considered; these are referred to as the Similar Sequence Model and the Multiple Pathways Model. The Similar Sequence Model suggests a universal and invariant sequence in the development of cognition, morality, and language. Utilizing this model, a Piagetian approach (1952) emphasizes that knowledge develops through a sequence of progressively complex patterns of behavior and thinking, with new patterns being organized from simpler ones that are present in earlier phases of development. Learning occurs through interaction with both the material and the social environment. Piaget's approach has been documented as pertinent to the study of sensorimotor development in cross-cultural studies. Yet the speed of development and acquisition of Piaget's stages may be influenced by environmental experience. Other authors emphasize that besides a similar sequence model that is universal and invariant, development can also be variable, there being multiple pathways to reach developmental goals.

Both the universal developmental sequence and the individualized developmental pathways models are pertinent for persons with intellectual disability. Neurobiologically based development ordinarily follows a universal sequence in the absence of brain damage, assuming an average expectable environment is provided; thus, there may be an invariant sequence for cognitive development or language development in normal development. Subsequent achievements, such as internalized language and social, cognitive, and moral development, may follow with the expected emergence of higher cognitive functions over time. Still, higher cognitive functions may be influenced by interpersonal contacts and social stimulation. If this is correct, then earlier cognitive development may be universal and neurobiologically based, but later, more sophisticated cognitive development may vary with social and cultural experiences (Hodapp, Burack, and Zigler, 1990). Yet there will be differences for a person with intellectual disability and its pattern of associated features, based on the specific syndrome, in how social experiences are internalized.

The development of children with intellectual disability may aid in understanding the universal sequence of development because there are differences in the sequence of development in a variety of syndromes. Biologically based developmental lines may be highly canalized and resistant to environmental input, resulting in a universal sequence of development. Yet other areas of development may be, to a greater degree, dependent on life experiences and individual differences in brain development among syndromes.

It was once assumed that there were universal deficits in persons with intellectual disability in areas such as the verbal mediation of thought and in focusing and sustaining attention. Thus, children with intellectual disability were thought to differ basically in their development from children who were not. In contrast to this view, other authors hypothesized that development involves the same processes in intellectually disabled persons as in the normal population but proceeds differently based on disorder-specific cognitive processes. If children with intellectual disability show the same sequence or a similar sequence in development as normally developing children, identical performance to that of normally developing children of similar mental age on information processing tasks and other tasks measuring cognition might be expected, although reduced cognitive efficiency must be considered. Similar performance of intellectually disabled persons of similar mental age and normally developing persons on such tests suggests that similar structures are involved in information processing. Similar sequence indicates a constant and invariant order of acquisition of increasingly complex cognitive capabilities. Structure refers to how different behavioral manifestations show a developmental or stage-like relationship to one another and may share common mechanisms.

Most research on the similar-sequence hypothesis has focused on sensorimotor development in children. Sensorimotor development refers to qualitative changes in psychological functioning in infants that takes place from birth to the beginning of symbolic and representational thought. The study of sensorimotor development derives from a psychobiological model of child development that emphasizes the infant's capacity to acquire, integrate, store, and act on information gained from both social and nonsocial experiences.

Dunst (1990) reports that there is strong evidence for the sequential acquisition in the development in children with Down syndrome and children with mixed etiologies of intellectual disability. He found that age-related changes do occur and that children who are intellectually disabled acquire more difficult test items in each of the six sensorimotor domains at later stages than they acquire items that are easier. Dunst found a strong relationship between the extent of sensorimotor acquisitions and increasing mental age and chronological age. He found that when the same children with intellectual disability were tested five to nine times over a span of years, sequential development could be demonstrated in individual cases. However, some groups of intellectually disabled children may show variability across domains and regressions and spurts or lags at different phases in their development. Despite the unevenness of development, in some individuals with Down syndrome the sequential acquisition of skills model is supported. Overall, these findings are in keeping with the suggestion that the more neurobiologically related areas in infant development show invariant sequences across cultures, whereas later and more culture-determined achievements show variability.

Moral Development: Is It Sequential?

Studies of moral development have not clearly demonstrated a sequential development model. Some evidence does support sequential moral development, yet Mahaney and Stephens (1974) found that results depended on the type of moral question asked. Moral development questions that dealt with a group's taking collective responsibility for the actions of group members did advance during a two-year observation period. However, when moral development questions were asked that involved understanding the difference between the consequences of an action and the consequences of one's intent, the group with intellectual disability did not progress and, in some instances, showed regression. For example, children with intellectual disability did not advance and continued to interpret stealing and lying in terms of their consequences rather than considering the intention of the person who was showing this behavior. There was variability in regard to sequential acquisition of moral stages. However, the study of moral development is complicated because there are differences of opinion in categorizing moral development stages. Some authors (e.g., Kohlberg, 1974), emphasize moral judgment and present a series of moral dilemmas to solve. Others (e.g., Hogan and Busch, 1984) emphasize mercy and ask how a person would respond to another in distress. If cognitive development and moral reasoning develop concurrently, then moral judgment may depend on cognitive processes. However, it is less clear whether the sense of mercy is so confined to mental age and the cognitive level achieved. As an example of compassionate behavior by persons with intellectual disability, the following episode is said to have occurred at the Special Olympics. It is reported that at the Seattle Special Olympics, nine contestants, all with physical or mental disability, assembled at the starting line for the 100-yard dash. At the gun, they all started out, not so much in a dash, but with the desire to run the race to the finish line and win. All, that is, except one little boy who stumbled on the asphalt, tumbled over a couple of times, fell, and began to cry. The other eight heard him cry, slowed down and looked back. Then every one of them turned around and went back. A girl with Down syndrome bent down and kissed him and said, "This will make it better." Then all nine linked arms and walked together to the finish line. Everyone in the stadium stood and cheered their compassion and solidarity.

In summary, the issue of sequential stages of moral reasoning continues to be unsettled for intellectually disabled persons. New studies on moral development should look to Kohlberg's (1969, 1974) stages of moral development and Hogan's measures of socialization, empathy, and autonomy (Hogan and Busch, 1984).

Implications of the Developmental Sequence Model

The view that persons with intellectual disability show similar sequences of development as do normally developing children is relevant to the treatment of intellectually disabled persons. It allows for greater confidence in setting goals for the next steps in treatment. It confirms that prerequisite skills are necessary for further development in other domains. Similar sequence findings are also important in terms of the type of psychometric instruments used for testing. Severely and profoundly intellectually disabled children are often difficult to test and show variable profiles on Stanford-Binet and WISC III-R assessments. However, tests based on sensorimotor development, such as the Uzgiris and Hunt (1975) test based on Piaget's model, can be adapted to test children with intellectual disability and other disabilities and may be more useful. These sensorimotor approaches help clarify that the child has the ability to understand and make use of basic concepts, which should be considered in planning interventions. Therefore, information about universal sequences in development is essential for both assessment procedures and the development of interventions.

Variations in Developmental Sequences

Both sensory and motor disabilities influence developmental progress. Some children may be blind or deaf and have absent limbs, yet their development proceeds in a universal manner if they are allowed to use other sensory modalities to compensate for their impairments. Still, not all developmental achievements follow a universal sequence. For example, in language development, semantic relations and grammatical morphemes do develop in a set order; however, pragmatic language functions may not follow fixed sequences. Children with autistic disorder show deviations in pragmatic language usage and may focus their attention on objects rather than on people in their early speech development. Yet later in their development, higher functioning children with autistic disorder may engage in more appropriate pragmatic social communication directed specifically toward others. In autistic disorder, the development from object-related to quasi-social to more social language follows a different pattern than that seen in normal development; these features are described in the DSM-IVTR definition. In contrast, in Down syndrome, pragmatic social communication emerges in the earliest phases of language communication. In both intellectually disabled and normally developing children, therefore, some behaviors have a lock-step sequence and others may follow a different course depending on the neurobiology of the specific disorder.

A developmental approach to intellectual disability emphasizes how development is organized even in those who are disabled. By comparing different etiologic groups, there is an opportunity to make comparisons about developmental organization that may elucidate mechanisms involved in normal developmental sequences. For example, children with Down syndrome may have reduced affective responsivity and difficulties in language development, yet they may have relatively high levels of social skills, whereas children with autistic disorder have severe social skills deficits, echolalia, and a different and deviant profile of language development. Behaviors also may show relationships across developmental domains. The study of behavior across domains is important to help clarify how various behaviors fit together in development. In the final stage of Piaget's sensorimotor development sequence, one object is used to retrieve another object; this stage can be demonstrated for normally developing children and for children with autistic disorder. An example of behavior that crosses domains is symbolic play, which may be important for early language development and is better developed in some syndromes, such as Down syndrome. Specific deficits can be investigated across domains, as shown by the study of how sequential processing deficits in fragile X syndrome affect cognitive, linguistic, and adaptive functioning. Knowledge of cross-modal problem solving can be applied to an intervention program to assist the child in adapting to his specific impairments.

The individual study of the various etiologies of intellectual disability takes into account the importance of individual impairments rather than simply targeting global differences in intelligence for intervention. Thus, when asking about developmental milestones during an interview, questions should focus on which specific functions are not developing. Adaptive behaviors are best studied based on which behaviors are specific for a given mental age. The Vineland Adaptive Behavior Scales provide a means to assess adaptive functioning and to contrast adaptive abilities with IQ score.

Development and Mastery Motivation

Mastery motivation is critical for the mastery of developmental tasks. How is mastery motivation related to both the delays and deficits in development? Mastery motivation paradigms define motivated behavior as behavior that is goal-directed and persistent in reaching a goal (Messer, 1993). The developmental course in Down syndrome is delayed in relation to normal development and is also disrupted. In many aspects, developmental progression follows the same stages and sequences as those in typically developing children. However, in other instances, development is linked to innate differences rather than to delayed development (Wishart, 1991, 1999). Individuals with Down syndrome might reach developmental landmarks following different pathways than those followed in typically developing children.

Studies that have investigated mastery motivation in Down syndrome at ages 6 months (MacTurk et al., 1985; Macturk, Morgan, and Jennings, 1995), 17 months (Ruskin et al., 1994a, 1994b), and 34 months (Landry, Miller-Loncar, and Swank, 1998) have demonstrated that when children with Down syndrome at these mental ages are compared to typically developing children of the same mental age, they show similar degrees of persistence in goal-directed behavior. Despite these findings, others have argued that motivation for young individuals with Down syndrome is delayed and fundamentally different (Wishhart, 1999) than that of typically developing children. In studies of operant learning, object concept development, and cognitive test performance, individuals with Down syndrome have shown task avoidant behaviors, lack of initiative, low persistence when difficult tasks are presented, and a lack of stability in their performance over time (Wishart, 1993). Others have suggested (Vietze et al., 1983) that although infants with Down syndrome show about the same degree of exploratory behavior as typically developing children of the same mental age (six months), their behavior is much less goal directed. Although mastery behavior has been shown to follow the same developmental course as typically developing children, it is delayed in comparison to those even of the same mental age. The issue is whether individuals with Down syndrome, compared to typically developing children, spend less time attending to tasks, are engaged in the task for a shorter period of time, and show limitations in integrating and generalizing motivational behaviors.

Another factor in the study of mastery motivation is observation of positive affect or positive emotional engagement during task-directed behavior (Morgan, Harmon, and Maslin-Cole, 1990). Evaluation of positive affect associated with goal mastery in children with Down syndrome may be difficult because children with Down syndrome may, in fact, show less affect overall. It should be noted that the lack of expression of emotion does not always mean that emotion has not been experienced. The majority of the studies conducted on mastery motivation have not included children with Down syndrome with a mental age of 24 months or more, which is an age when symbolic operations would be expected. Landry, Miller-Loncar, and Swank (1998) did investigate goal-directed play in children with Down syndrome who were four years to seven years of age and a group of typically developing children matched for mental age. They found that both groups spent the same amount of time in independent goal-directed activity involving the use of a circus toy.

Overall, young children with Down syndrome may show both similarities and differences in motivation when compared to typically developing children. It is not that infants and young children with Down syndrome are not persistent and goal-directed to a challenging task; it is more that differences have been found in sustained engagement to task, the level of mastery play, and parents' rating of the extent of mastery motivation. The issue of affective engagement is of concern since children with Down syndrome are generally noted to show less pleasure with task-directed behaviors in some studies. Therefore, to better understand the mastery motivation issues, it is important to consider that mastery motivation has both behavioral and emotional elements that are studied in terms of behavioral persistence and positive affect during goal-directed activity. It is generally assumed that mastery motivation reflects a person's general disposition to engage in tasks and is predictive of being confident later in life.

Gilmore, Cuskelly, and Hayes (2003) sought to clarify these important issues in mastery behavior for children with and without Down syndrome above a mental age of 24 months. They studied 25 children (15 girls and 10 boys) with Down syndrome, whose ages ranged from 4 years to 6 years and 8 months, and compared them with 43 typically developing children (20 girls) between 2 years and 3 years of age. Those with Down syndrome all had trisomy 21. The groups were matched for mental age (mean mental age = 30 months). Gilmore, Cuskelly, and Hayes (2003) used the instrument *Structured Mastery Tasks*, developed for 15–36-month-old mental age children (Morgan et al., 1992a), to study mastery motivation. The activities involved jigsaw puzzles and shape sorters with six levels of difficulty to clarify that the tasks were challenging for the children. In this study, the parents' perceptions of mastery motivation were examined, using The Dimensions of Mastery Questionnaire (Morgan et al., 1992b). The Object Persistence Scale and the Mastery Pleasure Scale were also used along with the Bayley Scales of Infant Development that were used to determine developmental age. The Bayley Scales include a rating "observations of behavior such as attention and persistence." The authors found that there were both similarities and differences in mastery behavior when children with Down syndrome were compared to typically developing children. There were similarities in task persistence and in displays of positive affect associated with persistence. There were differences in that individuals with Down syndrome showed higher across-task correlations of persistence, higher correlations of persistence and positive affect, and lower maternal ratings of persistence. Thus, although overall mastery behavior appeared the same for the two groups, there may be different processes associated with its development. In regard to differences, persistence does appear to be task-specific for typically developing children, but it is difficult to determine whether the differences across task in the group with Down syndrome are related to an undifferentiated intrinsic drive to mastery, compliance, or a disposition toward tasks that had developed through experience. The Down syndrome individuals, although the same mental age, were older chronologically and may have had different life experiences. Studies such as these must be evaluated carefully because of difficulties in assuming motives from observed behaviors in individuals. Still, this study in older children does provide some support for linking the two components of mastery motivation, persistence and emotional or affective engagement.

Finally, the issue for evaluating affective motivation is complicated in regard to what positive affect actually means. Is it intrinsic satisfaction in the mastery of tasks that is an important consideration when discussing mastery, or is it linked to social approval, or to both? Additional comparison groups are needed in future investigations that will take into account differences in years of life experience. Moreover, differences in environments, such as early intervention programs for those with Down syndrome, may also make a difference in terms of outcome. Early experience presents a challenge for those who study questions about developmental delay and developmental difference because the type of enrichment program may vary. It is particularly important to extend investigations beyond early childhood to middle childhood and later years. Clearly, longitudinal studies are important to continue to investigate the importance of mastery motivation as it impacts on children's development with Down syndrome and other developmental disorders.

Understanding mastery motivation may help caregivers facilitate development for individuals with Down syndrome. For example, finding ways to engage the child affectively may facilitate language development. When parents spent more time with children who have Down syndrome emphasizing joint attending to toys selected by the child and dialogue with the child, gains were noted in receptive language (Harris, Kasari, and Sigman, 1996). Gaining the attention of the child with Down syndrome and helping the child stay on task until the task is mastered may have long-term benefits.

Personality Development

Studies of persons with intellectual disability have focused primarily on intellectual and cognitive functioning and often have neglected social and personality development. Problems associated with cognitive functioning have often overshadowed a needed focus on adaptive and maladaptive personality features. However, personality and personal motivation are essential for predicting social and vocational adjustment. It is behavioral problems, poorly regulated emotion, and social deficits that most commonly lead to referral for their management.

Investigations of personality dysfunction in children and adolescents with intellectual disability should identify characteristics, such as overdependency, low ideal self-image, limited levels of aspiration, and an outwardly directed approach to problem solving (Zigler and Burack, 1989). These personality characteristics may have their origin in psychosocial experiences, such as repeated failure and disapproval, leading to doubts about one's capacity to succeed. Experiences of rejection and the lack of consistent social support may lead to excessive reliance on others for feedback and guidance. Out of a need for recognition by others, a person with intellectual disability may suppress the desire to become more independent.

Operant behavior modification programs may not address these personal needs. Such programs may not emphasize making choices but rather place primary emphasis on contingency management. As a result, the transition after completion of schooling to vocational programs may be more difficult because cognitive processes involved in making choices and in self-determination have not been emphasized in the school years. Consequently, a greater appreciation of the need to make choices has led to a greater emphasis on self-determination. During their adolescent years, persons with intellectual disability may experience parental restrictiveness and overprotection, peer rejection, and continuing low self-confidence that complicates their mastery of developmental tasks. These tasks involve the establishment of positive self-concept, sexual awareness, and identity. Adolescents with intellectual disability may view their lives as being less fulfilling than those of their peers because they commonly experience dissatisfaction with their physical appearance and become frustrated by their difficulty in controlling their impulses, emotions, and behavior. Such experiences may lead to social isolation, loneliness, and dysphoric mood. The failure to master developmental tasks is integral to producing maladaptive personality styles in adulthood. As many as one-half of adults with intellectual disability may have difficulties related to personality traits. Even though the diagnosis of personality disorder in persons with intellectual disability has been questioned, several personality disorder inventories that have adequate inter-rater and test-retest reliability have identified problematic personality traits and personality disorders in adolescents and adults with intellectual disability. The types of mal-adaptive personality characteristics found most commonly on these inventories include affective instability, explosive and disruptive behaviors, and introverted personality patterns (Reid and Ballenger, 1987). Menolascino (1988) reported that, among 543 admissions for psychiatric care for persons with intellectual disability over a 5-year period, 13% of those age 16 and over had a diagnosis of personality disorder; passive-aggressive and antisocial types were the most common. The presence of a seizure disorder, especially one involving the temporal lobes, may increase the risk for a personality disorder diagnosis among persons with intellectual disability.

AGING AND INTELLECTUAL DISABILITY

There are a number of misconceptions about aging in persons with intellectual disability. Among these are that people with intellectual disability are mentally ill, that people with intellectual disability do not survive to old age, that disabilities are the consequence of inappropriate behavior on the part of parents, that adults with intellectual disability may be cared for only in institutions, and that adults with intellectual disability are not capable to carry out everyday skills and to continue to be involved gainfully in the work force as they grow older (Hogg et al., 2000). However, these are all misconceptions. People with intellectual disability do live to old age and continue to work and, in many instances, live independently and make contributions in the community. Although persons with intellectual disability have a lower capability for self-determination, independent functioning, and the types of work and social environments in which they can participate, with adaptations they may continue to meet their potential as they age. Physical, sensory, and psychiatric impairments affect the individual to varying degrees that may be compensated for by treatment interventions, environmental enrichment, ongoing training, and special assistance and supports.

Aging is a continuous lifelong process, and there is no specific age that defines when a person has become old. In published reports, the sixth decade, a time when people with intellectual disability are in their fifties, has been chosen as the point to determine age-related changes. However, this may be unrealistic in some instances when there is premature aging and shortened life expectancy for individuals with some intellectual disability syndromes. Age-related changes are more likely in some persons with severe and profound intellectual disability with multiple disabilities and for some individuals with Down syndrome. However, life expectancy also may be reduced due to poor health status and inappropriate poor living conditions. Barriers continue to exist and biases about the nature and causes of disability may result in inadequate services and, in some instances, in government policies that do not provide adequate support, adequate health care, adequate mental health care, and appropriate mental health services. These barriers can be overcome through aggressive public policies, education of caregivers and professionals, continued advocacy and efforts to provide compensatory supports in the community.

During the twentieth century, there were considerable increases in life expectancy for persons with intellectual disability that came about because of advances in public health, medicine, education, technology and scientific research. Improvements in health care, increased longevity, and better services have resulted in greater numbers of persons with intellectual disability who are living longer.

Physical Health Concerns

Like others who grow older, those with intellectual disability have significant health needs. The U.N. International Plan of Action on Aging poses that each country respond to demographic trends in the population and the resulting changes "in the context of its own traditions, structures, and cultural values . . ." This applies to older people with intellectual disability and the general population. When addressing aging and intellectual disability, policies must be developed in a way to maintain and, hopefully, improve their individual situations as they grow older.

With growing numbers of persons with intellectual disability who reach older ages, additional functional impairments, morbidity, and even early death may occur as a result of early age–onset conditions, long-term illness progression, or interactions with disorders that emerge in the general population with aging. Therefore, the long-term consequences of therapeutic interventions must be taken into account. For example, with long-term use of neuroleptic medication, movement disorders may occur over time and bone demineralization may result from the chronic use of certain anticonvulsant medications. Consequently, continuing efforts are necessary to use medications that have fewer chronic effects and to recognize the effects of those medications that may lead to harmful consequences.

Still, many persons with intellectual disability are healthy and healthy people tend to live longer. Maintaining health and providing for equal opportunities to achieve old age with access to health care plans and social supports throughout the life span are critically important for persons with intellectual disability. The Surgeon General's Report on Health Disparities and Intellectual Disability (appendix C) lists six goals and action steps to meet them. These include the critical need to integrate health promotion into community settings where persons with intellectual disability live and to make health care routinely available.

Specific Health Risks

Particular intellectual disability syndromes have syndrome-specific health risks with increasing age. Individuals with specific syndromes make up a large segment of the adult population with intellectual disability. These syndromes may result from toxins, injuries, infections, and many genetic disorders that affect the central nervous system during the developmental period.

Persons with fragile X syndrome, the most common inherited disorder associated with intellectual disability, have higher rates of mitral valve prolapse, musculoskeletal disorders, early menopause, epilepsy, and visual impairments. Moreover, those with shorter repeat sequences who test in the mildly cognitively impaired or borderline range in early life may be at risk for central nervous system dysfunction in later age (Jacquemont et al., 2003). Those with premutation alleles (55-200 CGG repeats) are at risk not only for mild cognitive and/or behavioral deficits but also for premature ovarian failure and a neurodegenerative disorder in older adult carriers, the fragile X-associated tremor/ataxia syndrome (Hagerman and Hagerman, 2004).

Persons with Down syndrome, a common chromosomal disorder are at high risk for endocrine abnormalities such as hypothyroidism, infections, skin conditions, oral disorders, cardiac disorders, musculoskeletal and some other organ system dysfunction. They show higher rates of impaired vision and hearing problems that result from otosclerosis. Older individuals with Down syndrome are at greater risk for epilepsy and Alzheimer's disease. The longevity for persons with Down syndrome is 10 years to 20 years less than that of the general population of those with intellectual disability. In Prader-Willi syndrome, there is an increased risk of disorders related to obesity, especially diabetes and cardiac problems that result from obesity, particularly the Pickwickian syndrome.

Lifestyle and Choice

As individuals with intellectual disability, particularly those with mild cognitive impairment, have more choices, there are also risks associated with those choices. The opportunity for choice increases as the individual grows older. Some individuals with intellectual disability may be exposed to alcohol and tobacco use, violent behavior and abuse, and high-risk sexual activity (particularly the risk of AIDS). There are also risks for those who live in care facilities in that they may be exposed to neglect and possibly to infectious diseases. Other risks are related to lifestyle. A sedentary lifestyle with poor physical conditioning is a problem for adults with intellectual disability, as it is in the general population. Concerns about obesity are critical, since they may lead to coronary artery disease, hypertension, and diabetes if overweight is chronic. Monitoring is essential for those with intellectual disability who live in independent or semi-independent settings where lifestyle modifications may lead to greater health and quality of life, as well as functional capacity.

Overall, those with intellectual disability who receive supports have rates of adult and age-related disorders comparable to the general population, although in some instances for particular disorders, the rates may be higher. The interaction among biological, psychological and social aspects of aging is an important consideration for the later years of life. Hereditary factors and predispositions must be considered for individuals with intellectual disability just as they are for other family members.

Ongoing Health Assessment

Functional decline in older individuals with intellectual disability requires careful assessment. It should not be assumed that changes in functional status, particularly changes in behavior, are related to cognitive decline or dementia without a careful assessment (Hogg et al., 2000). Finding treatable conditions is critical; for example, mood and affective disorders, sensory impairment, delirium and medical conditions that were not previously diagnosed need to be considered at the time of evaluation. Moreover, these conditions may not present in a typical way. In persons with intellectual disability, communication difficulties and motor problems may make it difficult to conduct an adequate assessment. Furthermore, the medical history is generally provided based on the observations of the caregivers. These caregivers must be educated about the individual health needs of the person with intellectual disability for whom they care. The history should be obtained not only from the caregiver but also, to the extent possible, from the person with intellectual disability, and this history-taking may require time, so patience is needed.

Other barriers to completing assessments are behavioral problems or poor cooperation. Adults with intellectual disability may find it difficult to cooperate with certain examinations and diagnostic procedures. They may be fearful, confused or frustrated and need additional support during the assessment process. Time is needed to reassure them and help them to adapt to the examination setting. In order to complete examinations, conscious sedation may be necessary for many individuals who need diagnostic procedures. However, general anesthesia may be required to safely carry out certain types of examinations, especially neuroimaging procedures.

Following diagnosis, behavior must be carefully monitored, particularly during rehabilitation following an illness or an injury. Teaching the use of assistive devices, such as walkers, wheel chairs, braces, glasses and hearing aids, may require time and additional techniques. An individual must be helped in understanding and develop confidence in using health care service to assure care throughout the life span.

Consent to Treatment

Participation in medical procedures requires an understanding of that treatment and an agreement to participate. An individual's rights must be respected just as they are for individuals who are not disabled. Individuals with a disability must be informed about medical procedures or treatments and their assent or consent obtained. If the person is not able to consent, authorization must be obtained in a legally appropriate manner focused on the individual's best interests. Thus, health care and social service staffs require training to identify health care needs of adults with intellectual disability and experience, with community support, models that are developed to enhance older age and sustain health during aging.

AGING AND PSYCHOPATHOLOGY

Older persons with Down syndrome are at risk for clinical dementia and the neuropathological findings of Alzheimer's disease, although all persons with Down syndrome do not develop dementia. There is growing interest in clarifying the nature of clinical dementia in persons with intellectual disability of other etiologies. Advances in the clinical description in the assessment of dementia in intellectually disabled persons are ongoing. The diagnosis of dementia requires the demonstration of change in an individual's baseline functioning after excluding other physical or psychiatric disorders. Diagnoses that must be excluded include hypothyroidism, hearing impairment, and depression (Aylward et al., 1997).

The ICD-10 criteria for dementia provide greater emphasis on noncognitive aspects of dementia than do the DSM-IVTR criteria. The ICD-10 approach begins with describing the psychopathology of dementia and then excluding other possible causes of cognitive decline before making the diagnosis. One study reported on the assessment of 84 individuals with a mean age of 23.7 years and compared them to 84 older individuals with a mean age of 67.7 years. Both groups were institutionalized (Cherry, Matson, and Paclawskyj, 1997). Using the Diagnostic Assessment for the Severely Handicapped Scale, which includes a category of "organic syndromes," they found that 30 of the younger subjects and 36 of the older group had this diagnosis. An epidemiologic sample of 134 individuals (Cooper, 1997c) with intellectual disability, aged 65 years and older, using ICD-10 criteria, revealed the prevalence of dementia to increase in successive age cohorts (groups). The sample showed that 15.6% of those aged 65 years–74 years, 23.5% of those aged 75 years–84 years, and 70% of those aged 85 years–94 years received this diagnosis. The study included five individuals with Down syndrome, three of whom met criteria for dementia. Those with dementia were older and tended to have more poorly controlled epilepsy, as well as a larger number of other physical diagnoses. They were less likely to smoke and had lower scores on adaptive behavior scales than those without dementia. The same individuals were investigated to establish psychiatric symptoms of dementia (Cooper, 1997d). When symptoms occurred with onset during the dementing process, at least one psychotic symptom was demonstrated in 27.6%, persecutory delusions in 20%, and hallucinations in 20.7%. The most common type of hallucinations was visual hallucinations of strangers in the person's home. Other psychiatric symptoms were changed sleep pattern (69%), loss of concentration (69%), worry (41.4%), reduced quantity of speech (41.4%), change in appetite (31%), and increased verbal aggression (31%). Noncognitive symptoms were studied by comparing maladaptive behavior in 29 elderly people with dementia with 99 persons who did not have dementia (Cooper, 1997a). Seventeen of 22 maladaptive behaviors were documented in the group with dementia. Changes in behavior may be an early indicator of dementia.

The existence of noncognitive symptoms within dementia illustrates the need for psychiatric differential diagnosis across the spectrum of psychiatric disorders. When Cooper (1998) checked behavior checklist scores against psychiatric diagnoses in a group of 134 older individuals and 73 younger individuals, she found that a higher proportion scored positively on the behavior checklist. Caregivers described 35.8% of the older age group and 21.9% of the younger individuals as having behavior disorders; in 20.9% of the older group and 6.8% of the younger age group, the behavior disorder was symptomatic of a psychiatric illness. The higher rate of behavior problems among the elderly group was related to the diagnosis of dementia. Thus, an accurate diagnosis of dementia is essential when developing a treatment plan for older individuals with intellectual disability and cognitive decline.

Dementia in Down Syndrome

Sixty-seven adults with Down syndrome aged over 30 and 48 adults with other forms of intellectual disability were followed in a 4.5-year longitudinal study of adaptive behavior (Roeden and Zitman, 1995). Individuals with Down syndrome were 50 years of age and older and showed a decline in their mean adaptive behavior, except in written language, at the end of the 4.5-year period. The comparison group showed a similar trend but to a lesser extent. Dementia, rather than hearing or visual impairment, influenced the adaptive scores, intelligence scores, and scores on memory and motor function tests. A 5-year longitudinal study of adaptive behavior in 83 adults with Down syndrome, using the AAMR Adaptive Behavior Scales, showed that the scale scores were stable for young adults but decreased in middle and old age. Loss of skills was found in some domains in the group originally aged 40 years–49 years and in the majority of domains for those aged 50 years–59 years. There was loss of receptive language but not expressive language. The loss of receptive language may be an early change that occurs with age, and the ratio between expressive and receptive language may be pertinent, although further investigation is needed to confirm this.

In Down syndrome, there is a genetically programmed accumulation of Alzheimer's disease-like neuropathology after age 40, with the development of early dementia some years later. However, older nondemented adults with Down syndrome have been found to show normal rates of regional cerebral glucose metabolism at rest before the onset of dementia; thus, despite brain pathology, their neurons maintain function at rest. The authors hypothesized that an audiovisual stimulation paradigm, acting as a stress test, would reveal abnormalities in cerebral glucose metabolism before dementia in the neocortical parietal and temporal areas most vulnerable to Alzheimer's disease. Regional cerebral glucose metabolism was evaluated by means of positron emission tomography (PET) with [18F]fluorodeoxyglucose in eight younger (mean age = 35 years) and eight older (mean age = 50 years) healthy, nondemented adults with trisomy 21 Down syndrome (Pietrini et al., 1997). PET scans were performed at rest and during audiovisual stimulation in the same scanning session. Levels of general intellectual functioning and compliance were similar in the two groups. At rest, the two groups showed no difference in glucose metabolism in any cerebral region. However, during audiovisual stimulation the older subjects with Down syndrome had significantly lower glucose metabolic rates in the parietal and temporal cortical areas. Abnormalities in cerebral metabolism during stimulation were seen in the cortical regions typically affected in Alzheimer's disease. This stress test paradigm detected metabolic abnormalities in the preclinical stages of Alzheimer's disease even though there was normal cerebral metabolism at rest.

The importance of diagnosing depression in individuals with Down syndrome was illustrated in a study of 37 adults with Down syndrome, aged 40 years and over, referred because of loss of skills. There was a DSM-IVTR diagnosis of depression and associated dementia in 16 individuals and of a depression presenting as pseudodementia in four patients (Tsiouris et al., 2000). Of this group, 10 were treated with antidepressant medication (of these, 2 discontinued treatment early), 5 showed substantial improvement, and 3 showed a moderate improvement, illustrating the importance of diagnosing depression in individuals with Down syndrome and apparent cognitive decline and providing appropriate antidepressant treatment.

Management of Dementia

Older subjects tend to use health and social services less than younger individuals. One study confirmed this in 134 older individuals who were compared to 73 younger adults (Cooper, 1997b). Still, those with dementia and other psychiatric disorders were more likely to use health services. Those who lived in residential settings, day care or respite programs received services from a wide range of caregivers and providers. Failure of the older group to receive services was related to caregivers' assumption that mental symptoms are expected in an older age group, thus minimizing their importance or, if recognized, failing to appreciate their significance. Thus, symptoms in older individuals in residential and day care programs were commonly attributed to the person's intellectual disability and to old age. There is a need to be alert to the types of psychiatric problems that occur in older individuals with intellectual disability and, particularly, to appreciate the diagnostic criteria and natural history of dementia. Further work is necessary to establish better methods to diagnose and assess dementia in individuals with intellectual disability. This requires longitudinal studies of those with diagnosed dementia and additional investigations of the incidence of dementia and adaptive behavior decline. A better understanding of the genetics of dementia is also needed.

NORMALIZATION

A lifespan developmental approach must emphasize encouragement of normalization at all ages. Normalization refers to individuals with intellectual disability being entitled to services that are as culturally normative as possible to help them establish and maintain appropriate personal behavior (Wolfensberger, 1972). The normalization process continues throughout the life span as supports are provided to facilitate greater self-determination. Normalization emphasizes that persons with intellectual disability should live in community settings, attend regular schools, and seek competitive employment. Their behavior should be monitored to assist them to reach the standards for normally developing persons at a comparable developmental age. Persons with intellectual disability should be responsible for their behavior, and it should not be assumed their intellectual disability precludes their ability to take on this responsibility. Although intellectual disability is a chronic condition and is not curable, habilitation can be substantial and adaptation maximized for an IQ range. A developmental model of intellectual disability acknowledges the capacity for growth and emphasizes independent living. The developmental model specifically predicts that adaptive behavior may improve with habilitation. The developmental model constitutes an important aspect of normalization for persons with intellectual disability.

In developmentally based normalization programs for all age groups, communication skills, previous life experience, and any associated physical or behavioral disorders are considered. Special efforts may be needed to normalize communication, for example, teaching sign language and utilizing other approaches to facilitate communication. The nonverbal person with a physical disability, such as cerebral palsy, and intellectual disability may require a speech synthesizer or communication board, or picture cards to assist in communication. Normalization focuses on providing the opportunity for decision making and exposure to varied life experiences. For purposes of normalization, positive supports are needed as individuals grow older to allow them to maintain optimal functioning.

SUMMARY

In summary, a life span developmental approach to intellectual disability demonstrates that the same broad developmental sequences observed in normal development may be considered in developing age-appropriate interventions. However, the uniqueness of each individual and the type of intellectual, cognitive, language, and syndrome-specific development also must be specified in treatment planning. Particularly important is an emphasis on fluid intelligence, along with assessment of working memory, executive functioning, and cognitive processing efficiency. Understanding the mechanisms of learning that are used by persons with intellectual disability is critical in planning their care.

The term "developmental delay" is used to clarify which functions are not developing as expected, but it does not imply that the affected person will "catch up" and function normally. Instead, the term "normalization" is used to specify which personal supports are needed to allow an individual to function as closely as possible to his or her cognitive potential. Life transitions as the person moves from one support system to another (school entry, graduation, entry into a workshop or workplace) can be stressful and require careful preparation and ongoing personal supports.

Personality development requires adequate supports and appreciation of an individual's strengths and developmental differences. With advancing age, the individual must be engaged in treatment and provide assent and/or consent based on his or her level of understanding to facilitate self-determination. Specific health risks vary by syndrome, so physical and mental health assessment must be pertinent to individual needs and ongoing. Age-related psychopathology and health problems may occur; thus, family members and caregiving staff must be aware of the natural history of each intellectual disability syndrome.

KEY POINTS

1. A life span developmental approach considers the individual's developmental progress from infancy to old age, taking into account transitions from one developmental stage to the next.
2. Intelligence tests measure crystallized intelligence, knowledge that is already possessed. Fluid intelligence is involved in processing efficiency, utilization of working memory, executive functioning, and ongoing environmental adaptation.
3. The developmental perspective views development as the outcome of brain maturation, environmental engagement, and personal motivation to master developmental tasks at each phase of the life cycle.
4. Advances in the neurosciences to understand dendritic architecture, synaptic plasticity, brain circuit connectivity, and neuronal network formation may provide insight into the mechanisms involved in development.
5. Comparing brain development and mind/brain environmental interactions among neurogenetic syndromes is a promising approach to understand neurodevelopment.
6. Both the developmental sequence and the developmental pathway associated with intellectual disability should be considered, that is, both similar sequence and multiple pathway models.
7. Mastery motivation is a critical component in development and contributes to how reasoning is applied to problem solving and in consolidating new learning.
8. Mastery motivation entails not only cognitive process but also positive or negative affective engagement in task mastery. Thus, there are both behavioral and emotional components to task mastery.
9. Life transitions are a specific focus of intervention and require specific and personal supports to master transitions from one phase of development to the next one.
10. Self-determination for persons with intellectual disability involves understanding social and personality development. Adaptive features must be facilitated and maladaptive personality features addressed in treatment planning.
11. Greater life expectancy for persons with intellectual disability is the result of advances in public health, medicine, education, technology, and scientific research. With longer life come new opportunities to make choices about life styles that enhance health or endanger it.
12. Normalization refers to services being as culturally normative as possible in establishing and maintaining personal adaptive behavior.
13. Aging is a continuous lifelong process; no specific age defines old age. Still, there are age-related changes in both physical activity and mental life that must be considered in lifespan treatment planning.
14. Implementation of the Surgeon General's national blueprint to improve the health of persons with intellectual disabilities is essential to eliminate current disparities in healthcare.

References

Aylward, E.H., Burt, D.B., Thorpe, L.U., Lai, F., and Dalton, A. (1997). Diagnosis of dementia in individuals with intellectual disability. *Journal of Intellectual Disabilities Research,* 41:152–164.

Cherry, K.E., Matson, J. L., and Paclawskyj, T.R. (1997). Psychopathology in older adults with severe and profound mental retardation. *American Journal of Mental Retardation,* 101:445–458.

Cooper, S.A. (1997a). A population-based health survey of maladaptive behaviours associated with dementia in elderly people with learning disabilities. *Journal of Intellectual Disabilities Research,* 41:481–487.

Cooper, S.A. (1997b). Epidemiology of psychiatric disorders in elderly compared with younger adults with learning disabilities. *British Journal of Psychiatry,* 170:375–380.

Cooper, S.A. (1997c). High prevalence of dementia among people with learning disabilities not attributable to Down's syndrome. *Psychological Medicine,* 27:609–616.

Cooper, S.A. (1997d). Psychiatric symptoms of dementia among elderly people with learning disabilities. *International Journal of Geriatric Psychiatry,* 12:662–666.

Cooper, S.A. (1998). Clinical study of the effects of age on the physical health of adults with mental retardation. *American Journal of Mental Retardation,* 102:582–589.

Demetriou, A., Christou, C., Spanoudis, G., and Platsidou, M. (2002) The development of mental processing: Efficacy, working memory, and thinking. *Monographs of the Society for Research in Child Development,* 67(1, Serial No. 268):122–133.

Dunst, C.J. (1990). Sensorimotor development of infants with Down syndrome. In D. Cicchetti and M. Beeghly (eds.), *Children with Down syndrome: A developmental perspective.* Cambridge University Press, New York.

Durston, S., Hulshoff Pol, H.E., Casey, B.J., Giedd, J.N., Buitelaar, J.K., and van Engeland, H. (2001). Anatomical MRI of the developing human brain: What have we learned? *Journal of the American Academy of Child and Adolescent Psychiatry* 40(9):1012–1020.

Espy, K.A., Kaufmann, P.M., McDiarmid, M.D., and Glisky, M.L. (1999). Executive functioning in preschool children: Performance on A-not-B and other delayed response format tasks. *Brain and Cognition,* 41:178–199.

Fisher, K.W., and Dawson, T.L. (2002). A new kind of developmental science: Using models to integrate theory and research. Commentary on. Demetriou, A., Christou, C., Spanoudis, G., and Platsidou, M. (The Development of Mental Processing: Efficacy, Working Memory, and Thinking.) *Monographs of the Society for Research in Child Development,* 67(1, Serial No. 268):156–167.

Fossella, J.A., Sommer, T., Fan, J., Pfaff, D., and Posner, M.I. (2003). Synaptogenesis and heritable aspects of executive attention. *Mental Retardation and Developmental Disabilities Research Reviews,* 9: 178–183.

Giedd, J.N. (2004). Structural magnetic resonance imaging of the adolescent brain. *Annals of the New York Academy of Sciences,* 1021:77–85.

Giedd, J.N., Blumenthal, J., Jeffries, N.O., Castellanos, F.X., Liu, H., Zijdenbos, A., Paus, T., Evans, A.C., and Rapoport, J.L. (1999). Brain development during childhood and adolescence: A longitudinal MRI study. *Nature Neuroscience,* 2:861–863.

Gilmore, L., Cuskelly, M., and Hayes, A. (2003). A comparative study of mastery motivation in young children with Down's syndrome: Similar outcomes, different processes? *Journal of Intellectual Disability Research,* 47:181–190.

Gustafson, J.E. and Undheim, J.O. (1996). Individual differences in cognitive functions.

In D.C. Berliner and R.C. Calfee (eds.), *Handbook of Educational Psychology,* pp. 186–242. New York: MacMillan.

Hagerman, P.J., and Hagerman, R.J. (2004). The fragile-X premutation: a maturing experience. *American Journal of Human Genetics,* 74:803–816.

Harris, S., Kasari, C., and Sigman, M.D. (1996). Joint attention and language gains in children with Down syndrome. *American Journal of Mental Retardation,* 100:608–619.

Hodapp, R.M., Burack, J.A., and Zigler, E. (1990). *Issues in the developmental approach to mental retardation.* Cambridge University Press, Cambridge.

Hogan, R., and Busch, C. (1984). Moral action as autointerpretation. In W.N. Kurtines and J.L. Gerwitz (eds.), *Morality, Moral Behavior, and Moral Development.* Wiley, New York.

Hogg, J., Lucchino, R., Wang, K. Janicki, M.P., and Working Group (2000). *Healthy ageing—Adults with intellectual disabilities: Ageing and social policy.* World Health Organization, Geneva, Switzerland.

Inhelder, B. (1968). *The diagnosis of reasoning in the mentally retarded.* Day, New York.

Jacquemont, S., Hagerman, R.J., Leehey, M., Grigsby, J., Zhang, L., Brunberg, J.A., Greco, C., Des Portes, V., Jardini, T., Levine, R., et al. (2003). Fragile X premutation tremor/ataxia syndrome: Molecular, clinical, and neuroimaging correlates. *American Journal of Human Genetics,* 72:869–878.

Kohlberg, L. (1969). Stage and sequence: The cognitive-developmental approach to socialization. In D. Goslin (ed.), *Handbook of socialization theory and research.* Rand McNally, Chicago.

Kohlberg, L. (1974). Discussion: Developmental gains in moral judgment. *American Journal of Mental Deficiency,* 79:142–146.

Landry, S.H., Miller-Loncar, C.L., and Swank, P.R. (1998). Goal-directed behavior in children with Down syndrome: The role of joint play situations. *Early Education and Development,* 9:375–392.

MacTurk, R.H., Morgan, G.A., and Jennings, K.D. (1995). The assessment of mastery motivation in infants and young children. In R.H. MacTurk, and G.A. Morgan (eds.), *Mastery motivation: origins, conceptualizations and applications,* pp. 19–56. Ablex Publishing Corporation, Norwood NJ.

MacTurk, R.H., Vietze, P.M., McCarthy, M.E., McQuiston, S., and Yarrow, L.J. (1985). The organization of exploratory behavior in Down syndrome and nondelayed infants. *Child Development,* 56:573–581.

Mahaney, E., and Stephens, B. (1974). Two-year gains in moral judgment by retarded and non-retarded persons. *American Journal of Mental Deficiency,* 79:134–141.

Menolascino, F.J. (1988). Mental illness in the mentally retarded: Diagnostic and treatment issues. In J.A. Stark, F. J. Menolascino, M.H. Albarelli, and V.C. Gray (eds.), *Mental retardation and mental health: Classification, diagnosis, treatment, services.* Springer-Verlag, New York.

Messer, D.J. (1993). Mastery motivation: An introduction to theories and issues. In D. Messer (ed.), *Mastery motivation in early childhood: development, measurement and social processes,* pp. 1–16. Routledge, London.

Morgan, G.A., Busch-Rossnagel, N.A., Maslin-Cole, C.A., and Harmon, R.J. (1992a). *Individualized assessment of mastery motivation: Manual for 15–36-month-old children.* Fordham, University, New York.

Morgan, G.A., Harmon, R.J., and Maslin-Cole, C.A. (1990). Mastery motivation: Definition and measurement. *Early Education and Development,* 1:318–339.

Morgan, G.A., Harmon, R.J., Maslin-Cole, C.A., Busch-Rossnagel, N.A., Jennings, K.D., Hauser-Cram, P., and Brockman, L.M. (1992b). *Assessing perceptions of mastery motivation: The Dimensions of Mastery Questionnaire, its development, psychometrics and use.* State University, Human Development and Family Studies Department, Fort Collins, CO.

Palmen, S.J., Van Engeland, H., Hof, P.R., and Schmitz, C. (2004). Neuropathological findings in autism. *Brain*, 127 (pt. 12):2572–2583.

Paour, J. (2001) From structural analysis to functional diagnosis of reasoning: A dynamic conception of mental retardation. In A. Tryphon and J. Voneche (eds.), *Working with Piaget: Essays in Honour of Barbel Inhelder*, pp. 13–38. Psychology Press, Philadelphia, PA.

Pasnak, R., Willson-Quayle, A., and Whitten, J. (1998). Mild retardation, academic achievement, and Piagetian or Psychometric Tests of Reasoning. *Journal of Developmental and Physical Disabilities, 10*:23–33.

Piaget, J. (1952). *The origins of intelligence in children.* Norton, New York.

Pietrini, P., Dani, A., Furey, M.L., Alexander, G.E., Freo, U., Grady, C.L., Mentis, M.J., Mangot, D., Simon, E.W., Horwitz, B., et al. (1997). Low glucose metabolism during brain stimulation in older Down's syndrome subjects at risk for Alzheimer's disease prior to dementia. *American Journal of Psychiatry,* 154:1063–1069.

Reid, A., and Ballenger, B.R. (1987). Personality disorder in mental handicap. *Psychological Medicine, 17*:983–987.

Roeden, J.M., and Zitman, F.G. (1995). Ageing in adults with Down's syndrome in institutionally based and community-based residences. *Journal of Intellectual Disabilities Research, 39*:399–407.

Ruskin, E.M., Kasari, C., Mundy, P., and Sigman, M. (1994a). Attention to people and toys during social and object mastery in children with Down syndrome. *American Journal of Mental Retardation*, 99:103–111.

Ruskin, E.M., Mundy, P., Kasari, C., and Sigman, M. (1994b). Object mastery motivation of children with Down syndrome. *American Journal of Mental Retardation*, 98:499–509.

Schumann, C.M., Hamstra, J., Goodlin-Jones, B.L., Lotspeich, L.J., Kwon, H., Buonocore, M.H., Lammers, C.R., Reiss, A.L., and Amaral, D.G. (2004). The amygdala is enlarged in children but not adolescents with autism: The hippocampus is enlarged at all ages. *Journal of Neuroscience*, 24:6392–6401.

Tsiouris, J.A., Mehta, P.D., Patti, P.J., Madrid, R.E., Raguthu, S., Barshatzky, M.R., Cohen, I.L., and Sersen, E. (2000). Alpha2 macroglobulin elevation without an acute phase response in depressed adults with Down's syndrome: Implications. *Journal of Intellectual Disabilities Research*, 44:644–653.

Uzgiris, I., and Hunt, J. McV. (1975). *Assessment in infancy: Affect, cognition, and communication.* University of Illinois Press, Urbana.

Vietze, P.M., McCarthy, M., McQuiston, S., MacTurk, R., and Yarrow, L. (1983). Attention and exploratory behavior in infants with Down syndrome. In T. Field and A. Sosted (eds.), *Infants born at risk: physiological, perceptual, and cognitive processes*, pp. 251–268. Grune & Stratton, New York, NY.

Wishart, J.G. (1991). Taking the initiative in learning: A developmental investigation of infants with Down syndrome. *International Journal of Disability, Development and Education, 38*:27–44.

Wishart, J.G. (1993). The development of learning difficulties in children with Down's syndrome. *Journal of Intellectual Disabilities Research, 37*:389–403.

Wishart, J.G. (1999). Learning and development in children with Down's syndrome. In A. Slater and D. Muir (eds.), *Blackwell reader in developmental psychology*, pp. 493–508. Blackwell, Oxford.

Wolfensberger, W. (1972). *The principle of normalization in human services.* National Institute on Mental Retardation, Toronto, Ontario.

Woodward. M. (1959a). The application of Piaget's theory to research in mental deficiency. In N. R. Ellis (ed.), *Handbook of mental deficiency, psychological theory and research,* pp. 297–324. McGraw-Hill, New York.

Woodward, M. (1959b). The behaviour of idiots interpreted by Piaget's theory of sensori-motor development. *British Journal of Educational Psychology,* 29:60–71.

Woodward, M. (1979). Piaget's theory and the study of mental retardation. In N.R. Ellis (ed.), *Handbook of mental deficiency, psychological theory and research,* pp. 169–196. McGraw-Hill, New York.

Zigler, E., and Burack, J.A. (1989). Personality development and the dually diagnosed person. *Research in Developmental Disabilities,* 10:225–240.

9

Family, Psychoeducational, Behavioral, Interpersonal, and Pharmacologic Interventions

The capacity to adapt to disability and assist others with disability may have an evolutionary origin. De Waal (1996) describes assistance to an injured group member among primates as evidence of altruistic behavior. Mother monkeys will provide additional care to compensate for injuries, and other members of the group may "babysit" injured infants, as do other young of the group. If the risk of predation is low and food is adequate, handicapped animals may live to adulthood. In human evolution, Berkson (1993) described an adult Neanderthal male with severe arm and head injuries that occurred at an early age. Apparently, this individual adapted to the injury by using his teeth to hold objects. Other conditions, such as disabling arthritis, were found in Neanderthals as well. Thus, individuals with minor or even significant impairments in primate and human societies before the evolution of modern humans, in some instances, received adaptive assistance from other members of the group.

HISTORICAL BACKGROUND

Drawing on these possible evolutionary origins of assistance to others in need, this chapter reviews the historical background of care for persons with intellectual disability and discusses environmental provisions and supports, education and skill development, normalization and self-determination, and interventions for those with co-occurring mental and behavioral disorders (psychotherapy, behavioral interventions, and psychopharmacologic treatments).

Itard and the Beginnings of Care for Disabled Persons

The modern developmental approach to understanding learning and development began with Jean Itard, at the end of the eighteenth century. As a member of the medical staff at the Institute for Deaf Mutes in Paris, he considered the link between deafness and learning. Because of this background, he was asked to study a feral child discovered living alone in the wild in southern France. It was thought that this boy might approximate "man in the state of nature." Because the child was mute, he entered a school for the deaf in Paris although he was not deaf. Pinel (1809), the leading psychiatrist of the time, proposed that the boy, named Victor, was not teachable. Yet Itard, during the next five years, sought to instruct Victor, using approaches established for deaf persons. His approach was based on the work of Jacob Pereiere, whose teaching methods emphasized the interpretation by Rousseau of John Locke's view of sensationalist empirical psychology (Winzer, 1993). Itard individualized instruction and emphasized sensory stimulation, socialization, speech, concept development, and transfer of learning (Itard, 1802). He believed that Victor had experienced severe educational and social deprivation. Under Itard's tutorage, Victor developed limited speech but did not advance enough to be restored to society; he lived out his final days with a caretaker. Even though Itard felt that his intervention with Victor was unsuccessful, his intervention stimulated the interest of others to work with children with intellectual disability. Among them were Edouard Seguin and Maria Montessori, who refined the methods for intervention.

Institutional Placement

The systematic care of persons with developmental disabilities began at the beginning of the eighteenth century in Europe and during the nineteenth century in the United States. Samuel Woodward, superintendent of the Worcester State Hospital in Massachusetts, and Amariah Brigham at the Bloomingdale Center in New York proposed in 1845 that their respective states should make public education available for children with intellectual disability. Samuel Gridley Howe was appointed by the Massachusetts legislature to chair an epidemiological committee regarding intellectual disability. In this capacity, Howe carried out the first prevalence study of intellectual disability in the United States and made recommendations to establish an experimental school. Howe's school opened in October 1848 in Boston in a wing of the Perkins Institute for the Blind. In 1855, Wilbur became the superintendent of a new institution in Syracuse, New York, which was the first institution for people with intellectual disability that was constructed specifically for their care in the United States. (Fernald, 1917). Other states followed the leads of Massachusetts and New York in opening experimental schools. For example, in 1853, the Pennsylvania Training School for [intellectually disabled] Children opened in Elwyn, Pennsylvania. One consequence of the establishment of residential schools and institutional programs was the segregation of people with intellectual disability from those with mental illness.

Institutional programs for individuals with intellectual disability increased in size and number in the mid-1800s following the examples in Massachusetts and New York. It is reported that many of the training efforts were successful, and children with intellectual disability were returned to their communities as "productive workers" (Trent, 1995). With the onset of the Civil War and the economic recessions that followed it, there was less employment available for those with intellectual disability trained in residential settings. In some instances, their unpaid labor led to exploitation. By 1880, the training schools established by leaders such as Howe and Seguin had become custodial asylums with less emphasis on education and return to community life (Wolfensberger, 1976). There was a lack of supportive social services, family support, and work opportunities in the community. Negative attitudes toward people with intellectual disability persisted in the general public, and Wilbur (1888) suggested that lifelong protective custodial care was appropriate.

Samuel Gridley Howe opposed the trend toward lifelong institutionalization and, in a speech in 1866, stated that people with disabilities "should be kept diffused among sound and normal persons. Separation, and not congregation, should be the law of their treatment" (Wolfensberger, 1976). He proposed that the states should gradually dispense with custodial institutions. However, the states did not do so; they continued to build them, to expand them, and to emphasize their economical management and self-sufficiency. By 1900, the census of intellectual disability institutions in the United States was 11,800 persons (Fernald, 1917). Often the institutions were located in remote areas. In their institutional settings, residents were given work in laundries, on farmlands, and in workshops, contributing to the self-sustaining economy of the institution. However, Seguin (1870) did not support the growth of large institutions, stating "Let us hope that the State institutions for mentally retarded [intellectually disabled] persons will escape that evil of excessive growth . . . in which patients are so numerous that the accomplished physicians who have them in charge cannot remember the name of each."

By the beginning of the twentieth century, institutions for persons with intellectual disabilities were firmly established throughout the world. The first textbook on intellectual disability was written by Barr (1904). He completed an international survey stating that 21 nations operated 171 institutions for persons with intellectual disability. Twenty-five of these were in the United States. However, by the end of the twentieth century the practice of institutionalization had been substantially reversed and a national movement toward deinstitutionalization had successfully resulted in community placement, as described in detail in chapter 2. The sections that follow reflect current approaches to community treatment especially in regard to emotional and behavioral problems that affect community placement.

DIAGNOSIS, TREATMENT, AND COMMUNITY PLACEMENT

Intellectual disability is associated with a higher prevalence of behavioral, emotional, and mental disorders than that found in the general population, as described in chapter 4. Diagnosis of behavioral and mental disorders in intellectually disabled persons is 3 to 4 times that in the general population. With these higher rates of psychopathology, psychotropic drugs are increasingly being used, in combination with other treatments, in children, adolescents, and adults with intellectual disability. However, a major impediment to treating these disorders as effectively as in the general population is our inability to recognize mental health problems in persons with intellectual disability and developmental disorders. Assessment and diagnosis of emotional and behavioral disturbance is particularly difficult due to intellectual, adaptive, and verbal impairments that limit reliability or reporting of symptoms, and the presence of organic or environmental factors that either produce or exacerbate the specific forms of pathologic behavior, as described in chapter 6. Receipt of services is also frequently linked to the diagnosis of a specific condition or the severity of functional impairment relating to that diagnosis. As a consequence of difficulties with diagnosis and assessment, persons with developmental disorders may not receive effective treatments; the treatment they receive may actually be harmful, and they may be denied important services.

Behavioral phenotypes that are associated with neurogenetic syndromes resulting in intellectual disability include single-gene defects, microdeletion syndromes, and chromosomal aneuploidy. An understanding of the behavioral phenotype of a disorder, as described in chapter 7, is critical when considering psychiatric diagnoses. In addition, intellectual disability is associated with a variety of other medical and surgical conditions that require specific treatments of their own, as described in chapter 5. If treatment for associated conditions requires medication, then drug-drug interactions must be carefully monitored. Epilepsy is a diagnosis that is commonly associated with intellectual disability, co-occurring in as many as 40% of cases, especially in those who are more severely intellectually disabled. Because both psychoactive drugs and antiseizure medications are active in the central nervous system, the risk for adverse effects on central nervous system functioning is increased. For example, one medication may affect the metabolism of another. In addition, persons with intellectual disability may be at greater risk of developing side effects than the general population probably as a result of central nervous system dysfunction. Investigators (Aman et al., 1996; Handen et al., 1991; Handen, Johnson, and Lubetsky, 2000; Johnson et al., 1994) have reported a higher rate of tics, dysphoria, and lack of social responsiveness in children with both ADHD and intellectual disability on moderate doses of methylphenidate.

Intellectual disability, associated conditions, and the availability of positive supports all affect community placement.

MULTIMODAL TREATMENT

The framework for interventions in neurodevelopmental disorders is grounded in psychobiology, taking into account both psychological and neurobiological elements. Such interventions are based on a comprehensive assessment of the child and family, as outlined in chapters 5 and 6. The focus of intervention is on the active, adapting person with consideration given to mastery of developmental tasks that are consonant with the child's abilities, as discussed in chapter 8.

Case Formulation

A comprehensive evaluation is followed by a case formulation. The formulation is a concise summary that takes into account all the information available from the assessment process. It should begin with a brief statement of the current problem and be followed by a description of how the clinician understands the information that has been gathered. It is a synthesis of the assessment rather than a restatement of facts. The formulation provides an integration of the known biological, psychological, and social factors that contributed to the development of the current problem. It includes a discussion of the diagnosis and of the etiologic factors and conditions that are deemed important from a review of the course of the condition. It takes into account both the patient's current life situation and his or her background. It (1) supplements the formal diagnosis; (2) enriches the clinical data base by providing a synthesis that leads to hypotheses that are testable in part by clinical observation; and (3) provides an understanding of the history and examination, which is crucial to planning treatment.

Treatment Planning

Treatment planning involves determining the appropriate intervention based on the clinical formulation; this takes into account the multiple conditions that adversely affect the child and family. Treatment planning involves the selection of curative, corrective, ameliorative, or palliative approaches. A properly developed formulation suggests guides for appropriate intervention. The treatment modalities chosen should be the most efficacious, the least restrictive, and the most cost effective. Although treatment planning must take into account the problem areas identified in the clinical formulation, it must also take into account the patient's and family's strengths. It addresses problems in the individual (both psychological and physical), problems in the family, problems with peers, problems at school, and problems in the sociocultural environment. Treatment goals are developed for the individual child and his family, utilizing medical, interdisciplinary, individual psychodynamic, family systems, group, behavioral, pharmacological, and environmental approaches; these are incorporated into a multimodal intervention.

Treatment for children and adults with intellectual disability focuses on the individual and considers the complex interaction of neurobiological and psychosocial factors. A comprehensive and interdisciplinary approach is required. Consideration is given to the full range of treatments that are used with typically developing children and adults. Multimodal treatment designs seek to compare, contrast, and evaluate additive/interactive effects of several different modalities of treatment; the interventions must be carefully specified and independently monitored.

The AAMR's (Luckasson et al., 2002) multidimensional approach provides guidelines for those supports that facilitate development, education, interests, and personal well-being to enhance functioning. Such supports are provided through inclusive education for children and adolescents and supported living and supported employment for adults. Better environmental provision, cognitive and behavioral interventions, individual and family psychotherapy, and psychopharmacology are all applicable therapeutic approaches in the multidimensional approach. The efficacy of each of these interventions has been demonstrated when appropriately selected and implemented.

The goal of treatment is full habilitation and achievement of the best quality of life possible for a particular condition. Treatment begins with a conference to advise family members about the findings from the evaluation. If intellectual disability has been diagnosed, the first step is to work with the family to help them acknowledge the type of impairments that affect their family member. Typical questions (Kanner, 1953) asked by family members at the time of diagnosis have changed little over the past 50 years and are listed in table 9.1. However, with the mapping of the human genome, the questions of heredity and genetic counseling now receive greater emphasis (Holland and Clare, 2003).

The use of genetic screening and testing has an ethical dimension in regard to the impact of screening for genetic abnormalities and termination of pregnancy on the lives of individuals currently living with disabilities (Stainton, 2003). In one review, termination rates following prenatal diagnosis for Down syndrome, spinal bifida, anencephaly, Turner syndrome, and Klinefelter syn-

Table 9.1 Questions Commonly Asked by Parents Concerning a Child with Intellectual Disability

What is the cause of our child's intellectual disability?
Have we personally contributed to his condition?
Why did this have to happen to us?
What about heredity?
Is it safe to have another child?
Is there any danger that our normal children's offspring might be similarly affected?
How is his (or her) presence in the home likely to affect our normal children?
How shall we explain him (or her) to our normal children?
How shall we explain him (or her) to our friends and neighbors?
Is there anything that we can do to brighten him (or her) up?
Is there an operation that might help?
Is there any drug that might help?
Will our child *ever* talk?
What will our child be like when he (or she) grows up?
Can we expect graduation from high school? From elementary school?
Would you advise a private tutor?
Should we keep our child at home or place him (or her) in a residential school?
What specific school do you recommend?
If a residential school, how long will our child have to remain there?
Will our child become alienated from us if placed in a residential school?
Will our child ever be mature enough to marry?

From Kanner 1953.

dromes were reported. The termination rate varied with the condition; they were highest for Down syndrome (average = 92%) and lowest for Klinefelter syndrome (average = 58%) (Mansfield, Hopfer, and Marteau, 1999). The changing life expectancy for persons with intellectual disability impacts the life of the family and the community with both social and ethical implications for counseling. Finally, the meaning of disability from the standpoint of moral philosophy lends new importance to how disability in society is understood (Vehmas, 2004).

Each member of an interdisciplinary team discusses with the family what their role will be in treatment. This is followed by implementing the various elements of the treatment plan that are discussed in this chapter.

Goals of Treatment

Intellectual disability involves functional impairments. The overall goal of treatment is to reduce the effects of these impairments to reduce the extent of disability. Goals include the following:

1. Treatment of the underlying disorder that resulted in intellectual disability. If newborn screening has identified a genetic disorder, such as phenylketonuria, then dietary treatment is immediately initiated.
2. Treatment of any associated co-occurring conditions that may be present, physical, behavioral, or mental.
3. Interventions that are specifically focused on the functional impairments themselves. These include environmental provisions, educational interventions, provision of supports to facilitate self-determination, and psychological, behavioral, and pharmacological interventions based on the individuals' and families' specific needs.

An approach to treatment is based on the following supports and principles:

THE ENVIRONMENTAL PROVISION

Appropriate living conditions, vocational opportunities, and leisure time activities are essential environmental provisions for persons with intellectual disability. It is critical that the individual participate in society and have an opportunity to express preferences and make personal choices about living conditions, work, and recreational activities. When these issues receive attention and are handled well, an improved quality of life and a substantial reduction in maladaptive emotional and behavioral symptoms may result. When a child's parent is intellectually disabled, the parent requires particular support to provide for the child's needs (Accardo and Whitman, 1990). A well-designed home program provides access to preferred activities, offers choices with regard to household tasks, and schedules highly preferred tasks and activities immediately following nonpreferred (but essential) ones.

EDUCATIONAL INTERVENTIONS/SKILL DEVELOPMENT

A fundamental challenge in the care and treatment of persons with intellectual disability is to assist them in finding appropriate ways to interact with others. Emotional and behavioral disturbances commonly result from a lack of self-monitoring and adaptive control by the individuals over their inner lives and external environment. Communication deficits, learning difficulty, and limited educational experience may deprive them of the requisite skills needed for personal competence and social responsibility. Therefore, an educationally based program should emphasize social, communication, and vocational skills to reduce maladaptive behavior and improve self-control. Essential elements include independence training (teaching self-help and leisure skills), communication training (enhancing speech and nonverbal communication such as signing, gestures, and the use of picture/word boards), and self-management skill development (teaching strategies for self-monitoring and self-reinforcement). Social skills training offers concrete instructions, uses observation and modeling of effective behavior, provides reinforcement, and focuses on teaching appropriate behaviors. Social skills training emphasizes the enhancement of suitable interpersonal behavior in a variety of common social situations, such as being introduced to another person and properly responding, initiating and participating in social group activities, and learning to interpret and respond appropriately to verbal and nonverbal social cues. Successful social skills programs combine demonstration by instructors, modeling, role-play, social practice, constructive feedback, and positive reinforcement. The training may include initial instruction and practice in a therapeutic environment, followed by practice in natural community settings.

NORMALIZATION AND SELF-DETERMINATION

Normalization

Intellectual disability is a permanent condition and is not curable, although the degree of habilitation that can be accomplished for the person with intellectual disability can be substantial (Wolfensberger, 1972). Persons who are mildly cognitively impaired may not be categorized as intellectually disabled if they respond to early treatment; they may lose that designation after leaving their formal educational program. Deficits in current adaptive functioning are major targets for intervention. During the past 30 years, a focus on a developmental model that acknowledges the capacity for growth, developing independence in social skills, and new learning has been emphasized. The developmental model specifically addresses the fact that the intellectually disabled person's level of functioning is not static and that an individual's adaptive behavior may be improved through habilitation. Because a person with intellectual disability is capable of learning and adapting, legal approaches need to take into account that the person with intellectual disability may require additional education and, with instructional effort, can learn new information.

The focus on normalization (Wolfensberger, 1972) for persons with intellectual disability described in chapters 2 and 6 emphasizes the importance of intellectually disabled persons being entitled to services that are as culturally normative as possible to help them establish and maintain more appropriate personal behavior. Normalization emphasizes that persons with intellectual disability should live in the community, go to regular schools, seek competitive employment, and behave as closely as possible to the standards of the typically developing persons at a comparable developmental age. Furthermore, they should be responsible for their own behavior, and others should not assume that because they are intellectually disabled that they are not capable of doing so. Still, their differences and their need for individual assessment must be recognized to guarantee that services are provided (Simpson, 1998). For normalization, it is proposed not only that social competence is a critical focus in treatment programs but also that an ethical approach that recognizes interests, desires, and preferences of the individual is needed (Simpson, 1998). One risk is excessive programming for an individual with a lack of allowance for personal choices. Concern for personal choices is emphasized in the next section on self-determination.

Special features of persons with intellectual disability that need to be taken into account in normalization are their communication skills, previous life experiences, behavioral problems, and any associated physical disorders. Many people with intellectual disability have concurrent difficulties in language expression and articulation. Consequently, it may require a special effort to communicate with them, and in some instances, signing may be necessary to communicate. In other instances, the nonverbal intellectually disabled person with a physical handicap, such as cerebral palsy, may require a speech synthesizer or other language devices to assist in communication. The person with intellectual disability may because of poor programming lack certain life experiences that may influence his or her ability to respond to new situations. Finally, behavioral and physical disorders involving the brain and other organ systems that are quite commonly found in intellectual disability syndromes must be considered.

Self-Determination

Recognition of an individual's interests, desires, and preferences is central to normalization and is emphasized in programs to facilitate self-determination. It is proposed that self-determination is the culmination of the normalization and deinstitutionalization movements that started in the early 1970s. Self-determination is an essential aspect of special education and related services for people with disabilities. Self-determination can be taught and learned, and can make a difference in the lives of individuals with disabilities.

Self-determination has been defined as the combination of skills, knowledge, and beliefs that enable a person to engage in goal-directed, self-regulated, and autonomous behavior (Algozzine et al., 2001). Although the right to make decisions about one's own life and future is viewed as a basic civil right by American adults without disabilities, that right was not legally recognized for adults with disabilities (Wehmeyer et al., 2000) until the 1990s with the passage of disability legislation, that is, the Americans with Disabilities Act of 1990, the Individuals with Disabilities Education Act, 1990, 1997, and 2004, and the Rehabilitation Act Amendments of 1992 (Ysseldyke, Algozzine and Thurlow, 2000). Such legislation affirmed the right of individuals with disabilities to choose where and with whom they want to live, what jobs they want, and by what means they might achieve their personal goals and dreams. The U.S. Department of Education also has identified self-determination as an important outcome of the educational process for children and adults with disabilities and has committed significant resources to promote this concept by funding studies on self-determination (Wehmeyer and Schwartz, 1998a,b; Wehmeyer and Ward, 1995).

Recognition of the importance of self-determination for individuals with developmental disabilities became apparent when difficulties in making the transition from the final years of schooling to workshops and vocational programs were acknowledged. Thus, much of the literature on self-determination has focused on transitions for persons with disabilities from one type of program to another (e.g., Martin and Marshall, 1995; Wehmeyer, Agran, and Hughes, 1998; Wehmeyer, Agran, and Hughes, 2000; Wehmeyer and Ward, 1995). The needs of persons in specific disability categories, including learning disabilities (Field, 1996), intellectual disability (Wehmeyer, 1992; Wehmeyer, 1996), severe disabilities (Brown et al., 1998; Schloss, Alper, and Jyne, 1993), and autistic disorder (Field and Hoffman, 1999), have been studied. Although there are several components of self-determination, most commonly self-determination involves teaching choice making to individuals with moderate and severe intellectual disability and self-advocacy to individuals with mild intellectual disability.

Considerable effort is required to train children, youth, and adults with disabilities how to become self-determining persons. Concurrently, persons without disabilities must be taught to respect and honor the choices and decisions made by individuals with disabilities. Thus, both teaching and encouraging persons with disabilities to self-determine, as well as teaching those without disabilities to honor their choices and decisions, are essential.

Recommended strategies for promoting self-determination include involvement in the creation of an individualized education plan (IEP), transition planning, and person-centered planning to meet goals and direct teaching of self-determination skills. For Wehmeyer (1996), self-determination is (1) defined in relationship to characteristic features of a person's behavior; (2) considered an educational outcome; and (3) accomplished through lifelong learning, opportunities and experiences.

Self-determination refers to both interventions and outcomes for persons with intellectual disability. It includes (1) choosing goals based on an understanding of their interests, skills, and limits; (2) expressing their goals to help build support for themselves; (3) decision making with a plan to attain their goals; (4) evaluating their plan and actions toward achieving it; (5) adjusting their goal, plan, and actions for continued self-determination. Thus, problem-solving, self-awareness, and self-advocacy are encouraged (Martin, O'Brien, and Wray, 1999–2000).

Indeed, self-advocacy and choice making were the major intervention themes found in a meta-analysis of the self-determination literature in 51 studies reviewed by Algozzine et al. (2001). The most common interventions teach choice making to individuals with moderate-to-severe intellectual disability or self-advocacy to individuals with learning disabilities or mild intellectual disability. The majority of studies include individuals with intellectual disability or learning disabilities, although individuals with sensory impairments (Balcazar, Fawcett, and Seekins, 1991; Bowman and Marzouk, 1992; Hoffman and Field, 1995), autistic disorder (Fullerton and Coyne, 1999; Malette et al., 1992), emotional disturbance (Hoffman and Field, 1995; Wehmeyer and Lawrence, 1995) and traumatic brain injury (Prater, Bruhl, and Serna, 1998) have participated in self-determination programs. Self-advocacy knowledge and self-efficacy are aspects of self-determination that require further study.

Self-determination is taught using a variety of methods, including large group instruction (e.g., Abery and Zajac, 1996), individual conferences (Bowman and Marzouk, 1992), and one-to-one behavioral interventions with systematic prompting and feedback as the person practices the skill (e.g., Cooper and Browder, 1998). Interventions may be directed toward staff with concurrent measurement of changes for participants with disabilities (Ezell, Klein, and Ezell-Powell, 1999). Most studies focus on teaching self-determination skills; however, others have promoted self-determination through other forms of support, including using preference assessments to enhance choice making (Parsons, Reid, and Green, 1998) and person-centered planning to enhance goal setting (Everson and Zhang, 2000).

In addition to teaching choice making or self-advocacy to individuals with intellectual disability, other components of self-determination include goal setting and attainment, self-regulation, self-evaluation, and problem solving. Aune (1991) provides examples of how students can learn to set and attain goals ranging from daily objectives to long-term postsecondary goals. Van Reusen and Bos (1994; Van Reusen, Deshler, and Schumaker, 1989) demonstrate how students can participate in their own IEP meetings to recruit support for achieving these goals. Person-centered planning teams (Malette et al., 1992) and preference assessment (Parsons, Reid, and Green, 1998) provide options for supporting individuals with severe disabilities to have greater self-determination.

Previous research focusing on enhancing self-determination for adolescents or adults fits well with transition planning (Aune, 1991). Teaching such skills to younger students is receiving more emphasis. For example, Adelman et al. (1990) taught problem solving and decision making to children as young as five years of age. Others have studied choice making by children (Dattilo and Rusch, 1985). Brown and Cohen (1996) have emphasized that children all need opportunities to learn self-determination skills in age-appropriate ways. Most studies have participants with intellectual disability or learning disabilities; however, individuals with autistic disorder, emotional disturbance, and sensory impairments may require alternative approaches that are more appropriate to these disabilities.

Ongoing efforts are needed to help individuals make progress in a comprehensive self-determination curriculum. Focusing on more components of self-determination may yield more results either because there is a synergistic effect or because there is a great deal of overlap between some of these skills (e.g., problem solving and decision making). Algozzine et al. (2001) propose that maintaining employment requires using decision making, problem solving, goal attainment, self-regulation, and self-advocacy.

Promoting self-determination for school-age individuals involves not only teaching new skills but also creating opportunities to do so in environments in which they are encouraged to use those skills. Changing staff knowledge or behavior can be critical. Ezell, Klein, and Ezell-Powell (1999) had staff use portfolio assessments so that they would include students in planning and evaluating their own learning. Sigafoos et al. (1993) trained staff to provide more choice-making opportunities for students with severe disabilities. Crucially, two questions must be answered: Do staff who learn to teach a self-determination curriculum create opportunities for students to make their own decisions in the typical classroom routine? Do staff who learn to offer more classroom choices also create opportunities for choice making in other school or community settings?

In summary, there is now a foundation for promoting self-determination for students with disabilities in current school programs. Methods to teach choice making to individuals with moderate and severe disabilities and self-advocacy to individuals with learning disabilities or mild intellectual disability are ongoing.

Future research must accomplish the following (Algozzine et al., 2001):

1. *Demonstrate that self-determination can be taught by teaching more complex self-determination skills (e.g., self-advocacy and goal attainment) to individuals with severe disabilities.* There is minimal information on how to individualize this instruction for students with sensory impairments, autistic disorder, or emotional disturbance. Research on how to plan and implement a comprehensive self-determination curriculum as an individual progresses across grade levels is needed. What are the best ways to promote self-determination by redesigning the classroom and school climate? More specifics about best intervention practices must also be known. For example, are there benefits to providing instruction over a series of sessions versus several longer ones or to providing interventions that target the individual or the support staff?

2. *Demonstrate that self-determination can be learned.* There is strong evidence that individuals with intellectual disability can learn to make choices and solve problems, although this is based primarily on single-subject studies. There is modest evidence from group studies that individuals with mild intellectual disability and learning disabilities can learn to self-advocate. There is limited information about children acquiring self-determination skills that are specific to choice making. It is essential to demonstrate that individuals can master and use these skills.

3. *Demonstrate that self-determination makes a difference in the lives of individuals with disabilities.* Do any measures of outcomes of self-determination interventions in the lives of participants result in new opportunities for school,

employment, or leisure activities? Williams (1989) emphasized that life should be filled with rising expectations, dignity, responsibility, and opportunity. Future research requires outcome indicators to determine how specific interventions influence the quality of the lives of people with disabilities.

INTERVENTION STRATEGIES

Psychotherapy

Individuals with mild intellectual disability have been shown to benefit from individual, family, and group psychotherapy. Psychotherapeutic interventions are most effective in the treatment of emotional and behavioral disturbances in individuals who have experienced stressful or traumatic experiences that result in internalized conflict and maladaptive behavior. Repeated failure, social rejection, frequent losses, and dependency on others may result in feelings of inferiority, ambivalence, anxiety, and anger; each of these symptoms may be targeted for treatment. Family conflicts involving feelings of jealousy toward normally developing siblings and tension with parents regarding issues of emancipation and independence are other targets for intervention. For the adult, age-related issues, assisting with the transition to community life, bereavement, and dealing with exposure to dangers in the environment that come with community living are targets for intervention (Lynch, 2004).

Psychotherapeutic interventions tend to be underutilized in intellectually disabled persons because of misconceptions about their effectiveness despite the fact that these individuals are often good candidates for psychotherapy (Szymanski, 1980). They can be highly motivated to establish interpersonal relationships and often demonstrate a strong desire for enhancing their personal competence and independence. Beail (1998) carried out psychodynamic psychotherapy in 20 adults with intellectual disability and co-occurring mental disorders. They reported significant reductions in psychological distress, improved interpersonal functioning, and enhanced self-esteem. Modified forms of these treatment approaches have been used with individuals who test in the moderate-to-severe range of intellectual disability.

Attachment theory may provide a basis for psychotherapy with developmentally disordered persons. Attachment theory places its primary emphasis on interpersonal relationships whose evolutionary function is the protection of the young from danger. The early relationship between parent and offspring has its basis in interpersonal feedback and may provide a model for psychotherapy. Attachment models emphasize establishing a secure emotional base formed through the relationship with the therapist, resulting in affect regulation through interpersonal encounter. In the individual therapy situation, the affective interactions between the therapist and the individual in treatment involve modeling, as well as interpersonal modulation of affect. The psychotherapist working with an individual with a disability must openly accept the impaired individual as a person and develop a sense of respect for his individuality. The therapist appreciates the individual's relative strengths and takes satisfaction in small increments of change. The therapist must acknowledge their own negative thoughts, feelings, and attitudes toward the intellectually disabled person that may arise as a response to the individual's appearance or behavior.

The goals for psychotherapeutic treatment are similar to those for the general population and include the resolution of internalized conflict, improvement in self-esteem, and enhancement of personal competence and independence. Modifications of the usual treatment approaches that take into account the developmental level of the person are necessary. A supportive atmosphere, focused approaches by the therapist, and shorter, more frequent sessions may be needed. Modifications include simplifying language, using concrete language, regular checking for comprehension of conceptual information, providing information at a slower rate, and minimizing distractions. A more directive approach is required and caregivers may be involved to help in the generalization of skills and in making concepts more applicable to real world situations. More time should be allowed for verbal responses and nonverbal responses should be recognized. Overall, there should be more emphasis on being goal focused. Role-playing methods may enhance learning and provide an opportunity to demonstrate understanding. Recognition that the person may think of himself as a "disabled" person is important and may contribute to his excessive dependency on others. Persons in treatment may be outwardly directed in the sense that they look to others for cues in ambivalent situations rather than examining their own past experiences for ways to cope.

Cognitive-behavioral therapy has been utilized for persons with intellectual disability (Beail, 2003). There are two general approaches to cognitive-behavioral treatment: self-management approaches (Dagnan and Chadwick, 1997) and cognitive therapy. Self-management approaches assume that emotional and behavioral problems result from a lack of cognitive skills and include interventions to teach self-monitoring, self-control, problem solving/decision making, and anger management. Such methods are combined with relaxation techniques, skill acquisition procedures, and social skills training. Self-management strategies have been effective in improving anger management and enhancing self-concept and self-esteem (Rose, West, and Clifford, 2000). Cognitive-behavioral therapies have been utilized in both individual and group settings.

Cognitive therapy addresses cognitive distortions. Such distortions in the form of abnormal beliefs and inappropriate attributions or inferences about others actions may result from irrational emotions. The aim of treatment is to examine an individual's interpretations and understanding of the meaning of their experiences. There is limited evidence for the effectiveness of this approach in persons with intellectual disability, as it requires the development of self- and social awareness. However, one study successfully used this approach with men with intellectual disability who were involved in inappropriate sexual behavior with children (Lindsay et al., 1998).

Prout and Nowak-Drabik (2003) reviewed studies of psychotherapy in persons with intellectual disability conducted over a 30-year period and carried out a meta-analysis. They found a wide range of research designs and types of interventions (interpersonal, behavioral, desensitization, and skills training).

They reported moderate degrees of change in outcome measures and moderate effectiveness in regard to personal benefit, leading them to recommend that psychotherapy be considered routinely as part of the overall treatment program. Many of the studies reviewed were limited in scope; it is essential that new research continue to investigate the most effective forms of psychotherapy.

Behavioral Interventions

Behavioral approaches, the most widely used and best-studied treatment interventions for maladaptive behavior in persons with intellectual disability, begin with an applied behavior analysis. Applied behavioral analysis is based on the principles and methods of behavioral analysis and is intended to establish appropriate, functional skills and reduce problem behaviors. Even though behavioral interventions are based on the principles of learning theory (which posits that maladaptive patterns of behavior are the result of faulty conditioning), they can be effective for emotional and behavioral symptoms that result primarily from pathophysiological dysfunction. Behavioral procedures are used for improving adaptive behavior, reducing maladaptive behavior, and broadening skill development through direct training and education. Behavioral interventions may be specifically indicated for self-injurious behavior, self-stimulatory behavior, aggressive behavior, and habit training.

Behavioral approaches are generally grouped into those designed to enhance adaptive behavior and those designed to suppress maladaptive behavior. Behavior enhancement procedures are preferable because they reduce inappropriate behaviors by teaching adaptive solutions. This is accomplished by reinforcing appropriate behaviors and suppressing maladaptive ones.

Behavior Enhancement (Accelerating) Procedures

Behavior enhancement procedures may be subdivided into several types of differential reinforcement approaches. These include differential reinforcement of incompatible behavior, involves the direct reinforcement of preselected adaptive behaviors that compete with, and eventually replace, the target behaviors and differential reinforcement of alternative behavior that is an appropriate alternative to the problem behavior. For differential reinforcement of incompatible behavior, the competing behaviors are chosen because they are incompatible with the target behaviors (e.g., using one's hand to shake another's hand rather than to slap). These procedures are based on a careful determination of the characteristics of the maladaptive behaviors (e.g., frequency, duration, and intensity) and by establishing a variety of motivating reinforcers. Negative reinforcement is sometimes used to enhance behavior, for example, allowing the individual to avoid a predetermined punishment by engaging in desirable behavior.

Behavior Reduction (Decelerating) Procedures

These methods are used in combination with other techniques that are designed to promote alternative behaviors. The most commonly used method is the differential reinforcement of other behavior, in which the individual is rewarded for not exhibiting the target behavior. If the undesirable behavior does not occur within a specified time interval, positive reinforcement is provided. The time interval for positive reinforcement is determined based on the frequency of the target behavior. The time interval should be long enough to require some effort by the person to show self-control, but short enough to promote success. When the procedure is successful, the frequency of target behaviors decreases as the frequency of the more adaptive, competing behaviors (those which are reinforced) increases. For maladaptive behaviors that occur very frequently, differential reinforcement of low rates of behavior may be used. In this procedure, a predetermined frequency of the target behavior (lower than that occurring at baseline) is reinforced. This frequency is progressively lowered until the target behavior is eliminated. Behavior reduction procedures range from time-out to noxious stimulation. Behavior reduction procedures include (1) extinction, the elimination of reinforcing consequences of maladaptive behavior; (2) nonexclusionary and exclusionary time-out from positive reinforcement; (3) response cost, the loss of a previously earned reward; (4) overcorrection, restoring order after disrupting the environment or the repeated practice of an adaptive behavior (e.g., dressing); (5) physical or mechanical contingent restraint; and (6) visual screening. Among the behavior reduction strategies, extinction has been shown to result in the most consistent and rapid reversal effects on behavior with the fewest negative side effects.

Behavior reduction procedures can also provide unpleasant consequences immediately following the occurrence of the target behavior. Such contingent noxious stimulation procedures might include verbal reprimand, ammonia capsules, and mist spray. Although noxious stimulation procedures have short-term efficacy in suppressing maladaptive behaviors under certain circumstances, the stability and generalization of these effects is questionable. Such punishment procedures primarily suppress behavior rather than teach adaptive solutions. Such intrusive procedures typically have been reserved for the most dangerous behaviors (e.g., serious aggression and self-injury) and are rarely used. Punishment procedures have been sharply criticized and are the source of considerable controversy. Many states have enacted regulations that either ban or seriously restrict the implementation of such punishment procedures because of ethical concerns, but more important, because behavior suppression or punishment alone does not teach those self-regulation or problem-solving skills that enhance future adaptive responses to stress.

The National Institutes of Health sponsored a Consensus Development Conference on Treatment of Destructive Behaviors in Persons with Developmental Disabilities (NIH, 1990). A panel of nationally recognized experts in the field of developmental disabilities reviewed the available research and heard testimony from investigators and clinicians working with intellectually disabled persons with severe behavior disorders. The recommendations of the panel for the treatment of severely disruptive behavior included the following:

- Most successful approaches to treatment are likely to involve multiple elements of therapy (behavioral and psychopharmacologic), environmental change, and education.
- Treatment methods may require techniques for enhancing desired behaviors; for producing changes in social, physical, and educational environments; and for reducing or eliminating destructive behaviors.
- Treatments should be based on an analysis of medical and psychiatric conditions, environmental situations, consequences, and skill deficits. In the application of any of these treatments, an essential step involves a functional analysis of existing behavioral patterns.
- Behavior reduction procedures should be selected for their rapid effectiveness *only* if the exigencies of the clinical situation require such restrictive interventions and *only* after appropriate review. These interventions should *only* be used in the context of a comprehensive treatment program. (NIH, 1990).

Systematic research that identifies the specific behavioral interventions that are most efficacious for particular maladaptive behaviors is being conducted. However, most studies involve single-case designs with small sample sizes and may not include clinical factors that might affect treatment outcome (e.g., clinical psychiatric syndromes and disorders, family history, and psychosocial circumstances). Overall, positive behavioral interventions are useful for social skills deficits; mild punishment procedures (e.g., extinction, disapproval, or overcorrection) for psychophysiologic symptoms (e.g., enuresis or encopresis); and more intrusive punishment procedures (e.g., restraint or time-out) for initial management of destructive behaviors (e.g., aggression or self-injurious behavior). Self-stimulatory behaviors, psychophysiologic symptoms, and noncompliance are the most responsive to behavioral treatment (65%–75% success rate); destructive behaviors are next (45%–65% success rate), and inappropriate social interactions are the least responsive (35%–40% success rate). Overall, behavioral enhancement procedures have the best long-term outcome.

Multisensory Stimulation (Snoezelen Room)

Multisensory stimulation provided in a Snoezelen room can be used for persons with severe intellectual disability and behavioral and mental disorders to facilitate relaxation, inhibit challenging behavior (especially aggression and self-injury), and enhance quality of life. A Snoezelen room contains a variety of multisensory equipment to stimulate the senses. Among these are olfactory (aromatherapy diffuser and assorted scents), vibratory and tactile (vibrators and body massagers), auditory (electronic sound generators and stereophonic music), visual (laser light shows and interactive light panels), and vestibular (net swings and tumble form sitters) forms of stimulation. The stimulation should be individualized according to the needs of the person. A functional behavior analysis can be used to determine the best use of the equipment. For example, does the individual engage in maladaptive behavior to obtain sensory stimulation? The

Snoezelen room has been used successfully to reduce self-injurious behavior (Singh et al., 2004).

Positive Behavior Support

Behavior interventions have evolved into an approach referred to as positive behavior support. Positive behavior support describes a more comprehensive intervention that includes functional behavioral assessment and planned lifestyle enhancement. This approach was developed because traditional methods for dealing with serious behavior problems were often too narrowly defined. The traditional approach focused exclusively on consequences. Such intervention has been difficult to carry out in integrated settings and may be too intrusive and ineffective in helping people to accomplish meaningful changes in their behavior or lifestyle. Positive behavior support emphasizes designing positive and effective interventions that grow out of a more comprehensive assessment. (Horner et al., 1990; Ruef, Posten, and Humphrey, 1999). This approach is consistent with the 1997 amendments to the Individuals with Disabilities Education Act, which call for the use of functional behavioral assessment and positive supports and strategies (Tilly et al., 1998). The goal is to facilitate a better lifestyle with participation in community life by establishing satisfying relationships, expressing personal preferences, making choices, and developing personal competencies. Person-centered planning and the mobilization of natural supports are emphasized. A general support plan is developed and carefully monitored.

Psychopharmacology

Psychopharmacologic treatment can be an important treatment modality for children and adults with intellectual disability (Bregman, 1991; Reiss and Aman, 1998). The initiation of psychotropic medication trials requires a thorough psychiatric evaluation to identify a psychiatric disorder or a specific target behavior that may be responsive to medication. A drug-free baseline period in which the symptoms or behaviors identified for treatment are carefully defined and characterized (e.g., frequency, duration, and intensity) is strongly recommended. Valid and reliable behavior rating scales should be selected and used at appropriate intervals during the medication trial in order to monitor drug efficacy. Direct observational data and/or standardized rating scales should be used to monitor effects and potential side effects. The trial should include therapeutic doses of medication and should be conducted for an adequate length of time. Despite the frequent use of psychopharmacologic interventions for persons with intellectual disability, relatively few studies include appropriate control groups. Single-case reports and nonblind, open clinical trials make up the majority of these reports. Clinical reports often show evidence of methodological problems, such as reporting bias (underreporting of negative findings), retrospective rather than prospective, anecdotal data, and lack of inter-rater reliability. Moreover, the concurrent use of other psychotropic medications that may be changed during the course of the drug trial may confound the results. Studies should adhere to the basic guidelines for clinical trials, with random assignment of an adequate number of subjects to treatment conditions, double-blind, placebo-controlled procedures, treatment phases of adequate length, and valid and reliable methods for assessment at baseline and throughout the study.

Overall, psychotropic medications are effective in the treatment of a variety of psychiatric disorders, such as major depression, and behavioral problems, such as aggressive and destructive behavior, when combined with psychosocial interventions. Epidemiologic studies indicate that between one-fifth and one-half of persons with intellectual disability residing in institutions and one-fourth to one-third of those residing in community settings receive some type of psychotropic medication. One survey (Singh, Ellis, and Wechsler, 1997) showed that in the 1986 to 1995 period, typical prevalence rates in institutions ranged from 12% to 40% for psychotropics, 24% to 41% for anticonvulsants, and 44% to 60% for psychotropic and/or anticonvulsant drugs. In the same period, the prevalence rates in the community (for adults and children analyzed together) ranged from 19% to 29% for psychotropics, 18% to 23% for anticonvulsants, and 35% to 45% for psychotropic and/or anticonvulsant drugs. There are significant interinstitutional and interagency differences in prescribing patterns, ranging from under 10% in some settings to more than 40% in others.

One statewide population-based study showed that 22% of adults with intellectual disability were prescribed neuroleptics, 9.3% anxiolytics, and 5.9% antidepressants (Spreat, Conroy, and Jones, 1997). In both institutional and community settings, polypharmacy, or the use of multiple drugs, is common in both adults and children. Understanding pharmacotherapy and attitudes of staff members in community facilities are particularly important for adults, as well as for children.

The effects of pharmacologic medications on individuals with intellectual disability are generally no different from those that would be expected in typically developing persons. Still, one must take into account the diagnosis and type of intellectual disability when medications are prescribed. The drugs' effects may be influenced by associated medical and neurological disorders. Medications should be begun at a low dose and gradually increased. There may be increased sensitivities to some medications with particular intellectual disability syndromes, for example, anticholinergic medication in Down syndrome. In other instances, individuals with intellectual disability may be more sensitive to the sedative/hypnotic medications and become disinhibited following their use. Systematic studies are needed to clarify whether particular side effects occur with specific intellectual disability syndromes.

Medication choice is based on rational pharmacotherapy and following an accurate diagnosis. The risk-benefit ratio must be considered in prescribing medications for individuals with intellectual disability. Benefits are weighed with potential adverse effects. When medications are prescribed, their use is part of a comprehensive treatment plan. In some instances, service systems may seek medication treatment because of noncompliance in a living environment or work situation. Before prescribing medication, the source of the noncompliance must be investigated. Medications must be prescribed for specific indications, and the lowest effective dose should be used.

In 1997, the Health Care Financing Administration (HCFA) published *Psychopharmacological Medication: Safety Precautions for Persons with Developmental Disabilities* (HCFA, 1997). This publication is a manual for surveyors who assess a facility's compliance with the regulations regarding medication use. This manual interprets the original regulations in light of modern approaches to intellectual disability. The main points concerning psychotropic medication use are summarized in table 9.2.

Less information is available about safety and efficacy of psychotropic drugs in persons with intellectual disability, especially in children, than for the general population. Still, these medications are often prescribed off-label, based on knowledge obtained in other populations. To address questions about their use in persons with intellectual disability, an expert panel prepared *The International Consensus Handbook*, with guidelines for the use of psychotropic medications in developmental disabilities (Reiss and Aman, 1998). In addition, expert consensus guidelines for treatment of psychiatric and behavioral problems in intellectual disability have been published (Rush and Frances, 2000). These guidelines include issues of informed consent (noting that it is a process not a one-time discussion), general principles of medication treatment, selection of medications, managing inadequate response to initial drug treatment, and medication dosage. Moreover, there is an extensive series of questions posed to experts who list first-line, second-line, and third-line medication choices for the full range of diagnostic indications. The expert consensus guidelines have been summarized and updated by Aman et al. (2004).

Table 9.2 HCFA (Health Care Financing Administration) Guidelines for Psychotropic Medication Use in Persons with Mental Retardation

Prior to prescribing psychotropic medication
- Medical, environmental, and other causes of the behavioral problem must be ruled out
- A detailed description of symptoms and differential diagnosis is required
- Behavioral data should be collected
- The least intrusive and most positive interventions should be used including, as applicable, behavior therapy, psychotherapy, and habilitation/education; medications might be the least intrusive and most positive intervention in some cases

When medication is prescribed
- It should be an integral part of an overall individual active treatment program
- It should not diminish the patient's functional status
- The lowest effective dose should be used
- A gradual dose reduction should be periodically considered (at least annually) unless clinically contraindicated
- Adverse drug effects should be monitored
- Data documenting that the drug achieves the desired outcome (including patient's quality of life) should be collected

From Szymanski and King (1999). Reprinted by permission of the publisher, Lippincott, Williams & Wilkins, from Practice Parameters for the Assessment and Treatment of Children, Adolescents, and Adults with Mental Retardation and Comorbid Mental Disorders, *Journal of the American Academy of Children and Adolescent Psychiatry*, 38:12. American Academy of Child and Adolescent Psychiatry. Copyright © 1999.

In the guidelines, pharmacotherapy is recommended for defined psychiatric disorders such as major depression and obsessive compulsive disorder in individuals with intellectual disability. There is general consensus about its use in these individuals. However, there is less agreement about how these drugs should be prescribed for the control of aggression, disturbed behavior, hyperactivity, and stereotypical behaviors in the absence of a specific mental illness diagnosis (Santosh and Baird, 1999). However, psychopharmacologic treatment strategies are available for discrete behavioral symptoms with a proposed neurobiological substrate, such as impulsivity and anxiety. The neurochemical profiles have been described for a variety of psychotropic medications. When medications are used, their use involves complex interactions between neurochemicals, receptor systems, second messenger systems, protein synthesis, and gene expression. Neurotransmitters and neurohormones may modulate one another's actions. Therefore, care must be taken to understand the disorder being treated.

An approach to treatment that focuses on behavioral presentation assumes that the neurobiological underpinnings of psychopathology are dimensional rather than categorical. In practice, individuals will exhibit more than one target symptom, and more than one medication is commonly prescribed. Therefore, it is important to clarify whether the medication will have a positive effect on the chosen target symptom and also other co-occurring behavioral disturbances. If more than one medication is used, interactions of medications with one another must be considered.

Informed Consent/Ethical Considerations

Informed consent or assent must come from the person who is receiving treatment depending on the capacity to give it. The person with intellectual disability should always be engaged in the consent process and, if not consent, give assent before treatment. When a person with intellectual disability cannot give consent or assent, the parent or caregiver is actively involved in the decision-making process, and the decision must be discussed with the family in regard to the child or adult's best interest, especially in regard to risks and benefits. Otherwise, consent is obtained from a legally authorized representative. Informed consent is an ongoing process and is not provided in only one session. Informed consent must be voluntary after the individual is provided with the following information (Reiss and Aman, 1998): (1) description of the problem, (2) specific signs and symptoms that are targets of treatment, (3) description of the proposed treatment, (4) people involved in providing the treatment, (5) alternative treatments, (6) risk and adverse effects, (7) right to refuse proposed treatment, and (8) right to change one's mind about treatment.

Whenever medications are used, both the therapeutic effects and the side effect profile must be explained to the family and to the person receiving treatment. The capacity of an intellectually disabled person to understand and give consent must be assessed individually so that the information is provided at the appropriate developmental level.

Adjusting Medication Dosage

When medications are prescribed, they should be continued only as long as their benefits outweigh any side effects. Periodic trials of dose reduction and discontinuation of medication may be used to assess continuing need for medication. When medications are reduced or discontinued, this should be done gradually, especially because there may be withdrawal effects. In tapering medication, the rate of taper should be individualized. Generally, when a medication seems to show no identifiable benefit, or the risks are thought to outweigh its benefits, a more rapid taper of the medication is appropriate. If the medication is being tapered to establish a minimum effective dose when treatment effectiveness has been demonstrated, or if that individual has a history of withdrawal emergent symptoms, withdrawal should be more gradual.

Drug Interactions

It is not unusual for an individual with intellectual disability to be on multiple medications because of the coexistence of medical and psychiatric diagnoses. Thus, knowledge of psychotropics with other medications, particularly anticonvulsants, is critical since serious interactions are possible. For example, cimetidine inhibits the hepatic microsomal metabolism of psychotropic medications that have a phenothiazine structure. It also affects the metabolism of benzodiazepines that are metabolized by oxidation, thus resulting in increased plasma concentrations of the medication and greater risk for adverse effects. Carbamazepine, dilantin (phenytoin), and barbiturates may induce more rapid metabolism of tricyclic antidepressants, leading to a 50%–100% decrease in steady-state plasma concentrations so that the level would be reduced to below the minimum effective concentration for treatment. In addition, this combination may result in increased plasma concentrations of the anticonvulsant drugs. SSRIs, such as fluoxetine, have active metabolites, such as norfluoxetine, that are compounds with long half-lives. These active metabolites may continue to interact with other drugs for several weeks after the discontinuation of fluoxetine because of continued inhibition of a cytochrome enzyme. Antibiotics (tetracycline and ampicillin) may interfere with the renal clearance of lithium salts, resulting in possible lithium toxicity. The cytochrome and psychotropic drug interactions require particular attention. In using psychotropic medications, polypharmacy (multiple drug use) should be avoided if possible. However, if more than one medication is used, an awareness of drug interactions is particularly important.

Medication Side Effects

Careful follow-up is needed for side effects, such as tardive dyskinesia, akathisia, and extrapyramidal symptoms. Side effect monitoring must take into account that persons with intellectual disability may be unable to provide a self-report of their symptoms. Regular examination for involuntary movements, using scales such as the abnormal involuntary movement scale, is necessary. Stereotypies that occur in association with intellectual disability syndromes must be differentiated from tardive dyskinesia. The use of videotaping can be useful in establishing a baseline before beginning treatment. Table 9.3 lists side effects of commonly used medications.

Antidepressants. Neuroleptics, stimulant medications, and tricyclic antidepressants have the potential of lowering the seizure threshold even if there is no history of epilepsy. Clomipramine and bupropion also have been linked to precipitating seizures in higher doses. With tricyclic antidepressants, there are concerns about cardiac side effects, especially in children. If there is a significant increase in the QTc interval on the electrocardiogram or an increase in heart rate above 110 beats a minute, then the dose of the tricyclic should be reduced or the medication stopped.

The long-term side effects of selected serotonin reuptake inhibitors in children are unclear at this time. However, there are suggestions that, in the short-term, the side effects are relatively self-limiting. Gastrointestinal side effects have been observed in children and, on occasion, hyponatremia that is induced by inappropriate secretion of antidiuretic hormone has resulted from the selected serotonin reuptake inhibitors. Rarely, the serotonin syndrome may result from increased serotonin tone at the $5HT_{1A}$ receptor in the brain and spinal cord. The serotonin syndrome is associated with the use of multiple serotonergic drugs and can be potentially fatal. It is responsive to discontinuation of the drugs. However, 5HT antagonists, such as methysergide and propranolol, may be used for treatment. Monoamine oxidase inhibitors are problematic for individuals with intellectual disability who may find it difficult to understand and follow the dietary restrictions needed to prevent hypertensive reactions to certain foods when these medications are taken.

Anticholinergic Agents. These agents are indicated only for extrapyramidal symptoms from neuroleptic use. In high doses, these compounds may produce confusion and deterioration in behavior. Additionally, anticholinergic effects of psychotropic medications may lead to blurred vision and dryness of the mouth.

Anticonvulsants. Carbamazepine may cause a benign pruritic (itching) rash in 10%–15% of those treated within a few weeks of its introduction. The Stevens-Johnson syndrome and toxic epidermal necrolysis are rare complications of this medication. Carbamazepine rarely exacerbates behavioral problems and may result in delirium and hypernatremia that result from a syndrome of inappropriate secretion of antidiuretic hormone. Sodium valproate is hepatotoxic (liver toxicity) in a small portion of individuals. There have been some reports that link sodium valproate to polycystic ovarian disease, particularly in adolescent females. Vigabatrin may lead to myoclonus and can cause severe behavioral problems, agitation, and thought disorder in susceptible individuals. Visual defects also may occur and must be monitored. Topiramate also has behavioral and cognitive side effects and may result in renal stones in up to 3% of individuals who take it. This medication is also an appetite suppressant.

Table 9.3 Psychotropic Medications: Side Effects and Monitoring*

Formulation	Side Effects	Monitoring	Contraindications
Selective Serotonin Reuptake Inhibitors			
Fluoxetine	Nausea, dry mouth, somnolence, insomnia, tachycardia, hypotension, migraine, paresthesia, weight change, poor concentration, amenorrhea. Rarely, hyponatremia, SIADH, activation of mania/hypomania "serotonin syndrome" characterized by myoclonus, hyperreflexia, tremor, increased muscle tone, fever, sweating, shivering, diarrhea, delirium, and, rarely, coma	Baseline CBC, AST/ALT, ECG	MAOI or thioridazine use. Caution with sumatriptan and tramadol. Adjust dose for liver impairment
Paroxetine	See fluoxetine Withdrawal effects are often seen with the cessation of SSRIs especially paroxetine. Symptoms include dizziness, lethargy, parethesias, nausea, vivid dreams, irritability, and depressed mood. Patients should be tapered off over a week of longer	See fluoxetine	MAOI or thioridazine use. Caution with sumatriptan and tramadol. Adjust dose for liver impairment
Atypical Antidepressant			
Venlafaxine	Nausea, anorexia, sedation, dizziness, dry mouth, insomnia	BP	MAOI use. Adjust dose for liver and renal impairment
Anticonvulsants			
Carbamazepine	Sedation, ataxia, dizziness, diplopia, aplastic anemia, neutropenia, urinary retention, nausea, impaired liver function, SIADH, and Stevens-Johnson syndrome	LFTs, CBC, drug levels initially and at regular intervals	MAOI use, bone marrow suppression, hypersensitivity to TCA, pregnancy. Adjust dose for liver and renal impairment
Valproic acid Divalproex sodium	Sedation, GI side effects, hair loss, abnormal LFTs, potentially fatal hepatotoxicity, inhibition of platelet aggregation, weight gain, rash, neural tube defects if used in pregnancy. Should be tapered off over a week or longer to avoid withdrawal symptoms	LFTs, CBC, drug levels initially and at regular intervals	Liver disease, pregnancy, age under 2 years
Gabapentin	Dizziness, ataxia, somnolence, nystagmus, weight gain Moodiness, oppositional behavior, and anger outbursts reported at higher doses Should be tapered off over a week or longer	Baseline CBC AST/ALT	Adjust dose for renal impairment

Formulation	Side Effects	Monitoring	Contraindications
Benzodiazepine			
Clonazepam	Drowsiness, ataxia, confusion, behavioral inhibition, increased bronchial secretions, thrombocytopenia, leukopenia, hypotension, coma	LFTs, CBC	Liver disease, narrow angle glaucoma, pregnancy. Should be avoided in patients with history of substance abuse
α-Adrenergic Blocker			
Clonidine	Sedation, hypotension, and cardiovascular effects (such as bradycardia), dizziness, dry mouth, stomachache, nausea, vomiting, constipation, rebound hypertension, depression, contact dermatitis (patch) Must be tapered gradually over a week or more to avoid significant hypertensive sequelae	BP	Severe coronary insufficiency, conduction disturbances, recent myocardial infarction, cerebrovascular disease, chronic renal failure
β-Blocker			
Propranolol	Bradycardia, hypotension, vivid dreams, depression, fatigue, peripheral vasoconstriction, bronchospasm, diarrhea Should be tapered to avoid rebound hypertension	BP, ECG initially and with dose changes Mood	History of bronchospasm, congestive heart failure, cardiac shock, heart block, Raynaud's disease, or depression

Source: Adapted from Pao, 2003. Reprinted with permission from *Contemporary Pediatrics*, Vol. 20, October 2003, pp. 43–57.

AST/ALT = aspartate/alarine aminotransferase; BP = blood pressure; CBC = complete blood count; ECG = electrocardiogram; GI = gastrointestinal; LFT = liver function test; MAOI = monoamine oxidase inhibitor; SIADH = syndrome of inappropriate antidiuretic hormone; SSRI = selective serotonin reuptake inhibitor; TCA = tricyclic antidepressant.

*For more information about these drugs, see the following:

Web sites for consumers:

(1) www.fda.gov/cder/consumerinfo/default/htm

(2) www.fda.gov/opacom/morecons.htlm

Web sites for health professionals:

(1) www.fda.gov/oc/oha/default.htm (information on drugs)

(2) www.fda.gov/cder/pediatric/index.htm (pediatric drug development)

(3) www.fda.gov/cder/approval/index.htm (new and general drug approvals)

(4) www.pdr.net/pdrnet/librarian/action/command (Physicians Desk Reference online search for drugs and drug interactions)

Neuroleptics. Neuroleptics should be used for specific indications, such as psychosis, Tourette's disorder, and in some instances, uncontrolled aggression. Neuroleptic drugs should be used in low doses following baseline assessment and gradually increased. Older neuroleptics, such as phenothiazine, are used much less commonly since the introduction of the atypical antipsychotic medications. The phenothiazine group has increased anticholinergic, noradrenergic, and antihistaminic effects. Chlorpromazine particularly results in photosensitivity so that sunscreen should be used and time in the sun limited when on this medication. Atypical neuroleptics, such as risperidone, olanzapine, and quetiapine have less extrapyramidal side effects. When using neuroleptic drugs that block dopamine receptors, there is an increased risk of prolactin release that may result in breast enlargement, amenorrhea, and galactorrhea. Pimozide, a medication used to treat tic disorders or Tourette's disorder at higher doses has cardiac effects, and electrocardiogram monitoring is necessary. Clozapine has side effects that include agranulocytosis, hypersalivation, and sedation. Because of these side effects and the need for repeated blood samples to monitor them, this medication is rarely used in persons with intellectual disability. Risperidone and olanzapine both may result in substantial weight gain, sedation, and hypotension, and there is risk for diabetes for those at risk when taking olanzapine.

Neuroleptics may cause tardive dyskinesia and, in some cases, may impair learning. Tardive dyskinesia, as well as tardive akathisia, is an important side effect of neuroleptic medications that is clinically significant and may result in medico-legal difficulties. Several studies have investigated the prevalence, clinical presentation, and risk factors associated with the development of tardive dyskinesia among intellectually disabled individuals treated with neuroleptics. Prevalence figures range between 15% and 35% across studies. The clinical manifestations of the disorder are essentially identical to those manifested by typically developing individuals, although orofacial dyskinesias may be more prevalent. Several potential risk factors have been identified, including advanced age, cumulative dose, and length of exposure. The severity of cognitive impairment and the presence of other neurological conditions may increase the risk of tardive dyskinesia according to some, but not all, studies. Findings with atypical neuroleptics, such as risperidone, are more promising.

To monitor for tardive dyskinesia, baseline assessments of abnormal involuntary movement are essential before starting neuroleptic agents. This is of importance because involuntary movements may be seen in some individuals with intellectual disability at baseline. Most often, dyskinesias associated with dopamine blockade are linked to neuroleptic withdrawal and can be managed by very gradual withdrawal of the medication. Akathisia should be considered if a person with intellectual disability taking the neuroleptic shows a change in their behavior, particularly increased motor restlessness. This side effect is sometimes confused with hyperactivity or increased irritability.

Akathisia may be treated with propranolol, clonidine, or clonazepam to determine whether or not the symptoms resolve. Finally, neuroleptic malignant syndrome is a very serious and rare complication of psychotropic drug use. It is managed by stopping the neuroleptic drug, providing adequate hydration, and typically using a dopamine agonist, such as bromocriptine, or a muscle relaxant, such as dantrolene.

Stimulants. Side effects from methylphenidate occur at a greater frequency than reported in the general population (especially among nonresponders to treatment for attention deficit disorder). Side effects include irritability, lethargy, internal preoccupation, social withdrawal, increased motor stereotypy, and overly inclusive attention.

Drug Treatment for Specific Disorders

Attention Deficit/Hyperactivity Disorder (ADHD)

As many as 40% of children and adolescents with intellectual disability exhibit a high activity level, impulsive behavior, and inattentiveness. Epidemiologic studies show that for 10%–15% of individuals, these symptoms are severe enough to warrant the diagnosis of an attention deficit disorder (Gillberg et al., 1986). Central nervous system stimulants are among the most frequently prescribed psychotropic medications for children with intellectual disability, with statistics showing that 6%–8% of such children receive them. Yet systematic studies of efficacy in specific intellectual disability syndromes are limited and the findings are mixed (Aman, Buican, and Arnold, 2003; Gadow, 1985). Still, the stimulants are useful for children and adolescents, particularly those with mild intellectual disability who meet diagnostic criteria for attention deficit/hyperactivity disorder. Approximately 50%–75% of this group of children demonstrates a significant decrease in hyperactivity, impulsivity, and inattention and an increase in on-task behavior following drug treatment. Some studies have documented significant improvements in laboratory measures of attention, memory, and learning (e.g., continuous performance tasks, matching-to-sample tasks, and paired associate learning). However, there is little evidence that the stimulants improve behavior, learning, or performance among children with intellectual disability who do not meet diagnostic criteria for attention deficit/hyperactivity disorder (Aman, 1982).

Overall, symptoms of attention deficit/hyperactivity disorder can be treated successfully in children with intellectual disability, and higher doses of methylphenidate (0.6 mg/kg bid) may be more effective. These improvements were not accompanied by increases in symptoms such as staring, social withdrawal, or anxiety (Pearson et al., 2003). Successively higher doses (0.6 mg/kg bid) led to consistent gains in cognitive task performance, with optimal performance at the highest dose. At the highest dose, 55% of the children showed substantial behavioral gains and 46% made substantial gains in cognitive task performance. In another study (Aman, Bucan, and Arnold, 2003) 90 children with intellectual disability who received the same dose regimen of methylphenidate and three independent, placebo-controlled studies were evaluated. Both teachers and parents rated the children as being improved on subscales assessing attention, overactivity, and conduct problems. Of these, 44% of the subjects showed at least a 30% reduction compared with placebo on teacher rating scales. Methylphenidate improved accuracy on several cognitive tests, response speed was increased, and seat activity declined for one of three tests; heart rate was mildly increased (3.9 beats/minute). Analyses of IQ and mental age suggested that lower functional level (especially lower IQ) might be associated with a less favorable response to methylphenidate. Children with low IQ and ADHD respond to methylphenidate, but their rate of response is less and more varied than that of normal-IQ children. Different attentional mechanisms may moderate response to psychostimulants in various syndromes. Attention deficit disorder has been described in a several neurogenetic syndromes and treated successfully with methylphenidate; among them are fragile X syndrome, Williams syndrome, velocardiofacial syndrome, and Tourette's syndrome (Tourette's Syndrome Study Group, 2002).

Schizophrenia

Community epidemiological studies confirm that schizophrenic disorders occur in 1%–2% of persons with intellectual disability. The available literature documents the usefulness of neuroleptic medication for psychotic symptoms manifested by affected intellectually disabled patients. Treatment responsiveness is similar to that found in typically developing persons (Menolascino et al., 1986). Atypical neuroleptics are most commonly prescribed to those who are compliant with oral medication. For those who are noncompliant, long-acting, depot antipsychotic medication may be indicated.

Velocardiofacial syndrome (22q11.2 deletion syndrome) has been identified as a high-risk factor for developing adult onset schizophrenia, and antipsychotic medications have been instituted in treatment for psychotic symptoms. The behavioral manifestations of 22q11.2 deletion syndrome might result from haploinsufficiency of the catechol-O-methyltransferase (*COMT*) gene, located within the 22q11 region, resulting in excessive extraneuronal catecholamine concentrations. COMT has been implicated in schizophrenia through its roles in monoamine neurotransmitter metabolism and its impact on prefrontal cognition. One study (Sanders et al., 2004) evaluated eight markers spanning *COMT* and included portions of the two immediately adjacent genes, thioredoxin reductase 2 and armadillo repeat gene deletes in velocardiofacial syndrome (*ARVCF*). *ARVCF*, a member of the catenin family, has a potential role in neurodevelopment. These findings support previous association signals of schizophrenia with *COMT* markers and suggest that *ARVCF* might contribute to this signal.

Mood Disorders

Major depression and dysthymic disorder occur among individuals with intellectual disability. A number of reports support the efficacy of antidepressants. Moreover, mood disorders are being diagnosed more commonly. In one study (Hurley, Folstein, and Lam, 2003), 100 adults with mild intellectual disability, 100 patients with moderate, severe, or profound intellectual disability, and 100 matching normal controls were studied. For all groups, depressive disorders were the most frequent class of diagnoses. For those with intellectual disability, mood stabilizers were used in 28% and antidepressants in 27%. The normally intelligent individuals were most frequently prescribed antidepressants (40%) and anxiolytics (22%). In contrast to previous studies, outpatient providers frequently diagnosed depression, and the prescribing pattern showed increased usage of antidepressants and mood stabilizers for persons with intellectual disability. In another study from the state of Oklahoma, the use of antidepressant medication increased dramatically from 1994 to 2000, apparently due to increased use of SSRI medications (Spreat, Conroy, and Fullerton, 2004).

Individuals with clinical symptoms of bipolar disorder have been shown to have significantly more DSM-IVTR mood-related and non–mood-related symptoms, as well as functional impairments, than do individuals with major depression, depression with psychosis, or schizophrenia/psychosis NOS (not otherwise specified). Behavioral profiles of those with bipolar disorder differed significantly from patients in the other three groups, indicating that bipolar disorder can be readily distinguished from other behavioral and psychiatric diagnoses in individuals with intellectual disability, and DSM-IVTR criteria can be applied to make the diagnosis. Mood stabilizing agents (e.g., lithium carbonate, valproate) have been studied for the treatment of bipolar disorder and the control of aggressive behavior. Several open trials and two controlled studies reported lithium to be effective in treating acute manic episodes and in reducing the frequency and duration of affective cycles. "The Expert Consensus Guideline Series" (Rush and Frances, 2000) recommended valproic acid or lithium for classic, euphoric, manic disorder and valproic acid for mixed or rapid cycling mania. For major depression, an SSRI was recommended as a first-line medication. Mood Disorders have been described in several syndromes such as Down syndrome in which SSRI medications have been effective in treatment. Affective psychosis is associated with Prader-Willi syndrome.

Treatment with SSRIs can be associated with increased aggression, suicidal ideation, and mood switching from depression to mania. Because of the risk of increased suicidal ideation, the Food and Drug Administration provides a "black box" warning and patient guidelines for children in regard to the use of these medications. Although suicidal ideation may be more difficult to elicit in persons with intellectual disability, careful monitoring of behavior is advised, particularly in the first weeks following prescription of these medications. The combination of psychotherapy, behavior therapy, and antidepressant medication is the most effective treatment and provides the best opportunity to monitor aggressive behavior and suicidal ideation.

Disruptive and Aggressive Behavior

Behaviors are described as challenging based on their intensity, frequency, or duration and the fact that physical safety of the individual or others may be placed in jeopardy. Or challenging behavior may be behavior that disrupts access to and participation in community programs, for example, aggressive behavior and self-injurious behavior. These behaviors occur at a higher rate in those who are most severely intellectually disabled. They are more common in males than in females. Such challenging behaviors require initial behavioral interventions, with medications used as adjuncts as appropriate.

Aggression that occurs in the context of a psychiatric disorder that responds to medication, such as attention deficit disorder, psychotic disorder, bipolar disorder, and postictal behavior following seizures, is more likely to respond to the medications prescribed for the underlying condition; if the primary condition improves, the aggression may as well. If a specific diagnosis is not made, the behaviors involved with the aggression, such as impulsiveness, fearfulness, and irritability, may be targeted. However, there is limited evidence of efficacy of conventional neuroleptic drugs on behavioral disturbances in the absence of classic psychiatric symptoms. Still, the neuroleptics have been studied in clinical trials. Some studies have documented significant reductions in aggressive behavior, others have not. However, the atypical neuroleptics (e.g., risperidone and olanzapine) have resulted in improvement in behavioral disturbance in individuals with autistic disorder (McCracken et al., 2002) and in others with hostility, aggression, irritability, agitation, self-injury, hyperactivity, and autistic-like behaviors.

Self-Injurious Behavior

Self-injurious behavior is a severe and complex problem in persons with intellectual disability, particularly those whose intellectual disability is severe or profound. It may occur in 5%–10% of people with intellectual disability. Self-injurious behavior and other forms of destructive behavior are responsible for a disproportionate amount of the cost in the public health care of people with intellectual disability. The cost to the individual is significant as it may lead to disfigurement and even death. In examining mortality and avoidable death in individuals with self-injury, a higher-than-expected death rate was found; in 12% of cases, death was attributed to self-injurious behavior (Niessen and Haveman, 1997). Self-injurious behavior commonly results in placement in highly restrictive environments (Symons and Thompson, 1997). In one study of hospital admissions of persons with intellectual disability, it was the reason for referral in 36% of 251 cases.

The term "self-injury" applies to several different forms or topographies. Assessment involves an appreciation of the type or topography of self-injury when considering etiology and treatment. In the study of 29 school-age children and adolescents, the most common locations for self-injury were the head and hand (Symons and Thompson, 1997). The Timed Self-Injurious Behavior Scale has been introduced to record and discriminate the frequencies of the 16 most common types of self-injurious behavior (Brasic et al., 1997).

Self-injurious behavior is more common in individuals with co-occurring autistic disorder and intellectual disability (Schroeder, Rojahn, and Reese, 1997). Bhaumik et al. (1997) studied 2,200 adults with varying degrees of intellectual disability. Autistic features were found in those with severe intellectual disability, and self-injurious behavior was documented in 60% of those who had four or more autistic traits but only 9% of those with milder degrees of intellectual disability and no autistic traits. Those who live in institutional settings have a higher prevalence of self-injurious behavior.

Illness Associated with Self-Injurious Behavior. When self-injurious behavior occurs, an underlying medical condition should be sought. In one study, 25 patients with self-injury, ranging in age from 3 to 35, were referred during one year to an inpatient service. Charts were reviewed to determine medical conditions that were diagnosed and treated. Constipation, duodenal ulcer, otitis media, and dysphasic aspiration were identified. Twenty-eight percent of these individuals had previously undiagnosed medical problems that might be related to pain or discomfort. All but one of these individuals showed reduction in self-injury when the medical condition was treated (Bosch, Dyke, and Smith, 1997). Other cases of self-injury related to otitis media have been reported (O'Reilly, 1997). However, others have not documented a specific relationship between behavior and physical illness. Of 62 adults with profound intellectual disability who lived in a community setting in an intermediate care facility, sluggishness was the only behavior identified in a four-day period surrounding an episode (McDermott et al., 1997). Thus, self-injurious behavior more commonly is associated with psychiatric illness rather than physical disorders. Self-injury has been linked to mood disorders and, particularly, with depression (Davis, Judd, and Hermann, 1997a,b; Marston, Perry, and Roy, 1997). Aggressive behavior and self-mutilation are sufficiently common in individuals with depression and intellectual disability that they should be considered among diagnostic criteria for depression for those with this disorder. Self-injury may also occur in the context of stereotypical movement disorder and in individuals with disturbance in sleep. These associations were reported by Matson et al. (1997), using the Diagnostic Assessment for the Severely Handicapped (DASH-II). Pharmacotherapy of self-injurious behavior is considered in the next section.

Self-Injurious Behavior and Intellectual Disability Syndromes. Certain topographies of self-injury are associated with a specific genetic syndrome. In Lesch-Nyhan disease, finger and lip biting is the most common presentation (Anderson and Ernst, 1994). Prader-Willi syndrome is associated with skin picking (Hellings and Warnock, 1994). Nail pulling is associated with Smith-Magenis syndrome (Dykens, Finucane, and Gayley, 1997). In Cri du Chat syndrome (5p-), self-injury is commonly seen (Dykens and Clarke, 1997). Self-injury has also been described in an intellectual disability syndrome that involves the terminal deletion of chromosome 3 (3q27-q29) (Davies and Mathew, 1997). Because patterns of self-injury are associated with particular syndromes, the underlying etiology for a particular pattern may be determined through studies of the particular syndrome. New knowledge derived from the study of these syndromes may help to identify underlying mechanisms. A significant reduction in basal ganglia volume and reduced NAA in the striatum and prefrontal cortex in Lesch-Nyhan disease suggest dysregulation of a brain circuit that may control impulsive behavior (Harris et al., 2002). In Lesch-Nyhan disease, abnormalities in dopamine and serotonin metabolism also may be linked to self-injurious behavior. The skin picking that occurs in Prader-Willi syndrome may potentially be linked to an abnormality in serotonin and influence pain perception.

Behavioral Treatment for Self-Injurious Behavior. Treatment of self-injurious behavior is a continuing focus of interest. A treatment program for self-injury requires not only medication but also a comprehensive approach that involves both medical and psychiatric assessment before the initiation of any drug trials. Self-injurious behavior may be conceptualized as a stress-related behavior disorder. The utility of behavioral approaches, including noncontingent reinforcement (Fischer, Iwata, and Mazaleski, 1997) and intermittent punishment (Lerman et al., 1997), are under investigation. A 35-year review (1964–2000) (Kahng, Iwata, and Lewin, 2002) of behavioral treatments of self-injurious behavior revealed 396 published reports (706 participants). The authors found that the use of reinforcement-based interventions has increased, while the use of punishment-based interventions has decreased. These trends coincide with the increase in the use of functional behavioral assessments. The majority of individuals studied were males diagnosed with severe/profound intellectual disability. Overall treatment has been successful, but relapse after the initial intervention commonly occurs. For severe cases combined behavioral and medication treatment can be successful.

Pharmacologic Treatment for Self-Injurious Behavior. Serotonergic dysfunction has been hypothesized to underlie some forms of destructive behavior. Reduced central nervous system levels of serotonin have been reported in association with violent and impulsive behavior. Pharmacologic interventions, such as the use of antidepressants like paroxetine and other SSRIs, are being explored (Davanzo et al., 1998). These drugs (for example, fluoxetine) have been demonstrated to be effective in pathological skin picking in individuals without intellectual disability (Simeon et al., 1997). Both case reports and controlled studies have reported that lithium (which enhances serotonin synthesis) can reduce both aggressive and self-injurious behavior. These findings are supported by open clinical trials involving other medications that reportedly increase serotonergic activity, including buspirone, trazodone, and fluoxetine.

Among neuroleptic agents, the atypical agents such as risperidone and olanzapine may be beneficial in the treatment of self-injury. The potential involvement of dopaminergic mechanisms in self-injurious behavior is supported by studies in animals and humans. Animal models suggest that D_1 dopamine antagonist medications may be helpful (Allen, Freeman, and Davis, 1998). A large single injection of pemoline, an indirect dopamine agonist, results in stereotypical self-biting in the rat. Self-biters could be discriminated from controls based on differences in cortically stimulated depolarizing postsynaptic potentials elicited in neostriatal neurons in the presence of dopamine (Cromwell, King, and Levine, 1997). These findings are consistent with dopamine-glutamate interactions linked to self-injury in the pemoline model. The D_2 dopamine receptor subtype has been described by several investigators (Yokoyama and Okamura, 1997) as increased in the substantia nigra in a rat model of self-injury, to the extent that ventral mesostriatal dopamine system damage is linked to a predisposition to self-biting. However, differences in the D_2 dopamine subtype binding sites do not discriminate biters from nonbiters. Apparently, stimulation of both D_1 and D_2 receptor subtypes is needed to stimulate self-injury. Caffeine, theophylline, and clonidine are adenosine antagonists that act indirectly to increase dopamine activity; they are also known to exacerbate self-injurious behavior. Conversely, adenosine itself has been shown to block L-dopa-induced self-injurious behavior in an animal model. These data collectively indicate that self-injurious behavior might be successfully treated by medications that reduce dopamine transmission.

The GABAergic system may play a role in destructive behavior. However, medications that affect GABA functioning (e.g., benzodiazepines) do not appear to have consistent effects on aggression and self-injury. Some studies have reported that benzodiazepines reduce destructive behavior; others have reported an exacerbation of aggression and self-injurious behavior. Paradoxical excitement has also been reported.

Several lines of evidence implicate the endogenous opioid system in the pathogenesis of destructive behavior, especially self-injurious behavior. Two major hypotheses have been offered to explain the potential role of the endogenous opioid system. Preliminary studies suggest that some patients have elevated peripheral (and perhaps central nervous system) levels of endogenous opioids, leading to a high pain threshold and a tendency to persist in self-injurious behavior. Self-inflicted injury itself may cause endogenous opioid levels to rise resulting in stress-induced analgesia. Opioid antagonists have been recommended as treatment either to increase the perception of pain (thereby serving as a natural deterrent to self-injurious behavior) or to extinguish the theoretically reinforcing effects of self-injurious behavior-induced elevations in endogenous opioid levels. Several methodologically sound, controlled investigations have assessed the efficacy of opioid antagonists (e.g., naloxone and naltrexone) in the treatment of intellectually disabled individuals with self-injurious behavior. Sandman et al. (1997) demonstrated that a group of patients with self-injury had elevated plasma levels of b-endorphin shortly after an episode of self-injury. The subgroup with this elevation was significantly more responsive to naltrexone (2 mg/kg four times a day) and showed reductions in self-injury. Subsequently, the same authors studied the long-term use of naltrexone for self-injurious behavior (Sandman et al., 2000). Additional investigations, employing larger subject samples, are needed to identify the types of patients likely to benefit from such treatment.

Finally, there is evidence that increased noradrenergic activity may lead to aggressive behavior, perhaps secondary to anxiety or a state of heightened arousal. Several case reports and open clinical trials suggest that both centrally and peripherally acting beta-adrenergic blockers (e.g., propranolol and nadolol) may be helpful in reducing the frequency and intensity of explosive episodes of aggression. Mood stabilizing medications such as lithium, valproic acid, carbamazepine, and gabapentin have been effective in individuals with self-injurious behavior and mood instability.

Stereotypic Behavior

Study of the etiology and treatment of stereotypic behavior in children and adults with intellectual disability is of long-standing interest. Both preclinical and clinical studies suggest involvement of the dopaminergic system (perhaps via postsynaptic dopaminergic supersensitivity) in the etiology of some forms of stereotypy. Dopamine agonists are known to induce stereotypic behavior, a response that can be blocked by treatment with dopaminergic antagonists; neuroleptics may reduce stereotypic behavior among persons with intellectual disability.

Inappropriate Sexual Behavior

Some individuals with intellectual disability may be involved in inappropriate sexual behavior. This might include accusations of molesting children or genital exposure. In many instances, persons with intellectual disability who commit sexual offenses do not appreciate what constitutes acceptable sexual behavior. Sexual education programs may be utilized to establish gaps in knowledge of both the patients and their families about dealing with sexual behavior. Psychological treatments, especially behavioral treatments, may be beneficial in treating these difficulties.

In some instances, psychopharmacologic treatments including antilibidinal agents may be considered. However, there are no large control studies of antilibidinal agents with clearly defined outcome measures. Still, some individuals may benefit from the administration of antilibidinal drugs. Before such medications are prescribed, permission must be sought. If the individual cannot give informed consent, then the guardian or family members must give consent. Cyproterone acetate is the most widely used antiandrogenic drug. It decreases serum testosterone and is reported to reduce masturbation, indecent exposure, and some types of sexually inappropriate behavior in men with intellectual disability (Clarke, 1989). Cyproterone may be hepatotoxic in large doses; therefore, liver function testing must be done on a regular basis. Medroxyprogesterone acetate is another antiandrogenic agent that may be utilized. When assessing individuals with abnormal sexual behavior, past history of abuse must be considered.

Sleep Disorders

Pharmacotherapy for sleep disorders is an issue for some individuals with intellectual disability. In those with sensory impairments, such as deafness and blindness, sleep disorders may be particular problems. Initial approaches to treatment include sleep hygiene and anxiety management; antihistamines such as benadryl are commonly prescribed. In general, benzodiazepine should be avoided in the treatment of sleep problems due to the possibility of dependence, as well as the risk of worsening behavior by producing confusion or paradoxical aggression. Chlorohydrate (30 mg/kg/dose–50 mg/kg/dose) is the most commonly used sedative; however, paradoxical excitation may occur in some individuals when this medication is prescribed. If sleep problems persist, then sedative antidepressants such as trazodone (50 mg at night) may be helpful. In some instances, melatonin has been used successfully to treat sleep disorders; however, there have been concerns expressed about its effect on changing the seizure threshold in those with seizure disorders. The first approach should be the use of behavioral treatments before moving on to pharmacological treatments.

Seizure Disorders

Seizure disorders are the most common medical problem in individuals with intellectual disability. Seizures are reported in 8%–18% of those in the mild range of intellectual disability and 30%–36% of those in the severe range. Anticonvulsant medications are the most commonly used psychoactive drugs in persons with intellectual disability. In one study, active seizure disorder (one or more seizures in the past five years) occurred in 44% of children with IQ scores below 50 but only 0.5% in the general population (Steffenburg, Gillberg, and Steffenburg, 1996). Moreover, 59% of the children in the study had at least one psychiatric disorder.

Management of seizure disorder in people with intellectual disability includes the following: (1) accurate diagnosis and classification of the type of seizure disorder; (2) examination for other medical conditions that may be associated with seizure disorder, particularly tuberous sclerosis complex; (3) provision of information and support for individuals, family, and other caregivers; (4) careful monitoring of medications; and (5) emphasis on understanding educational work and socially related issues (Santosh and Baird, 1999).

In persons with intellectual disability, psychogenic seizures, episodic dyscontrol syndrome, and self-induced seizures are reported. For those testing in the severe range of intellectual disability, stereotypy and involuntary movements can at times be difficult to distinguish from a seizure disorder, requiring direct observation and/or video electroencephalography.

For the treatment of seizures, monotherapy is preferred based on the seizure type. Carbamazepine is recommended for partial seizures and valproate for generalized seizures. Lamotrigine, clobazam, vigabatrin, and topiramate are newer anticonvulsants. These medications may result in less cognitive impairment, fewer idiosyncratic reactions, and fewer long-term side effects. However, each of these drugs must be monitored carefully because when side effects occur, they may be severe. The newer drugs may be used as adjuncts to current treatments or as single therapies.

Delirium

Persons with intellectual disability are at risk for delirium because of the presence of central nervous system disease or metabolic disorders. Treatment with anticonvulsants, antidepressants, neuroleptics, benzodiazepines, and compounds with anticholinergic activity all may lead to cognitive difficulties. Therefore, vigilance is necessary, and the clinician should be alert to rule out delirium as a cause of behavioral deterioration, particularly when multiple medications are being prescribed.

SUMMARY

In summary, treatment is multimodal and based on a comprehensive medical, psychiatric, and functional assessment. It includes provision of positive environmental supports, educational interventions, and skills development with the goal of normalization and self-determination for persons with intellectual disability. Specific interventions for mental, emotional, and behavioral disorders are tailored to the needs of the individual. These include individual and family psychotherapy, behavior interventions, and pharmacotherapy. The overall goal of treatment is to help each person with intellectual disability reach his or her potential.

KEY POINTS

1. The first institutions for the care of individuals with intellectual disability were established in the United States in the mid-1800s. Thus, persons with intellectual disability were placed in separate institutions from those with mental illness.

2. Samuel Gridley Howe (1866) opposed lifelong institutionalization and insisted that people with impairments should be kept among "sound and normal" persons; he opposed custodial institutions. Despite this plea, by the beginning of the twentieth century, institutions for persons with intellectual disability were firmly established the world.

3. In the 1960s, deinstitutionalization was initiated in the United States, and in the twenty-first century, family and community care are the norm.

4. Community-based, multidimensional treatment programs must address habilitation and community integration, associated medical illnesses, mental disorders, and maladaptive behaviors.

5. Self-determination by a person with intellectual disability is an essential goal. Self-determination refers to the recognition of interests, desires, and preferences of an individual; it is the culmination of the normalization and deinstitutionalization movements.

6. Self-determination requires adequate supports that will vary according to the extent of impairment.

7. Specific environmental, educational, behavioral, psychotherapeutic, and psychopharmacologic interventions are tailored to individual needs so as to facilitate adaptation.

8. Behavioral and psychiatric disorders are major obstacles to full participation in educational, community, and habilitation programs.

9. Self-injurious behavior and aggressive behaviors are sometimes referred to as challenging behaviors and are a major focus of intervention, especially for those with severe intellectual disability.

10. Treatments are available for major psychiatric disorders, such as attention deficit disorder, mood disorders, and schizophrenia.

11. When psychotropic medications are used, careful monitoring is needed for drug-related effects and side effects.

12. The overall treatment plan is based on a comprehensive medical diagnosis, educational, and functional assessment, as well as behavioral and psychiatric evaluation. Specific interventions are tailored to meet the needs of the individual and to help that person reach his or her potential.

References

Abery, B., and Zajac, R. (1996). Self-determination as a goal of early childhood and elementary education. In D. Sands and M. Wehmeyer (eds.), *Self-determination across the lifespan: Independence and choice for people with disabilities,* pp. 169–196. Brookes, Baltimore.

Accardo, P.J., and Whitman, B.Y. (1990). Children of mentally retarded parents. *American Journal of Diseases of Children,* 144:69–70.

Adelman, H.S., MacDonald, V.M., Nelson, P., Smith, D.C., and Taylor, L. (1990). Motivational readiness and the participation of children with learning and behavior problems in psychoeducational decision making. *Journal of Learning Disabilities,* 23:171–176.

Algozzine, B., Browder, D., Karvonen, M., Test, D.W., and Wood, W.M. (2001). Effects of interventions to promote self-determination for individuals with disabilities. *Review of Educational Research,* 71:219–277.

Allen, S.M., Freeman, J.N., and Davis, W.M. (1998). Evaluation of risperidone in the neonatal 6-hydroxydopamine model of Lesch-Nyhan syndrome. *Pharmacological and Biochemical Behavior,* 59:327–330.

Aman, M.G.. (1982). Stimulant drug effects in developmental disorders and hyperactivity—toward a resolution of disparate findings. *Journal of Autism and Developmental Disorders,* 12:385–398.

Aman, M.G., Buican, B., and Arnold, L.E. (2003). Methylphenidate treatment in children with borderline IQ and mental retardation: Analysis of three aggregated studies. *Journal of Child and Adolescent Psychopharmacology,* 13:29–40.

Aman, M.G., Crismon, M.L., Frances, A., King, B.H., and Rojahn, J. (2004). *Treatment of psychiatric and behavioral problems in individuals with mental retardation: an update of expert consensus guidelines.* Postgraduate Institute for Medicine, Englewood, CA.

Aman, M.G., Pejeau, C., Osborne, P., Rojahn, J., and Handen, B. (1996). Four-year follow-up of children with low intelligence and ADHD. *Research in Developmental Disabilities,* 17:417–432.

Anderson, L., and Ernst, M. (1994). Self-injury in Lesch-Nyhan disease. *Journal of Autism and Developmental Disorders,* 24:67–81.

Aune, E. (1991). A transition model for post-secondary-bound students with learning disabilities. *Learning Disabilities and Research,* 6:177–187.

Balcazar, F.E., Fawcett, S.B., and Seekins, T. (1991). Teaching people with disabilities to recruit help to attain personal goals. *Rehabilitation Psychology,* 36:31–41.

Barr, M.W. (1904). *Mental defectives.* P. Blakiston's Sons, Philadelphia.

Beail, N.(1998). Psychoanalytic psychotherapy with men with intellectual disabilities: A preliminary outcome study. *British Journal of Medical Psychology,* 71:1–11.

Beail, N. (2003). What works for people with mental retardation? Critical commentary on cognitive-behavioral and psychodynamic psychotherapy research. *Mental Retardation,* 41:468–472.

Berkson, G. (1993). *Children with handicaps: A review of behavioural research.* Earlbaum, Hillsdale, NJ.

Bhaumik, S., Branford, D., McGrother, C., and Thorp, C. (1997). Autistic traits in adults with learning disabilities. *British Journal of Psychiatry,* 170:502–506.

Bosch, J., Van Dyke, C., Smith, S.M., and Poulton, S. (1997). Role of medical conditions in the exacerbation of self-injurious behavior: An exploratory study. *Mental Retardation,* 35:124–130.

Bowman, O.J., and Marzouk, D.K. (1992). Using the American with Disabilities Act of 1990 to empower university students with disabilities. *The American Journal of Occupational Therapy,* 46:450–456.

Brasic, J.R., Barnett, J.Y., Ahn, S.C., Nadrich, R.H., Will, M.V., and Clair, A. (1997). Clinical assessment of self-injurious behavior. *Psychology Reports,* 80:155–160.

Bregman, J.D. (1991). Current developments in the understanding of mental retardation: II. Psychopathology. *Journal of the American Academy of Child and Adolescent Psychiatry,* 30:861–872.

Brown. F., and Cohen, S. (1996). Self-determination and young children. *Journal of the Association for Persons With Severe Handicaps,* 2:22–23.

Brown. F., Gothelf., C.R., Guess, D., and Lehr, D.H. (1998). Self-determination for individuals with the most severe disabilities: Moving beyond chimera. *Journal of the Association for Persons With Severe Handicaps,* 23:17–26.

Clarke, D.J. (1989). Antilibidinal drugs and mental retardation: A review. *Medical Science and Law,* 29:136–146.

Cooper, K J., and Browder, D.M. (1998). Enhancing choice and participation for adults with severe disabilities in community-based instruction. *Journal of the Association for Persons With Severe Handicaps,* 23:252–260.

Cromwell, H.C., King, B.H., and Levine, M.S. (1997). Pemoline alters dopamine modulation of synaptic responses of neostriatal neurons in vitro. *Developmental Neuroscience,* 19:497–504.

Dagnan, D., and Chadwick, P. (1997). Cognitive-behavioral therapy for people with learning disabilities: Assessment and intervention. In B.S. Kroese, D. Dagnan, and K. Loumidis (eds.), *Cognitive behavior therapy for people with learning disabilities,* pp. 110–123. Routledge, London.

Dattilo, J., and Rusch, F.R. (1985). Effects of choice on leisure participation for persons with severe handicaps. *Journal of the Association for Persons With Severe Handicaps,* 10:194–199.

Davanzo, P.A., Belin, T.R., Widawsk, M.H., and King, B.H. (1998). Paroxetine treatment of aggression and self-injury in persons with mental retardation. *American Journal of Mental Retardation,* 102:427–37.

Davies, J.L., and Mathew, G. (1997). Behaviour disorder in an adolescent with terminal deletion of chromosome 3. *Journal of Intellectual Disabilities Research,* 41:278–280.

Davis, J.P., Judd, F.K., and Herrman, H. (1997a). Depression in adults with intellectual disability. Part 1: A review. *Australia New Zealand Journal of Psychiatry,* 31:232–42.

Davis, J.P., Judd, F.K., and Herrman, H. (1997b). Depression in adults with intellectual disability. Part 2: A pilot study. *Australia New Zealand Journal of Psychiatry,* 31: 243–51.

De Waal, F. (1996). *Good natured: The origins of right and wrong in humans and other animals.* Harvard University Press, Boston.

Dykens, E.M., Finucane, B.M., and Gayley, C. (1997). Brief report: cognitive and behavioral profiles in persons with Smith-Magenis syndrome. *Journal of Autism and Developmental Disorders,* 27:203–211.

Dykens, E.M., and Clarke, D.J. (1997). Correlates of maladaptive behavior in individuals with 5p- (Cri du Chat) syndrome. *Developmental Medicine and Child Neurology,* 39:752–756.

Everson, J.M., and Zhang, D. (2000). Person-centered planning: Characteristics, inhibitors, and supports. *Education and Training in Mental Retardation and Developmental Disabilities,* 35:36–43.

Ezell, D., Klein, C.E., and Ezell-Powell, S. (1999). Empowering students with mental retardation through portfolio assessment: A tool for fostering self-determination skills. *Education and Training in Mental Retardation and Developmental Disabilities,* 34:453–463.

Fernald, W.E. (1917). The growth of provision for the feebleminded in the United States. *Mental Hygiene,* 1:34–59.

Field, S. (1996). Self-determination instructional strategies for youth with learning disabilities. *Journal of Learning Disabilities,* 29:40–52.

Field, S., and Hoffman, A. (1999). The importance of family involvement for promoting self-determination in adolescents with autism and other developmental disabilities. *Focus on Autism and Developmental Disabilities,* 14:36–41.

Fischer, S.M., Iwata, B.A., and Mazaleski, J.L. (1997). Noncontingent delivery of arbitrary reinforcers as treatment for self-injurious behavior. *Journal of Applied Behavior Analysis,* 30:229–234.

Fullerton, A., and Coyne, P. (1999). Developing skills and concepts for self-determination in young adults with autism. *Focus on Autism and Other Developmental Disabilities,* 14:42–52.

Gadow, K. (1985). Prevalence and efficacy of stimulant drug use with mentally retarded children and youth. *Psychopharmacology Bulletin,* 21:291–303.

Gillberg, C., Persson, E., Grufman, M., and Themner, U. (1986). Psychiatric disorders in mildly and severely mentally retarded urban children and adolescents: Epidemiological aspects. *British Journal of Psychiatry,* 149:68–74.

Handen, B.L., Feldman, H., Gosling, A., Breaux, A.M., and McAuliffe, S. (1991). Adverse side effects of methylphenidate among mentally retarded children with ADHD. *Journal of the American Academy of Child and Adolescent Psychiatry,* 30:241–245.

Handen, B.L., Johnson, C.R., and Lubetsky, M. (2000). Efficacy of methylphenidate among children with autism and symptoms of attention-deficit hyperactivity disorder. *Journal of Autism and Developmental Disorders,* 30:245–255.

Harris, J.C., Wong, D.F., Jinnah, H.A., Schretlen, D., and Barker, P. (2002). Neuroimaging studies in Lesch-Nyhan syndrome and Lesch-Nyhan variants. In S.R. Schroeder, M.L. Oser-Granite, and T. Thompson (eds.), *Self-injurious behavior: gene-brain-behavior relationships,* pp. 269–278. American Psychological Association, Washington, DC.

Health Care Financing Administration. (1997). *Psychopharmacological Medication: Safety Precautions for Persons with Developmental Disabilities.* Health Care Financing Administration, Washington, DC.

Hellings, J.A., and Warnock, J.K. (1994). Self-injurious behavior and serotonin in Prader-Willi syndrome. *Psychopharmacology Bulletin,* 30:245–250.

Hoffman, A., and Field, S. (1995). Promoting self-determination through effective curriculum development. *Intervention in School and Clinic,* 30:134–141.

Holland, A., and Clare, I.C.H. (2003). The Human Genome Project: Considerations for people with intellectual disabilities. *Journal of Intellectual Disability Research*, 47: 515–525.

Horner, R.H. (1999). Positive behavior supports. In M. Wehmeyer and J. Patton, (eds.), *Mental Retardation in the 21st Century,* pp. 181–196. Pro-Ed, Austin, TX.

Hurley, A.D., Folstein, M., and Lam, N. (2003). Patients with and without intellectual disability seeking outpatient psychiatric services: diagnoses and prescribing pattern. *Journal of Intellectual Disability Research*, 47:39–50.

Itard, J.M. (1802). *The wild boy of Aveyron*. Richard Phillips.

Johnson, C.R., Handen, B.L., Lubetsky, M.J., and Sacco, K.A. (1994). Efficacy of methylphenidate and behavioral intervention on classroom behavior in children with ADHD and mental retardation. *Behavior Modification,* 18:470–487.

Kahng, S., Iwata, B.A. and Lewin, A.B. (2002). Behavioral treatment of self-injury, 1964 to 2000. *American Journal of Mental Retardation.* 107:212–221.

Kanner, L. (1953). Parent's feelings about retarded children. *American Journal of Mental Deficiency*, 39:479–489.

Lerman, D.C., Iwata, B.A., Shore, B.A., DeLeon, I.G. (1997). Effects of intermittent punishment on self-injurious behavior: An evaluation of schedule thinning. *Journal of Applied Behavior Analysis*, 30:187–201.

Lindsay W.R., Neilson C.Q., Morrison F., Smith A.H. (1998) The treatment of six men with a learning disability convicted of sex offences with children. *British Journal of Clinical Psychology,* 37(Pt 1):83–98

Luckasson, R., Borthwick-Duffy, S., Buntinx, W.H.E., Coulter, D.L., Craig, E.M., Reeve, A., Schalock, R.L., Snell, M.E., Spitalnik, D.M., Spreat, S., and Tasse, M.J. (2002). *Mental retardation: Definition, classification, and systems of supports,* 10th ed. American Association on Mental Retardation, Washington, DC.

Lynch, C. (2004). Psychotherapy for persons with mental retardation. *Mental Retardation*, 42:399–405.

Malette, P., Mirenda, P., Kandborg, T., Jones, P., Bunz, T., and Rogow, S. (1992). Application of a lifestyle development process for people with severe intellectual disabilities: A case study report. *Journal of the Association for Persons with Severe Handicaps,* 17:179–191.

Mansfield, C., Hopfer S., and Marteau, T.M. (1999). Termination rates after prenatal diagnosis of Down syndrome, spina bifida, anencephaly, and Turner and Klinefelter syndromes: A systematic literature review. European Concerted Action: DADA (Decision-making After the Diagnosis of a fetal Abnormality). *Prenatal Diagnosis*, 19:808–812.

Marston, G.M., Perry, D.W., and Roy, A. (1997). Manifestations of depression in people with intellectual disability. *Journal of Intellectual Disability Research,* 41:476–480.

Martin, J., O'Brien, J., and Wray, D. (1999–2000). *Teaching self-determination.* University of Georgia Interactive Teaching Network, Athens, GA.

Martin, J.E., and Marshall, L.H. (1995). Choicemaker: A comprehensive self-determination transition program. *Intervention in School and Clinic,* 30:147–156.

Matson, J.L., Hamilton, M., Duncan, D., Bamburg, J., Smiroldo, B., Anderson, S., and Baglio, C. (1997). Characteristics of stereotypic movement disorder and self-injurious behavior assessed with the Diagnostic Assessment for the Severely Handicapped (DASH-II). *Research in Developmental Disabilities,* 18:457–469.

McCracken, J.T., McGough, J., Shah, B., Cronin, P., Hong, D., Aman, M.G., Arnold, L.E., Lindsay, R., Nash, P., Hollway, J., et al. (2002). Risperidone in children with autism and serious behavioral problems. *New England Journal of Medicine,* 347: 314–321.

McDermott, S., Breen, R., Platt, T., Dhar, D., Shelton, J., and Krishnaswami, S. (1997). Do behavior changes herald physical illness in adults with mental retardation? *Community Mental Health Journal*, 33:85–97.

Menolascino, F.J., Wilson, J., Golden, C., and Ruedrich, S. (1986). Medication and treatment of schizophrenia in persons with mental retardation. *Mental Retardation*, 24: 277–283.

National Institute of Health. (1990). *Consensus conference on treatment of destructive behaviors in persons with developmental disabilities*. U.S. Government Printing Office, Washington, DC.

Nissen, J.M., and Haveman, M.J. (1997). Mortality and avoidable death in people with severe self-injurious behaviour: Results of a Dutch study. *Journal of Intellectual Disability Research*, 41:252–257.

O'Reilly, M.F. (1997). Functional analysis of episodic self-injury correlated with recurrent otitis media. *Journal of Applied Behavioral Analysis*, 30:165–167.

Pao, M. (2003). Managing pain: An exploration of psychotropic medications. *Contemporary Pediatrics*, 20:43–57.

Parsons, M.B., Reid, D.H., and Green, C.W. (1998). Identifying work preferences prior to supported work for an individual with severe disabilities including deaf-blindness. *Journal of the Association for Persons with Severe Handicaps*, 23:329–333.

Pearson, D.A., Santos, C.W., Roache, J.D., Casat, C.D., Loveland, K.A., Lachar, D., Lane, D.M., Faria, L.P., and Cleveland, L.A. (2003). Treatment effects of methylphenidate on behavioral adjustment in children with mental retardation and ADHD. *Journal of the American Academy of Child and Adolescent Psychiatry*, 42:209–216.

Pinel, P. (1809). *Traité médico-philosophique sur l'aliénation mentale*, 2nd ed. J.A. Brosson, Paris.

Prater, M.A., Bruhl, S., and Serna, L.A. (1998). Acquiring social skills through cooperative learning and teach-directed instruction. *Remedial and Special Education*, 19: 160–172.

Prout, H.T., and Nowak-Drabik, K.M. (2003). Psychotherapy with persons who have mental retardation: An evaluation of effectiveness. *American Journal on Mental Retardation*, 108:82–93.

Reiss, S., and Aman, M.G. (eds.). (1998). *Psychotropic medications and developmental disabilities: The International Consensus Handbook*. Ohio State University Nisonger Center, Columbus, OH.

Rose, J., West, C., and Clifford, D. (2000). Group interventions for anger in people with intellectual disabilities. *Research in Developmental Disabilities*, 21:171–181.

Ruef, M., Posten, D., and Humphrey, K. (1999). *PBS: Putting the "positive" into behavioral support: An introductory training packet*. University of Kansas, Beach Center on Families and Disability, Lawrence, KS.

Rush, A.J., and Frances, A. (eds.) (2000). The Expert Consensus Guideline Series. Treatment of psychiatric and behavioral problems in mental retardation (Issue 3, Special Issue). *American Journal of Mental Retardation*, 105:159–228.

Sanders, A.R., Rusu, I., Duan, J., Molen, J.E., Hou, C., Schwab, S.G., Wildenauer, D.B., Martinez, M., and Gejman, P.V. (2004). Haplotypic association spanning the 22q11.21 genes *COMT* and *ARVCF* with schizophrenia. *Molecular Psychiatry*, 10: 353–365.

Sandman, C.A., Hetrick, W., Taylor, D.V., Marion, S.D., Touchette, P., Barron, J.L., Martinezzi, V., Steinberg, R.M., and Crinella, F.M. (2000). Long-term effects of

330 intellectualDisability

naltrexone on self-injurious behavior. *American Journal of Mental Retardation,* 105: 103–117.

Sandman, C.A., Hetrick, W., Taylor, D.V., and Chicz-DeMet, A. (1997). Dissociation of POMC peptides after self-injury predicts responses to centrally acting opiate blockers. *American Journal of Mental Retardation,* 102:182–199.

Santosh, P.J., and Baird, G. (1999). Psychopharmacotherapy in children and adults with intellectual disability. *Lancet,* 354:233–242.

Schloss, P.J., Alper, S., and Jayne, D. (1993). Self-determination for persons with disabilities: Choice, risk, and dignity. *Exceptional Children,* 60:215–225.

Schroeder, S.R., Rojahn, J., and Reese, R.M. (1997). Brief report: Reliability and validity of instruments for assessing psychotropic medication effects on self-injurious behavior in mental retardation. *Journal of Autism and Developmental Disorders,* 27: 89–102.

Seguin, E. (1870). *New facts and remarks concerning idiocy, being a lecture before the New York Medical Journal Association,* October 15, 1869. William Wood, New York.

Sigafoos, J., Roberts, D., Couzens, D., and Kerr, M. (1993). Providing opportunities for choice making and turn taking to adults with multiple disabilities. *Journal of Developmental and Physical Disabilities,* 5:297–310.

Simeon, J.G. (1997). Challenges to pediatric psychopharmacology. *Journal of Psychiatry and Neuroscience,* 22:15–17.

Simpson, M.K. (1998). The roots of normalization: A reappraisal. *Journal of Intellectual and Developmental Disabilities Research,* 42:1–7.

Singh, N.N., Ellis, C.R., and Wechsler, H. (1997). Psychopharmacoepidemiology of mental retardation: 1966 to 1995. *Journal of Child and Adolescent Psychopharmacology,* 7: 255–266.

Singh, N.N., Lancioni, G.E., Winton, A.S., Molina, E.J., Sage, M., Brown, S., and Groeneweg, J. (2004). Effects of Snoezelen room, Activities of daily living skills training, and vocational skills training on aggression and self-injury by adults with mental retardation and mental illness. *Research in Developmental Disabilities,* 25:285–293.

Spreat, S., Conroy, J.W., and Fullerton, A. (2004). Statewide longitudinal survey of psychotropic medication use for persons with mental retardation: 1994 to 2000. *American Journal of Mental Retardation* 109: 322–331.

Spreat, S., Conroy, J.W., and Jones, J.C. (1997). Use of psychotropic medication in Oklahoma: A statewide survey. *American Journal of Mental Retardation,* 102:80–85.

Stainton, T. (2003). Identity, difference and the ethical politics of prenatal testing. *Journal of Intellect Disability Research,* 47:533–539.

Steffenburg, S., Gillberg, C., and Steffenburg, U. (1996). Psychiatric disorders in children and adolescents with mental retardation and active epilepsy. *Archives of Neurology,* 53:904–912.

Symons, F.J., and Thompson, T. (1997). Self-injurious behaviour and body site preference. *Journal of Intellectual Disabilities Research,* 41:456–468.

Szymanski, L., and King, B.H. (1999). Practice parameters for the assessment and treatment of children, adolescents, and adults with mental retardation and comorbid mental disorders. American Academy of Child and Adolescent Psychiatry Working Group on Quality Issues. *Journal of the American Academy of Child and Adolescent Psychiatry,* 38(12 suppl.): 5S–31S.

Szymanski, L.S. (1980). Individual psychotherapy with retarded persons. In L.S. Szymanski and P.E. Tanguay (eds.), *Emotional disorders of mentally retarded persons.* University Park Press, Baltimore, MD.

Tilly, W.D., Knoster, T.K., Kovaleski, J., Bambara, L., Dunlap, G., and Kincaid, D. (1998). *Functional behavioral assessment: Policy development in light of emerging research and practice.* National Association for State Directors of Special Education (NASDSE), Alexandria, VA.

Tourette's Syndrome Study Group. (2002). Treatment of ADHD in children with tics: A randomized controlled trial. *Neurology,* 58:527–536.

Trent, J.W. (1995). *Inventing the feeble mind: A history of mental retardation in the United States.* University of California Press, Berkeley.

Van Reusen, A.K., Deshler, D.D., and Schumaker, J.B. (1989). Effects of a student participation strategy in facilitating the involvement of adolescents with learning disabilities in the Individualized Education Program planning process. *Learning Disabilities,* 1:23–34.

Van Reusen, A.K., and Bos, C.S. (1994). Facilitating, student participation in individualized education programs through motivation strategy instruction. *Exceptional Children,* 60:466–475.

Vehmas S. (2004). Ethical analysis of the concept of disability. *Mental Retardation,* 42: 209–222.

Wehmeyer, M.L. (1992). Self-determination and the education of students with mental retardation. *Education and Training in Mental Retardation and Developmental Disabilities,* 27:302–314.

Wehmeyer, M.L. (1996). Self-determination as an educational outcome: Why it is important to children, youth, and adults with disabilities. In D. Sands and M. Wehmeyer (eds.), *Self-determination across the lifespan: Independence and choice for people with disabilities,* pp. 17–36. Brookes, Baltimore.

Wehmeyer, M.L., Agran, M., and Hughes, C. (1998). *Teaching self-determination to students with disabilities: Basic skills for successful transition.* Brookes, Baltimore.

Wehmeyer, M.L., Agran, M., and Hughes, C. (2000). A national survey of teachers' promotion of self-determination and student-directed learning. *Journal of Special Education,* 34:58–68.

Wehmeyer, M.L, and Lawrence, M. (1995). Whose future is it anyway? Promoting student involvement in transition planning. *Career Development for Exceptional Individuals,* 18:69–83.

Wehmeyer, M.L., Palmer, S.B., Agran, M., Mithaug, D.E., and Martin, J.E. (2000). Promoting causal agency: The self-determined learning model of instruction. *Exceptional Children,* 66:439–453.

Wehmeyer, M.L, and Schwartz, M. (1998a). The relationship between self-determination and quality of life for adults with mental retardation. *Education and Training in Mental Retardation and Developmental Disabilities,* 33:3–12.

Wehmeyer, M.L., and Schwartz, M. (1998b). The self-determination focus of transition goals for students with mental retardation. *Career Development for Exceptional Individuals,* 21:75–86.

Wehmeyer, M.L., and Ward, M. (1995). The spirit of the IDEA mandate: Student involvement in transition planning. *The Journal for Vocational Special Needs Education,* 17:108–111.

Wilbur, C.T. (1888). Institutions for the feebleminded. *Proceedings of the 15th national conference of charities and correction,* 17:106–113.

Williams, R.R. (1989). Creating a new world of opportunity: Expanding choice and self-determination in lives of Americans with severe disability by 1992 and beyond. In

R. Perske (ed.), *Proceedings from the National Conference on Self-Determination,* pp. 16–17. Institute on Community Integration, Minneapolis, MN.

Winzer, M.A. (1986). Early developments in special education: Some aspects of Enlightenment thought. *Remedial and Special Education (RASE),* 7:42–49.

Wolfensberger, W. (1972). *The principle of normalization in human service.* National Institute on Mental Retardation. Toronto, Canada.

Wolfensberger, W. (1976). On the origin of our institutional models. In R. Kugel and A. Shearer (eds.), *Changing patterns in residential services for the mentally retarded,* rrevised ed., pp. 35–82. President's Committee on Mental Retardation, Washington, DC.

Yokoyama, C., and Okamura, H. (1997). Self-injurious behavior and dopaminergic neuron system in neonatal 6-hydroxydopamine-lesioned rat: 1. Dopaminergic neurons and receptors. *Journal of Pharmacology and Experimental Therapeutics,* 280:1016–1030.

Ysseldyke, J.E., Algozzine, B., and Thurlow, M.L. (2000). *Critical issues in special education,* 3rd ed. Houghton Mifflin, Boston.

10 _____

Ethics and Spirituality

This chapter considers ethical and spiritual issues related to intellectual disability. Consideration of the meaning of life of an intellectually disabled person must take into account how society defines and responds to individual differences. There are ethical and religious concerns regarding prenatal diagnosis and questions of how to teach ethical behavior to persons with intellectual disability. Participation in religious practices in the community and in group home settings is important for families and persons with intellectual disability. This chapter reviews these issues in detail.

HISTORICAL PERSPECTIVE

In biblical times, there were edicts about disability that offer insight into attitudes toward disabled people. There is an Old Testament injunction: "Thou shalt not curse the deaf, put a stumbling block before the blind, nor maketh the blind wander out of a path" (Leviticus 19:14). This may be the first Western command to legislate for the protection of the deaf and handicapped. Moreover, deaf persons without speech were viewed as children and provided the same protections as children. Yet, the threat of disability was also an element in biblical injunctions: "If you do not follow his commandments and decrees . . . all these curses will become upon you and overtake you: The Lord will afflict you with madness, blindness, and confusion of mind. At midday, you will grope around like a man in the dark" (Deuteronomy 28:15). Although help for those with disabilities was seen as a charitable obligation, disability was perceived potentially as a punishment from God. Ancient people often believed that illness was inflicted by a deity or supernatural power (Rosen, 1968). In records dating back before 2000 B.C., the birth of children with congenital impairments were used to predict the future of the community. In Babylonia, those who prophesized about the future kept a list of birth deformities and the specific meaning and prophecy that these disabilities foretold. Although a disability was viewed as a portent of things to come (Braddock and Parish, 2002) or punishment for immorality, there also existed the attitude that the disabled should be treated with compassion.

The New Testament provides insight into how attitudes about disability evolved. Mark reports Jesus healing a blind man by spitting and laying hands on the man's eyes. Healing of people with paralysis, leprosy, epilepsy, mental illness, and blindness is also recorded (Black, 1996). The tales of healing were sometimes interpreted to suggest that people "have disabilities . . . to show the power of God" (Black, 1996). When Jesus was asked whether a blind man's sins or his parents' sins caused the blindness, he replied that it was neither, but rather a mechanism for "God's work [to be] revealed to him" (Black 1996; John 9:3).

In the Middle Ages, there were various beliefs about disability. Some disabilities, particularly deafness, epilepsy, and mental disabilities, were proposed to have demonological origins, resulting in persecution of people with these disabilities. On the other hand, persons with disability were thought to be part of the natural order like people who were poor. The latter view led people with disabilities to networks of support to survive when times were difficult. Both views coexisted, and there was no clear interpretation and universal definition of disability at this time.

In the United States, views on the religious meaning of disability have been traced to Puritan New England, where, on the one hand, the goodness of the simple spirit humbled by affliction was confirmed, while on the other, severe intellectual disability reflected the depths of spiritual desolation (Wickham, 2001).

In summary, in the long historical span from antiquity to Puritan New England, there were many attitudes toward disability. The writings of the Old Testament suggested, on the one hand, that society should be generous and kind toward individuals who were impaired, but also declared that impairment may be a mark of the wrath of God. There was a similar complexity in Greece and Rome, where the killing of newborns with congenital impairments existed, and society perceived the birth of a child with congenital anomalies as an indication of the anger of the gods. Still, the provision of pensions to soldiers injured on the battlefield was part of Athenian life, and individuals with impairments were known to work at different trades. At the time of Christ, impairment had different meanings, offering redemption opportunities for kind strangers but also signifying superstitious beliefs about causation. Overall, in antiquity, impairment was accepted as one aspect of the course of life. In the Middle Ages, confusion about causes continued, but attitudes toward individuals with disabilities were often supportive. Similarly, both compassionate support and divine retribution continued as themes among the pilgrims who immigrated to North America.

PARENTAL BELIEF SYSTEMS: COPING WITH INTELLECTUAL DISABILITY

The role of ethical understanding and religious beliefs in coping with the stresses of managing an intellectually disabled child is of growing importance. Haworth, Hill, and Glidden (1996) used the Fewell Religiosity Scale, a 12-item self-report questionnaire concerning religious beliefs and participation, with 204 families who were raising at least one child who had or was at risk for a developmental disability. Mothers interviewed made mostly positive statements about religion and spoke of how their beliefs helped them with coping. Religious connectedness has been studied in African Americans by Rogers-Dulan (1998), who assesses religious socialization, religious media, and participation in religious groups. The author's 19-item questionnaire on religious connectedness provides a means to assess the importance of religious life in other ethnic groups.

MINISTERING TO PERSONS WITH INTELLECTUAL DISABILITY

During the past 20 years, there has been a major expansion in ministries and services for persons with intellectual disability. There has been an increase in the kinds of ministries and services that are offered, in the variety of religious organizations that have become engaged, and in the numbers of both professionals and laypersons involved in engaging persons with intellectual disability in spiritual endeavors. The traditional questions and the traditional models for ministry with people with intellectual disability have changed as the service system has understood the need for greater services and greater supports.

The trend in working with persons with intellectual disability has shifted from an emphasis on whether they have the capacity to believe and articulate their understanding of their faith to a focus on the emotional and spiritual importance of belonging and to their participation as members in a faith community. Special religious education programs developed for persons with intellectual disability are moving toward inclusive ministries that emphasize how people with and without intellectual disability may engage one another in a faith community.

In the past, the questions raised dealt with whether persons with intellectual disability could understand religious instruction. Consequently, their participation in religious services was a major concern. How could individuals with intellectual disability participate in the religious service in a meaningful way? Questions were raised in the Christian tradition about whether or not persons with intellectual disability should receive communion, and in the Jewish community questions were raised about whether a bar mitzvah or bat mitzvah could be meaningful. Thus, as adolescence approached, the issue of membership in a faith community became important to family members who emphasized inclusion in the community. Such concerns emphasized the ability of a person with intellectual disability to reason or to express often-abstract beliefs in the way that the general faith community does.

A large number of special spiritual education programs were developed in response to concerns about cognitive functioning and abstract understanding. Such specialized curricula focused on teaching persons with intellectual disability about their community and the faith traditions chosen by their families. In residential settings, religious staff adapted worship and education programs to their special needs. With deinstitutionalization, fewer people with intellectual disability live in residential settings; consequently, community services are developing to provide greater inclusion. Community leaders ask how a congregation might not only provide special education programs but also provide for greater inclusion in the life of the specific faith community.

As community members of the various religious affiliations became more aware of the needs of individuals with intellectual disability and sought to befriend them, it became apparent that religious practice was meaningful in the lives of persons with intellectual disability and their expressions of faith were valid. With this new understanding, the question about persons with intellectual disability shifted from whether or not they could understand to how they might best be provided the opportunity to participate in a faith community. The emphasis gradually shifted to considerations of how "different" behavior might be appreciated by community members and that participation might facilitate understanding. How could persons with intellectual disability who had often been excluded and had not grown up in a religious tradition be engaged? Their understanding might be enhanced by participating in practices in the faith community rather than discussing their meaning in greater detail. Special religious ministries and education programs would continue to play an important role, but they could not be the only form of ministering. Thus, inclusion in preschool programs, in faith community recreation programs, in day programs, in youth groups, and confirmation or bar/bat mitzvah training were initiated. Respite care, supported by a religious community that also supports social programs, families, and groups, was provided. Moreover, participation in spiritual activities that include music, choir, and service activities received greater emphasis. Finally, as an approach to normalization, individuals with intellectual disability could act as ushers and participate as others their age might in a religious program.

Gaventa (1993) suggests milestones toward inclusion in religious communities have emerged during the past 20 years. He indicates that:

1. National networks have developed that connect people who are involved in religious services for people with intellectual disability and their families. Such networks may be initiated at the local level by parents, by laypeople, by clergy, and by educational services to professionals who are working with religious groups. Such networks of services may include group home support and consultation advice to families, congregations, and service providers. The religious division of the American Association on Mental Retardation (AAMR), the National Apostolate of Persons with Mental Retardation, and other national groups hold annual conventions and provide newsletters and share information.
2. Resource materials on pertinent topics are now available to assist congregations for inclusion of persons with intellectual disability. Such

resource materials are available on religious education, ethics, theology, sacraments, family support, and respite care. Curricula are available for special religious instruction along with guides to help teachers adjust the religious curriculum so that adults and children with intellectual disability can be included.

3. In some settings, rather than a chaplain or educator who works with a segregated population of affected individuals, a "spirituality coach" may be involved. Analogous to the job coach who works with inclusion in the workplace, the "spirituality coach" provides support and facilitates participation in services. Rather than having separate programs, linkages are facilitated among people living in group homes and community religious residences. Regional offices may be available to assist congregations in religious education and services.

4. Services for individuals with intellectual disability and their families are increasingly provided through religious agencies. Both group homes and other residential options are supported. Such service organizations include Catholic Charities, Martin Luther Homes, The Jewish Foundation for Group Homes, and The Southeast Methodist Agency for Rehabilitation. Moreover, almost every faith has agencies of this kind. Their expansion is a needed response for parents for long-term care that will continue to affirm the importance of the religious life for individuals with intellectual disability as they grow older.

SPIRITUALITY AND THE AAMR DEFINITION

The AAMR classification manual (1992) provides a definition of intellectual disability that shifts the focus from descriptions of cognitive-level and adaptive functioning to a multidimensional approach. This multidimensional approach highlights the development of supports for persons with intellectual disability to normalize their lives (Luckasson et al., 2002). Spiritual support, in addition to environmental support, is needed for meaningful inclusion in the community (Gaventa, 2003). An interdisciplinary dialog between individuals in the community, ministries, and people with intellectual disability may be facilitated by using a multidimensional approach. In addressing classification, professionals who work in scientific settings must engage with the religious community and consider the different frameworks and languages that they use to communicate. When normalization is considered, individuals in the service system should consider what is meant by normal in regard to religious practice for individuals with intellectual disability. In this sense, diagnostic descriptions must be understood to focus on needed community supports. The AAMR definition focuses on inclusion, self-advocacy, self-choice, and the importance of community support and friendships within the community. This focus may bridge gaps in understanding between scientific and religious communities. Preparation for participation is ongoing, and it requires considerable sensitivity and understanding. Families struggle with inclusion in this area as they do in others. Some testify to the essential importance of their children's engagement in their faith. Others have experienced insensitivity in having received lip service regarding the provision of the treatment but not the actual needed support.

Although there is improved programming for individuals with intellectual disability, provision of adequate supports, sufficient staff, and combating negative attitudes must be addressed. It is tragic when the easy way out has been to do nothing, even though resources and supports are increasingly available but may not be utilized. The issue of belief is less focused on the understanding of individuals with intellectual disability than it is on what people in the religious community and service system believe about spirituality and faith for those individuals. These groups need to work together to increase opportunities and supports that take into account and respect the faith tradition involved as well as the preferences of persons with intellectual disability. The critical element is an opportunity for involvement along with the availability of staff, such as spirituality coaches, who can provide support to the individual and background knowledge about intellectual disability to the community. With the establishment of new resources, the issue is whether families believe that spiritual life for people with intellectual disability is important and advocate the opportunity for their engagement in a faith community. Finally, the individual with intellectual disability must speak for himself or herself and then be helped to make informed choices. When they are made, the person with intellectual disability must be provided with the necessary supports.

AAMR MULTIDIMENSIONAL CLASSIFICATION

An enhanced quality of life for a person with intellectual disability implies full integration into the community. There are ethical issues when carrying out assessment, providing supports, and offering treatment (Wolfensberger, 1979, 1982). Cultural traditions about which actions are right and which are wrong, assumptions about the meaning of human life, how one values the life of a person with intellectual disability, and political beliefs about the social contract between the government and service provision may shape our engagement with specific individuals, our views of social policy, and the allocation of resources. Spiritual assumptions and beliefs impact how ethical decisions are made in assessment and caregiving.

The AAMR multidimensional classification system allows for an affirmation for the value of life for each person. Spirituality is an important support. In a sense, persons with intellectual disability are "at risk" spiritually in that they may lack an opportunity to experience love in a community, to be connected with sources of hope, and to fully participate in a community of faith. A central issue is how to instill spiritual awareness and supports and to routinely include these spiritual supports as part of a multidimensional approach.

Any discussion of spirituality starts with "the fundamental affirmation that all human beings have within them a spark of divinity" (Gaventa, 2003). In Judeo-Christian terms, each individual is created in the image of God. To assess a person with intellectual disabilities and adaptive limitations from a spiritual point of view requires consideration of fundamental concerns about what it means to be human and the role of the sacred in the life of the person with the handicapping condition and in the life of his or her parents. Parents must consider whether there is a difference between their own religious practice and the one in which their child can participate. An assessment raises questions about the meaning of suffering experienced by a person with intellectual disability and the purpose of that individual's life. It also raises questions about how we are connected in a spiritual sense to those with intellectual disability. The AAMR definition of intellectual disability asks questions that are linked to values in regard to the independence, the productivity, and the role in life of persons with intellectual disability. To consider the spiritual life of a person with intellectual disability is to reflect on the nature of human experience and to plan for a means to organize support to facilitate growth toward his or her further spiritual development. From this perspective, one must look upon spirituality as a basic dimension of human life.

Not only should the dimensions included in the multidimensional approach to diagnosis and classification and supports be implemented but also spiritual considerations should be included. Spirituality has been defined as "the dimension of life that reflects the need to find meaning in existence and in which we respond to the sacred" (Fitchett, 1993a). A functional approach to spiritual assessment of individuals is needed that emphasizes finding and making meaning in one's life, rather than specifying what that meaning is. This implies that the family and professionals working with the person with intellectual disability emphasize how that individual's life can be or might become meaningful to them, to their family and to the community.

Spirituality may be experienced and expressed within or outside a specific faith community. In this way, it is a broader term than religion. When conducting an assessment of a person with intellectual disability, it is not simply a question of whether one attends a religious institution, such as a church, synagogue, or mosque, and has the necessary supports to do so. More specifically, the focus is on carrying out a spiritual assessment of the individual and the spiritual dimension of his or her life. There are seven elements or dimensions that must be considered in an assessment of spiritual life (Fitchett, 1993b, 1996). These include basic beliefs and meanings (sense of purpose, affiliation), vocation and obligations (a calling or duty), experience and emotion (experience of the sacred or demonic and interpretations of those feelings), courage and growth (openness to change in beliefs based on experience), ritual and practice (the specific rituals and practices associated with belief), community (formal participation in a community with shared beliefs and type of participation), and authority and guidance (the source of authority for beliefs and practices and where one looks for guidance within oneself or outside oneself).

In developing supports for persons with intellectual disability, these elements must be considered individually. Spirituality is often equated with doctrine or intellectual understanding. Yet, how might spirituality be approached when considering intellectual functioning and adaptive skills in persons with intellectual disability, particularly since spirituality is expressed through religious practice?

Moreover, spiritual practices may be linked to mental health (Carder, 1984; Larson and Larson, 1994). Spirituality may impact physical health in regard to "a sense of wellness," in the facilitation of recovery from illness, and in coping with physical illness.

Spirituality is a dimension separate from the other dimensions that must be considered when implementing the AAMR multidimensional definition of mental retardation (intellectual disability). When addressing spirituality, several issues should be emphasized. First, individuals with intellectual disability can grow and develop because of their spirituality (spirituality as a dimension of life and growth). Second, spirituality is a major way to find meaning in life and to be motivated to master tasks (spirituality as meaning and purpose). Third, spirituality links individuals with intellectual disability to communities (spirituality and culture). Fourth, spirituality honors the choice of the individual and empowers them to make a choice (spirituality as choice and self-determination). Hoeksema (1995) proposes that self-determination includes recognition of spirituality in the sense that self-determination is based on freedom of choice and individual responsibility for one's actions.

Rationale for Including Spirituality in the AAMR System of Supports for Persons with Mental Retardation (Intellectual Disability)

1. *Spirituality as a dimension of life and growth.* Westerhoff (1976) and Fowler (1981) have considered spirituality in a developmental sense. The importance of spirituality in the lives of typically developing children has been explored by Robert Coles (1990). Webb-Mitchell (1993) has further examined the same issues that Coles raised in children with developmental disabilities. When one considers the dimension of spirituality and spiritual growth, faith arises as love and trust are experienced and celebrated. Subsequently, affiliative faith emerges and is linked to a sense of emotional attachment to a set of beliefs in a particular community of faith. As affiliative faith deepens, there is a period of searching characterized by questioning and experimentation in beliefs and, finally, the emergence of an "owned faith" through spiritual practice and participation in a shared community. Elaborations of these stages of faith to individuals with different levels of intellectual disability are provided, for example, by Schurter (1994), who has utilized levels of support to establish how persons with intellectual disability deal with grief, death, and dying.

An evaluation of spiritual life may be based on those elements in spirituality that are (1) distancing from religious belief and (2) those that are confirming. Elements that are distancing include fear, alienation, guilt, and despair, as described in table 10.1.

For the person with intellectual disability, fear may be experienced as mistrust, victimization, or helplessness; alienation experienced as social stigma, rejection, and estrangement; guilt experienced from a sense of internalized stigma and self-blame; and despair experienced when life seems meaningless, leading to withdrawal. When afraid, the individual asks "Am I safe?" When alienated,

Table 10.1 Tools for Spiritual Diagnosis

Spiritual Diagnosis	Image of God	Experience	Existential Question	Experience	Image of God	Spiritual Diagnosis
Fear	Unpredictable; Capricious; Chaotic	Mistrust; Victimization; Helplessness; Passivity	"Am I safe?" "Is my world a threat or opportunity?"	Hope, Courage; Active Agency; Opportunity	Trustworthy; Reliable	Faith
Alienation	Vengeful; Derisive	Social Stigma; External Judgment; Rejection; Estrangement	"Do I belong"	Social Acceptance; Communication Embracement	Loving; Inclusive	Community
Guilt	Punishing; Judgmental	Internalized Stigma; Personal responsibility for illness	"Am I worthy?"	Grace; Repentance	Merciful; Compassionate	Reconciliation
Despair	Withholding; Silent; Absent	Meaninglessness Death Anxiety; Nonbeing	"Am I valued?" "Do I have a legacy?" "Did my life make a difference?" "Am I content?" "Regretful?"	Vocation; Purpose; Creativity; Meaning	Blessing; Affirming; Revealing	Providence

Modified by Gaventa, 2003. From Landau-Stanton, et al. (1993). Spiritual, cultural, and community systems in AIDS: Health and mental health: A primary source book (eds.) J. Landau-Stanton and C. Clements, pp. 267–298. Brunner/Mazer, New York. Reprinted by permission of publisher from *What is Mental Retardation? Ideas for an Evolving Disability*. American Association on Mental Retardation, Washington, DC. Copyright © 2003.

"Do I belong?" When guilty, "Am I worthy?" When despairing, "Am I wanted? Does my life matter?" The religious response to fear is the establishment of hope and courage associated with the emergence of faith and a trustworthy and reliable spiritual image of God. Alienation is rectified through social acceptance, through communion and embracement, and the experience of being loved and included as a member of a community. Guilt is resolved through repentance and grace, with the experience of a merciful religious image of God that leads to reconciliation; and despair is dissolved with the emergence of a sense of purpose and meaning, an image of God that provides affirmation and blessing and providence. This author proposes that this framework may be applied to all individuals, including those individuals with intellectual disability. But how does this transformation occur? Prins (1994) assessed spiritual strengths and needs, and outlined ways for experiences of safety, hope, and trustfulness to occur that might enhance a sense of belonging. The goal is full acceptance into a community to deepen experiences of self-worth and to strengthen personal values and meaning. Religious activities may be used to encounter these distancing elements but must take into account the individual's level of understanding and capacity for spiritual practice; capacity for religious participation may vary from one person to the next. However, awareness of transcendent love is mediated and experienced in temporal love through loving relationships. Thus, it may be in the quality of our relationships rather than the quantity of our intellect that the image of a compassionate god is established (Swinton, 1997).

2. *Spirituality as meaning and purpose in coping.* Gaventa (2003) notes that spiritual assessment instruments consider how people utilize spirituality and religious faith as a means for coping with stress. Most research on coping and spirituality has studied aging, hospice practice, addiction programs, and programs for the mentally ill rather than for persons with intellectual disability. Research on developmental disabilities has focused on the spiritual needs of families coping with a family member with intellectual disability (Haworth, Hill, and Glidden, 1996). An expanded focus on persons with intellectual disability may utilize the approaches of Fitchett (1996) and Landau-Stanton and colleagues (1993) outlined above.

3. *Spirituality and culture* (Heifitz, 1987). A culturally competent program for persons with intellectual disability should provide services and supports for spirituality. The belief system of the individual and family and that of the community should be considered. One must ask, "What does it mean to have a disability in a particular community? Will a community provide a place for an individual who has cognitive limitations? How will an individual who is cognitively impaired participate in spiritual rituals and practice, including specific religious holidays, and how will religion be used to help with transitions and life changes?" Effective involvement in the community requires that the community apply the ethic of inclusion to include spiritual practices.

4. *Spirituality as choice and self-determination.* As a community begins to provide supports in community life, not only should the spiritual needs of the person with intellectual disability be affirmed but also these needs should be supported in practice to facilitate self-determination through flexibility and en-

couragement of individual choices (Nerney and Shumway, 1996). One obstacle is the overregulation of programs attended by persons with intellectual disability. Establishing specific goals and objectives may lead to such intensive programming that individuals are "overprogrammed" and not allowed sufficient choices or opportunities to contribute to the life of that community. For self-determination to occur, the individual must be encouraged to be more independent and productive; staff members and community members in faith communities should facilitate and provide supports that lead to full inclusion and integration in the program. Thus, Hoeksema (1995) points out that a respectful attitude is needed for religious freedom and choices; specific policies are needed to facilitate self-determination in family settings, in group homes, and in community systems. The self-determination approach encourages spiritual expression and provides support for choices. Moreover, there is a need for freedom to choose one's own supports, for example, to make a choice whether to attend a religious service or not. In community agencies, community supports do enhance quality of life when they address spiritual needs.

The inclusion of spirituality among essential AAMR systems of support for persons with intellectual disability may impact the attitudes of caregivers and family members in a profound way. If one considers a person with intellectual disability as having particular gifts and strengths and being part of the spiritual life of the family, a more nurturing environment may be established. By exploring religious vocation and responsibility and supporting choices, engagement in the community may be enhanced. Including a spiritual perspective among systems of support allows greater respect for the meaningfulness of the life of a person with intellectual disability. Although spiritual understanding may be difficult to classify in observable and measurable terms, this does not diminish the possibility of meaningful experiences in ways that are not measurable. The term "assessment" (Hilsman, 1997) comes from the Latin "to sit next to." Assessment means sitting next to the individual to try to understand what is real for him or her, to be with the person, and listen, observe, and plan with him or her. This type of assessment appreciates the impact of experiences on the person observed and seeks to use the observer's understanding to engage the person with intellectual disability in a community of practice.

Including a spiritual emphasis within the system of needed support services acknowledges the role of the personal experience in the life of a person with intellectual disability. This is a continuing task and one that impacts the future of the individual and those around him or her. The importance of including spiritual supports becomes apparent in an existential sense. It involves the process of discerning meaning and purpose in human experience and recognizing the role of spirituality in the community. It acknowledges the person with intellectual disability's right to make choices and how these choices must be respected. It deals with how family and staff members facilitate "adaptive spirituality" and what it means to be "spiritually competent." In a broader sense, Gaventa (2003) asks, "What does it mean to be 'spiritually retarded' or 'spiritually disabled'?" How are the elements of spiritual distancing linked to a "disabled spirituality?" (Landau-Stanton et al., 1993). "Disabled spirituality" involves despair, a lack of experience of love and affirmation, and an absence of trust. Yet, with appropriate supports, spiritual disability can be overcome. Moreover, persons with intellectual disability who may view the world in less complicated ways may provide spiritual strength for others.

More research and more emphasis placed on the integration of the spiritual in caregiving for persons with intellectual disability are essential. Increasingly, religious groups emphasize inclusion with support systems. Advocates and friends engage with persons with intellectual disability and their families and work to provide them a voice in a community that allows spiritual identity and a journey into the spiritual and religious dimension of life. Diagnostic and support planning processes are best served if spirituality is included and considered in every assessment for support services performed. Spiritual supports may be offered not only by religious organizations but also through each of the specialists who work with persons with intellectual disability to help them find meaning in their lives, for example, through medicine, social work, occupational therapy, psychology, and psychiatry. The crucial issue is that each of these professions appreciates the spiritual needs of the individual and family. A religious or spiritual coach can be helpful, just as job coaches are available for employment. A "spiritual clinician" may have a place in the mainstream for professional assessment. Professionals from many fields emphasize diagnosis and classification to carry out treatment. Longer term supports to sustain individuals in the community are enhanced if spiritual supports are provided. Finally, the inclusion of spiritual issues in each assessment may contribute to a greater understanding of individuals, families, and communities and add a new emphasis on meaningfulness to treatment planning.

SUMMARY

In summary, since antiquity there has been an ongoing struggle to make sense and to find meaning when there is an unexpected occurrence. In the case of intellectual disability, fear and superstition have often resulted in ostracism, neglect, and even death. In modern times, these residual attitudes result in stigma and avoidance. Yet, there has always been compassionate concern for those who suffer and are impaired physically and cognitively. In all religions and humanistic belief systems, respect for life is a central element. For persons with intellectual disability, such respect is shown when positive supports are provided to normalize, as much as possible, the life of the disabled person. This means removing both physical and psychological barriers to allow that person to make choices and have some degree of self-determination.

Religious beliefs and a "spiritual" attitude provide succor for parents and the opportunity for loving reception of the intellectually disabled person in community life. The AAMR multidimensional model allows a place for spiritual supports. Within various religious and secular humanistic belief systems, the focus is increasingly on giving meaning, rather than simply finding meaning, to the life of the person with intellectual disability through inclusion in all aspects of community life.

KEY POINTS

1. Ethical attitudes and religious beliefs impact the emotional development of persons with intellectual disabilities.
2. Historically, kindness and generosity toward persons with intellectual disability have been widely encouraged, yet fear and superstition have, at times, prevailed.
3. Impairment has been viewed as providing each of us with an opportunity for redemption through acts of kindness and compassionate support or, conversely, as a basis for the belief that the impairment is a mark of the wrath of God or an evil omen.
4. Parental coping with intellectual disability may be aided through religious beliefs and connectedness to faith communities.
5. There is a shift in focus from an emphasis on the cognitive capacity to believe and articulate those beliefs to an emphasis on the emotional and spiritual importance of belonging, being loved, and participating in spiritual practices.
6. Hope, embracement of belief, repentance, and spiritual meaningfulness are sought in response to fear, alienation, guilt, and despair.
7. Quality of life means full integration in the community. Gaventa has proposed an extension of the AAMR multidimensional approach that emphasizes supports for normalization to include spiritual support, in addition to environmental support, to emphasize meaningful inclusion in the community.
8. The spiritual "coach," like the job coach in other settings, may provide support and facilitate participation in a meaningful life in a faith community.
9. The essential emphasis is on giving meaning to the life of a person with intellectual disability through full inclusion into the life of the community.

General References

Matthews, D., Larson, D., and Barry, C. (1993). *The faith factor: An annotated bibliography of clinical research on spiritual subjects.* National Institute for Healthcare Research, Rockville.

Moran, M., and Weiner, K. (1991). *Spiritual and faith community integration needs of catholic developmentally disabled adults.* Bureau for Exceptional Children, Inc., Holyoke, MA.

References

American Association on Mental Retardation. (1992). *Mental retardation: Definition, Classification and Systems of Support,* 9th ed. Author, Washington, DC.

Black, K. (1996). *Healing homiletic: Preaching and disability.* Abington, Nashville, TN.

Braddock D., and Parish, S.L. (2002). An institutional history of disability. In D. Brad-
    dock (ed.), *Disability at the dawn of the 21st century and the state of states.* Amer-
    ican Association on Mental Retardation, Washington, DC.

Carder, M. (1984). Spiritual and religious needs of mentally retarded persons. *The Jour-
    nal of Pastoral Care*, 38 no. 2.

Coles, R. (1990). *The spiritual life of children.* Houghton Miffon, Boston.

Fitchett, G. (1993a). *Assessing spiritual needs: A guide for caregivers.* Augsburg/Fortress
    Press, Minneapolis.

Fitchett, G. (1993b). *Spiritual assessment in pastoral care: A guide to selected resources.*
    Journal of Pastoral Care Publications, Inc., Decatur.

Fitchett, G. (1996). The 7x7 model for spiritual assessment. *Vision*, March:10–11.

Fowler, J. (1981). *Stages of faith. The psychology of human development and the quest
    for meaning.* Harper and Row, San Francisco.

Gallimore, R., Wesiner, T., Kaufman, S., Bernheimer, L. (1989). The social construction
    of ecocultural niches: Family accommodation of developmentally disabled children.
    American Journal on Mental Retardation, 94:216–230.

Gaventa, W.C. (1993). From belief to belonging to belief: Trends in religious ministries
    and services with people with mental retardation. *Disability Rag/Resource*, Septem-
    ber/October:27–29.

Gaventa, W.C. (2003). Defining and assessing spirituality and spiritual supports: Moving
    from benediction to invocation. In H. Switzky and S. Greenspan (eds.), *What is
    mental retardation? Ideas for an evolving disability*, Chapter 11. HTML e-BOOK.
    AAMR Books, Washington, D.C.

Haworth, A., Hill, A., and Glidden, L. (1996). Measuring the religiousness of parents of
    children with developmental disabilities. *Mental Retardation*, 34:271–279.

Heifitz, L. (1987). Integrating religious and secular perspectives in the design and delivery
    of disability services. *American Journal of Mental Retardation*, 25:127–131.

Hilsman, G. (1997). Spiritual pathways: One response to the current standards challenge.
    Vision, June:8–9.

Hoeksema, T. (1995). Supporting the free exercise of religion in the group home context.
    Mental Retardation, 33:289–294.

Larson, D., and Larson, S. (1994). *The forgotten factor in physical and mental health:
    What does the research show?* National Institute of Healthcare Research, Rockville.

Laundau-Stanton, J., Clements, C., Tartaglia, A., Nudd, J., and Espaillat-Pina, E. (1993).
    Spiritual, cultural, and community systems. In J. Landau-Stanton and C. Clements
    (eds.), *AIDS: Health and mental health, a primary sourcebook*, pp. 267–298. Bruner/
    Mazel, New York.

Luckasson, R., Borthwick-Duffy, S., Buntinx, W.H.E., Coulter, D.L., Craig, E.M., Reeve,
    A., Schalock, R.L., Snell, M.E., Spitalnik, D.M., Spreat, S., et al. (2002). *Mental
    retardation: definition, classification, and systems of supports*, 10th ed. American
    Association on Mental Retardation, Washington, DC.

Nerney,T., and Shumway, D. (1996). *Beyond managed care: Self determination for people
    with disabilities.* University of New Hampshire, Concord, NH.

Prins, G. (1994). *Spiritual Life Plan.* AAMR National Conference, Boston.

Rogers-Dulan, J. (1998). Religious connectedness among urban African American fam-
    ilies who have a child with disabilities. *Mental Retardation*, 36:91–103.

Rosen, G. (1968). *Madness in society: Chapters in the historical sociology of mental
    illness.* University of Chicago Press, Chicago.

Schurter, D. (1994). Guidance for the journey—Fowler's stages of faith as a guide for
    ministry with people with mental retardation. In *A mutual ministry: Theological*

reflections and resources on ministry with people with mental retardation and other disabilities, pp. 35–53. Denton State School, Denton, TX.

Swinton, J. (1997). Restoring the image: Spirituality, faith, and cognitive disability. *Journal of Religion and Health*, 36:21–27.

Webb-Mitchell, B. (1993). *God plays the piano too: The spiritual lives of disabled children.* Crossroad, New York.

Westerhoff, J. (1976). *Will our children have faith?* Seabury Press, New York.

Wickham, P. (2001). Images and idiocy in Puritan New England. *Mental Retardation,* 39:147–151.

Wolfensberger, W. (1979). An attempt toward a theology of social integration of devalued/handicapped people. Information Service 8(1), Publication of Religion Division, AAMR, Washington, D.C.

Wolfensberger, W. (1982). An attempt to gain a better understanding: a Christian perspective of what "mental retardation" is. *National Apostolate with Mentally Retarded Persons Quarterly*, 13:2–7.

APPENDIX A
Intellectual Disability Resources

LOCAL SOURCES OF INFORMATION

Depending on the state, clinicians and families can obtain information on local services, other resources, and entitlement to services from the state department of mental retardation, the state department of public health, or the state department of education.

ASSOCIATION OF UNIVERSITY CENTERS ON DISABILITIES (AUCD)

These programs, located in all states, focus on provision of clinical services, training professionals, and research related to developmental disabilities. Clinicians might refer patients to such programs and/or use them as sources of information about services in their areas. The addresses and details about the AUCD may be obtained from:

Association of University Centers on
  Disabilities
8630 Fenton Street, Suite 410
Silver Spring, MD 20910-3803
(301) 588-8252
www.aucd.org

NATIONAL ORGANIZATIONS CONCERNED WITH SERVICES FOR PERSONS WITH DEVELOPMENTAL DISABILITIES AND THEIR FAMILIES

The offices below can provide addresses of the local chapters, which are good sources of information concerning local services. In addition, the Family Village Web site, based at the Waisman Center at the University of Wisconsin-Madison, brings together valuable information for parents of individuals who have disabilities. This site can be accessed via the Internet at www.familyvillage.wisc.edu/ (e-mail: familyvillage@waisman.wisc.edu).

American Association on Mental
  Retardation (AAMR)
444 North Capitol Street, N.W.
Suite 846
Washington, DC 20001-1512
(800) 424-3688
(202) 387-1968
(202) 387-2193 (fax)
www.aamr.org

The Arc of the United States
1010 Wayne Avenue
Suite 650
Silver Springs, MD 20910
(301) 565-3843
(301) 565-3843 (fax)
(301) 565-5342 (fax)
www.thearc.org

Autism Society of America
7910 Woodmont Avenue, Suite 300
Bethesda, MD 20814-3067
(301) 657-0881
(301) 657-0869 (fax)
www.autism-society.org

FRAXA Research Foundation
45 Pleasant Street
Newburyport, MA 01950
(978) 462-1866
(978) 463-9985 (fax)
e-mail: info@fraxa.org
Executive Director: Katie Clapp

The International Rett Syndrome
  Association
9121 Piscataway Road
Clinton, MD 20735
(800) 818-RETT
(301) 856-3334
(301) 856-3336 (fax)
e-mail: irsa@rettsyndrome.org
Founder and President: Kathy Hunter
e-mail: khunter@rettsyndrome.org

Lesch-Nyhan Syndrome Children's
  Research Foundation
210 South Green Bay Road
Lake Forest, IL 60045
(847) 234-3154
(847) 234-3136 (fax)
e-mail: cbtbct@aol.com

The National Association for the
  Dually Diagnosed (NADD)
132 Fair Street
Kingston, NY 12401
(800) 331-5362
(845) 331-4336
(845) 331-4569 (fax)
info@thenadd.org

National Down Syndrome Congress
1370 Center Drive
Suite 102
Atlanta, GA 30338
(800) 232-6372
(770) 604-9500
www.ndsccenter.org
e-mail: ndsccenter@aol.com

National Down Syndrome Society
666 Broadway
New York, NY 10012
(800) 221-4602
(212) 460-9330
(212) 979-2873 (fax)
www.ndss.org
e-mail: info@ndss.org

National Fragile X Foundation
P.O. Box 190488
San Francisco, CA 94119
(800) 688-8765
(925) 938-9300
(925) 938-9315 (fax)
www.nfxf.org
e-mail: natlfx@fragilex.org

The Prader-Willi Syndrome
   Association (USA)
5700 Midnight Pass Road
Sarasota, FL 34242
(800) 926-4797
(941) 312-0400
(941) 312-0142 (fax)
www.pwsausa.org/
e-mail: reception@pwsausa.org

Williams Syndrome Association
P.O. Box 297
Clawson, MI 48017-0297
(800) 806-1871
(248) 244-2229
(248) 244-2230 (fax)
www.williams-syndrome.org
e-mail: info@williams-syndrome.org

APPENDIX B
Special Olympics

The Special Olympics is the leading global organization that promotes and provides sports training and opportunities to compete for people with intellectual disability. Services are provided directly to individuals in more than 150 countries and in each of the 50 states. Over one million people with intellectual disability participate in Special Olympics training programs and in competition. Thus, the Special Olympics are uniquely situated to help individuals with intellectual disability develop a sense of personal responsibility.

Currently, the Special Olympics serve approximately 1.2 million athletes with intellectual disability annually in more than 150 countries. There are more than twenty thousand local, regional, and national events that are included and held each year. Success in the Special Olympics illustrates how sports may contribute to the lives of children and adults with intellectual disability. Moreover, the Special Olympics have helped to change societal perceptions regarding the accomplishments of persons with intellectual disability.

THE MISSION OF THE SPECIAL OLYMPICS

The Special Olympics provide year-round sports training and athletic competition for Olympic-type sports for children and adults with intellectual disability and afford them continuing opportunities to enhance their physical fitness. Individuals, through sports participation, can demonstrate courage in competition, experience success, and share their success with friends, family members, and others in the community. The Special Olympics were founded on the belief that individuals with intellectual disability, through encouragement and instruction, can benefit from participation in individual and team sports, that such participation may lead to physical, psychological, social, and spiritual development. Moreover, it was believed that families could be strengthened through their family member's participation and that the community, seeing them compete successfully, would cheer them on and be more understanding and less likely to stigmatize them.

HISTORICAL BACKGROUND

The Special Olympics began in 1963 with the summer camp that Eunice Kennedy Shriver began for children and adults with intellectual disability. Observing that individuals with intellectual disability were more capable in physical activities than generally believed, Shriver initiated the Special Olympics. In 1968, one thousand individuals from 26 states and Canada joined the first International Special Olympics Game that was held in Chicago's Soldiers' Field. By 1997, the Winter Games had been initiated in Steamboat Springs, Colorado. The European Games started on a regular basis in the 1980s. In 1999, the Special Olympics held the World Summer Games in Raleigh-Durham, North Carolina, which included 7,500 athletes from more than 150 countries. The next Special Olympics, the World Summer Games, will be held in 2003 in Ireland.

The Special Olympics provide an opportunity not only for the benefits that come to the individual and his or her family through participation but also for research. A Special Olympics Research & Evaluation Committee was established in 1996 to provide oversight and direction for research. At the 1999 World Games, research questions considered at a strategic research symposium considered proposals to study health outcomes, social-emotional functioning, and effects on families.

Over five hundred thousand volunteers contribute in programs in each of the 50 states and in 150 participating nations. The Special Olympics are supported by The Arc of the United States, the Council for Exceptional Children, and the American Association on Mental Retardation.

The Special Olympics enhance function, physical activity, and health and also help individuals with intellectual disability improve and adapt in society. Research findings that lead to enabling athletes to maximize their individual abilities are critical. Emphasis must be placed on furthering the social and emotional development of those who participate. Individuals who participated in the 1993 Special Olympics Winter Games were noted to have better social competence and adaptive skills and more positive self-perceptions (Dykens and Cohen, 1996; Dykens, Rosner, and Butterbaugh, 1998).

The Special Olympics is in a unique position to promote collaborative research and interdisciplinary studies of persons with intellectual disability. It is important to clarify how long social and emotional benefits last and how much participation is needed to maintain gains that occur in the Special Olympics; also, it is important to determine how the needs of those who participate change as they grow older, leave school, and become more independent.

A vital area of research into the benefits of the Special Olympics is mental health, that is, on better adaptive functioning and the social-emotional functioning of athletes. This encompasses self-esteem, self-concept, self-confidence, friendship development, and peer interaction. Moreover, the effect of the Olympics on maladaptive behavior must be understood to establish if Special Olympics' participation is an effective intervention. Physical health outcomes that may emerge from athletic participation include cardiovascular fitness, prevention of osteoporosis, development of positive health habits, reduction in obesity, and overall greater physical competence.

Of specific importance is how families of athletes enrolled in the Special Olympics mutually involve and affect one another. Specific experiences that families have in a variety of cultures and regions may provide a multinational knowledge base regarding the role of sports in the lives of persons with intellectual disability.

The headquarters of the Special Olympics is in Washington, DC, and those wishing to participate in research may contact the Research Coordinator at the following address:

The Special Olympics
133 19th Street, N.W.
Washington, DC 20036
(202) 628-3630
(202) 824-0200
www.specialolympics.org

References

Dykens, E.M., Rosner, B.A., and Butterbaugh, G. (1998). Exercise and sports in children and adolescents with developmental disabilities. Positive physical and psychosocial effects. *Child and Adolescent Psychiatric Clinics of North America,* 7:757–771.
Dykens, E.M., and Cohen, D.J. (1996). Effects of Special Olympics International on social competence in persons with mental retardation. *Journal of the American Academy of Child and Adolescent Psychiatry,* 35:223–229.

APPENDIX C

Closing The Gap: A National Blueprint to Improve the Health of Persons with Mental Retardation

Report of the Surgeon General's Conference on Health Disparities and Mental Retardation

> *Our national commitment to the health of every American is demonstrated most clearly in efforts to reach those whose circumstances in life are most difficult.*
> —Tommy G. Thompson, Secretary of Health and Human Services,
> Introduction to the Surgeon General's Report

From December 5–6, 2001, the Surgeon General of the United States sponsored a conference to address health disparities, both physical and mental, in persons with intellectual disability. The Surgeon General's conference followed a national Listening Session that was held on October 10, 2001. At that time, over 8,500 comments and suggestions were made that were utilized in planning the conference. Because persons with intellectual disability have been reported to have poorer health, less access to screening for health problems, and disparities in diagnosis and treatment, the meeting was called to better understand their needs and to face unmet needs. As a result of cognitive and language impairment, individuals with intellectual disability may have difficulty describing their health needs; critically, they must be empowered to participate in their treatment to improve their health. Families need guidance in finding the means and the emotional and financial support to carry through with treatments. The needs are broad and include basic screening and corrective treatment for vision, hearing, and oral health problems as well as diagnosis and treatment for both physical and mental illnesses.

Planning health care services, conducting appropriate research, finding sufficient resources, and monitoring physical and mental health care throughout the lifetime are major challenges for policy makers.

At the conference, important issues in physical and mental health were identified, and action steps were proposed to address them. Subsequently, plenary session presentations by experts in the field provided background information on what is currently known on the topics that were addressed. Eight conference work groups identified priority issues from those proposed during the planning process. Topics considered by the work groups included: (1) provider attitudes; (2) health care financing; (3) appropriateness of services throughout the lifetime; and (4) research needs and health promotion. Action steps and strategies were recommended after work group recommendations were developed to achieve six broad goals. Of particular concern is the need for health care services throughout life. During transitions from one life phase to another, loss of services can be devastating. This is most apparent in the transition from adolescence into adult life, when pediatric coverage is no longer available, and adult benefits are limited.

Providing adequate care requires recognition of the needs of individuals from all cultures and backgrounds within the United States. Multiple medical and behavioral problems may be associated with intellectual disability and are often disproportionately increased in low-income communities and among minority groups. Further complicating care is the issue of the health care provider who may lack direct clinical experience with intellectual disability or may feel inadequate to provide appropriate care. Unfortunately, persons with intellectual disability are often insufficiently valued, and their potential to contribute to their own health care is not appreciated.

Six goals were established to improve the health of persons with intellectual disability: (1) health promotion and community environments, (2) knowledge and understanding, (3) quality of health care, (4) training of health care providers, (5) health care financing, and (6) sources of health care. These six goals created an agenda for national, state, and local action in both private and public sectors to improve physical and mental health for persons with intellectual disability and to facilitate their inclusion in health care systems.

Behavioral and emotional health is a particularly serious concern as it relates to persons with intellectual disability and their families. A separate workshop was held November 29–December 1, 2001, prior to the Surgeon General's conference, to develop a comprehensive agenda for research on emotional and behavioral disorders and mental illnesses in persons with intellectual disability and developmental disabilities. The findings of that workshop were presented for the first time at the Surgeon General's workshop on health disparities in persons with intellectual disability. These co-occurring conditions are among the most common and least understood aspects of health care. Persons with intellectual disability are often excluded from research on mental disorders just as they are for other types of disorders. These exclusions are frequently on the basis of IQ rather than for safety reasons and need to be examined. Moreover, health care services may be organized in ways that deny access. At the workshop sponsored by the National Institutes of Health and the Joseph P. Kennedy, Jr. Foundation, research recommendations were made, and ethical considerations essential to participate in research were discussed. These topic areas included epidemiology, diagnosis and assessment, interventions, research design, and research training needs.

For both physical and mental health problems, a lifespan view emphasizes ways to enable individuals with disabilities to live in their communities and receive appropriate health care and mental health care services. Family support is particularly important to prevent "caregiver burnout." The need for community programs for individuals, for family support, for respite care, and for job training and job coaching is also pertinent to health care. The Health Resources and Services Administration (HRSA), working with the March of Dimes, the American Academy of Pediatrics, and Family Voices, has developed a 10-year plan for appropriate community-based services for children and youth with special health care needs (HRSA, *All Aboard the 2010 Express: A 10-Year Action Plan to Achieve Community-Based Service Systems for Children with Special Health Care Needs and Their Families,* December 2001).

The recommendations in the Surgeon General's report come at a time when the life expectancy of persons with conditions associated with intellectual disability has been extended because of the success of early treatment and intervention programs. Because of their longer life span, a renewed effort is necessary to provide lifetime health care. Moreover, instead of institutional care, more people with intellectual disability are remaining in the community or remaining with their families, with community supports. Despite these advances that have resulted in longer life and deinstitutionalization, many health professionals have not been trained to meet the new community needs of people with intellectual disability. Services are required for the specific and distinctive health care needs that are apparent in each stage in the life cycle. Throughout this process of intervention, the stigma of intellectual disability must be recognized and core values for the life of each individual appreciated.

BACKGROUND INFORMATION FOR THE SURGEON GENERAL'S REPORT

Prevalence of Intellectual Disability

To establish health care services and develop health care policies, accurate and consistent prevalence data on intellectual disability is needed. Estimates vary in the general population in regard to prevalence, with estimates ranging from 0.3% to 3.1% of the general population. Overall, about 1.1% of all children are diagnosed with intellectual disability. Definitions of intellectual disability vary, with some focusing on intellectual functioning, and others on intellectual functioning with adaptive behaviors, or intellectual functioning with an identifiable etiology. Prevalences vary depending on how classification is carried out. To address health disparities, more accurate estimates of rates of intellectual disability are needed based on better prevalence estimates. This requires using a standard definition of intellectual disability, utilizing population-based data for planning, and encouraging those in clinics to specifically identify adults and children with intellectual disability who come for their services.

In service settings, family members and self-advocates may encounter negative attitudes among health care providers. This requires professional education and the need for accessible, comprehensive family-centered care that is culturally competent, continuous, and well coordinated. Societal issues must be considered because adults with disabilities are three times more likely to live in poverty than other adults in the United States. Children with intellectual disabilities are twice as likely to live in poverty as other children. A further complication is that people with intellectual disabilities are less likely to have insurance than those in the general population. Individuals whose physicians are familiar with intellectual disability may provide excellent services. However, health care providers who lack expertise tend to be more reluctant to provide treatment. The provider's attitude influences access to services, and provider training affects the expertise of service delivery. Service provision is complicated further by problems in communication with persons with intellectual disability as well as problems in transportation.

Access to health care is a particular issue for individuals with behavioral and mental health concerns. Dr. Nancy King has outlined a community-based program to help with mental health–related needs. This program in Rochester, New York, has a crisis intervention team and a specialized psychiatric clinic. Crisis intervention means working with families and with group homes on a short-term basis to find appropriate care and to deal with emergency situations. This is accomplished by having staff on call for consultation 24 hours a day. For those who require ongoing care, specialized psychiatric clinics with staff who are trained to work with intellectual disabilities are provided. Both crisis intervention and specialized outpatient clinics prevent unneeded hospitalizations, facilitate appropriate community placements, and maintain good behavioral health. The consultation program enhances the expertise of staff working in the community by regular consultation and increased collaboration.

To address the issues raised by the plenary presenters and those raised by the conference work groups, participants deliberated to develop the six goals and action steps that are the primary recommendations from the Surgeon General's conference. These goals and action steps are listed below.

GOALS AND ACTION STEPS

Goal 1: Integrate Health Promotion into Community Environments of People with Mental Retardation (MR)

Health promotion programs should accommodate with MR. Examples include smoking cessation, weight control, fitness, safe sex, drugs, and alcohol.

As with other populations, health promotion and disease prevention are multifactorial for individuals with MR. They need to be empowered with adequate and understandable information and reinforcement to avoid health risks and maintain healthy personal habits. Their health care providers and the environments where they live, work, learn, and socialize should offer opportunities to inform, support, and reinforce healthy lifestyles. Routine preventive services, from periodic oral prophylaxis and restoration, to cancer screening, immunizations, and early intervention with emerging mental illness are critical to prevention of more serious conditions and secondary disability. Because of the potential for modeling behaviors, health-promoting knowledge and habits of personal care attendants and family members, coworkers, and others can help individuals with MR protect and maintain their health.

Action Steps

• *Wellness: Educate and support individuals with MR, their families, and other caregivers in self-care and wellness.*

Potential strategies: Adapt self-care and wellness programs designed for general populations and cultural, ethnic, and socioeconomic minorities to the needs of individuals with MR. When proven effective, replicate existing programs for individuals with MR, especially peer-designed programs for wellness, self-care, and mental health. Evaluate the use of assistive technology and different media in educating and reinforcing healthy behaviors in individuals with MR, their families, and their caregivers. Develop and disseminate models for health care provider counseling and reinforcement of wellness and healthy behaviors in individuals with MR, their families, and their caregivers.

Potential topics: Nutrition and weight control; exercise; oral health; family planning; safe sex; strategies for protection from rape, domestic violence, and sexual abuse; maintaining treatment regimens; avoiding medication errors; recognizing and seeking care for emerging disorders; and age-related changes in, and risks to, health status.

• *Caregiver support: Develop and implement strategies for reducing care burdens for families of individuals with MR, and reducing high rates of turnover in nonfamily caregivers.*

Potential strategies: Identify stressors and sources of resilience in individuals with MR, their families, and their caregivers, and support strategies to enhance resilience. Support respite care, case management, advance (lifetime) planning for transitions to different stages of life and age-associated health needs. Provide assistance in caring for individuals with dual diagnosis, including family and caregiver training in behavior management and advance planning for behavioral crises. Provide technical assistance to families in information technologies, including how to use the Internet. Explore compensation, including basic health coverage, for family caregivers whose care responsibilities prevent them from working outside the home.

Additional strategies: Provide training in health care, including supporting healthy habits, for personal care attendants and other caregivers. Create career tracks leading to certification of caregivers with regard to health-related competencies. Support basic health care coverage and increased compensation, commensurate with demonstrated health competencies, for caregivers.

• *Workplace: Protect the health of individuals with MR from occupational hazards.*

Potential strategies: Develop and disseminate modules to educate and train individuals with MR, their employment counselors and job coaches, their families and caregivers, their employers and potential employers, and occupational health and safety inspectors, in recognizing and eliminating hazardous working conditions that may require special accommodations for employees with MR. Potential accommodations include ensuring that employees with MR work in safe and healthful environments and understand how to avoid repetitive motion disorders and other occupational hazards.

• *Assessment: Assess the effects of health promotion and wellness activities for individuals with MR on their morbidity, secondary disability, mortality, life satisfaction, independent living, achievement of life goals, and cultural and ethnic identity.*

Goal 2: Increase Knowledge and Understanding of Health and Mental Retardation, Ensuring that Knowledge Is Made Practical and Easy to Use

> *We're invisible in the data. We can't make people believe we need more services if we don't have data to back us up.*

Credible scientific knowledge is considered essential to all goals in this blueprint, from establishing appropriate standards of health care, to training health care providers, to revising financing structures, and improving the capacity of individuals and their families to protect and maintain their health. For example, the lack of population-based data on prevalence of MR and the health status and service needs of this population impedes planning and allocating resources for their care. Failure to monitor the quality of their care hampers detection of prejudicial or inadequate treatment. Recent advances in neurosciences, genetics, psychopharmacology, and other fields of research could improve the diagnosis and treatment of individuals with MR and emotional, behavioral, or psychiatric disorders (dual diagnosis). At the same time, individuals, family members, and health care providers need easily accessible, scientifically accurate, culturally relevant, and understandable information for prevention and health promotion, as well as for diagnostic and treatment decisions. All aspects of health-related research, from biomedical and epidemiologic to health services and ethics, offer multiple opportunities to increase and improve the utility of scientific knowledge on health and MR.

Action Steps

• *Participation: Enable individuals with MR, their families, and their health care providers to partner with professional investigators in identifying health research priorities, and in designing and implementing research relating to health and MR.*

Potential strategies: Include individuals with MR, family members, and their primary and specialty health care providers in research advisory committees and planning groups to provide input into the development of research proposals and grant submissions. Offer training to lay advisors in identifying research questions and other technical matters. Encourage federally funded health researchers to develop partnerships in which persons with MR, their family members, and other caregivers, including health care providers, are consulted and participate in the planning and conduct of research relevant to MR.

• ***Research agenda:*** *Develop a national research agenda that identifies gaps in existing scientific knowledge related to health and MR, including methodological challenges, priorities, feasibility, and timetables for achieving priority research.*

Potential strategies: Develop specific agendas for basic, clinical, and translational research; for studies of the efficacy of wellness and treatment services and service models for people with MR; for legal and ethical issues, health care financing, and its relationship to outcomes; and for other matters identified by the community. Implement the December 2001 research agenda of the Workshop on Emotional and Behavioral Health in Persons with Mental Retardation/Developmental Disabilities (National Institutes of Health, Workshop on Emotional and Behavioral Health in Persons with Mental Retardation/Developmental Disabilities: Research Challenges and Opportunities, November 29–December 1, 2001) (see appendix E). Enhance research collaborations across multiple research agendas and disciplines.

• ***Data collection:*** *Collect data on the health status of persons with MR in relation to the utilization, organization, and financing of their health services.*

Potential strategies: Identify and evaluate existing data on health and MR. Add MR to population-based data collection on health status, health risks, health services utilization, and health care costs. Test methods of identifying patients with MR on Medicaid and other third-party payer claims for purposes of collecting data, while also protecting patient confidentiality. Conduct market research to determine attitudes toward MR of health care providers, and how to change negative attitudes. Survey individual practices, managed-care organizations, and localities and states to better understand the experiences of individuals with MR when they seek health care.

• ***Research subject protection:*** *Review current ethical and legal rules for protection of human research subjects as they relate to individuals with MR. Revise these rules as necessary to facilitate the participation of persons with MR in clinical trials and other types of research, with full protection of their autonomy, health, and safety. Ensure that individuals, their families, their health care providers, and their advocates participate as partners in reviews and revisions of these rules. Ensure their participation in Institutional Review Board (IRB) reviews of research proposals relating to MR.*

Potential strategies: Provide training in legal and ethical rules for protection of human research subjects to lay participants in review and the revision of these rules. Provide training in IRB standards and procedures.

• ***Understanding and use:*** *Provide assistance for individuals with MR, their families, and their health care providers in finding, evaluating, and using health research findings to help in the prevention, diagnosis, and management of medical (including psychiatric), psychological, and oral health conditions, and to inform treatment decisions by individuals and their families.*

Potential strategies: Establish, and keep current, a national clearinghouse, a Web site, and a list-serve to guide users in identifying and evaluating research, and to promote their exchange of information and opinions. Design science-based continuing-education curricula for licensed health care providers. Translate peer-reviewed journal information, reports of evidence-based best practices, and other findings for lay consumption, and disseminate information to provider groups, and state agencies that serve persons with MR, and provider trade journals.

• **Research capacity:** *Increase the number of investigators trained in health and MR research.*

Potential strategies: Fund undergraduate training and postdoctoral research fellowships at medical, dental, and other health professions schools and training programs targeted specifically at issues relevant to MR. Solicit proposals for multidisciplinary research. Solicit proposals from centers and programs that provide health care to individuals with MR, especially those living in their communities. Solicit joint proposals from these providers and investigators at medical, dental, and other health professions schools and programs.

• **Visibility:** *Enhance the visibility of health and MR research.*

Potential strategies: Increase and ensure appropriate use of funds to support research on health and MR, including expansion of studies on dual diagnosis and other disorders for which individuals with MR are at elevated risk. Create prizes and other awards for excellence in health and MR research. Endow chairs for health and MR research at health professions schools. Establish special interest sections in health research organizations. Support special plenary lectures on health and MR at national medical, dental, and other health professions meetings. Publish health and MR research findings in peer-reviewed medical (including psychiatric), dental, psychological, nursing, physician assistant, dental hygienist, and other health-related journals, as well as in health services research and policy journals.

Goal 3: Improve the Quality of Health Care for People with Mental Retardation

> *Encourage agencies and health care professionals to treat people with MR according to age and health needs, not just for their disability.*

The quality of health care for individuals with MR depends on the knowledge and skills of individual providers, particularly their capacity to engage these patients in their own health care, and on systemic factors. Such factors include monitoring the utilization of health care services and outcomes for people with MR, and correcting deficiencies in the quality of their care, such as medication error, underutilization of services, and failure to interact effectively with patients and family members. At both the individual provider and health systems levels, credible standards of health care, based on scientific evidence, are essential to improving the quality of health care for people with MR. Until an adequate science base is available, however, consensus standards that reflect the knowledge and experience of recognized experts (including the community of people concerned with health and MR), and are formulated in standardized procedures, are an important interim step. The potential for MR-specific standards to contribute to stigmatization must be balanced against the need for health care services that fully meet the needs of this population.

Action Steps

• **Priorities:** *Identify priority areas of health care quality improvement for persons with MR.*

Potential strategies: Consult with individuals with MR, their families, and their primary and specialty health care providers and researchers to identify priority areas for ensuring and improving the quality of their health care. Identify existing best practices that may be used system wide to improve the quality of care, and those areas in which better practices may be needed. Use these consultations, together with evaluations of existing and needed scientific knowledge, to establish priorities for improving the quality of health care for people with MR.

• **Standards of care:** *Identify, adapt, and develop standards of care for use in monitoring and improving the quality of care for individuals with MR.*

Potential strategies: Work with associations of health professionals that develop consensus- and science-based standards of care for populations with disabling conditions, for people with MR and for general populations. Identify and adapt standards developed with the support of the National Institutes of Health, the Centers for Disease Control and Prevention, the Centers for Medicare & Medicaid Services, and other federal agencies; consult with the National Committee for Quality Assurance and with contractors that develop health care standards for quality assurance in managed care. Identify existing strategies for adapting and developing additional standards of care for use with culturally diverse populations.

Additional strategies: Develop science-based standards on topics for which sufficient scientific knowledge exists. Develop interim, consensus standards on topics for which scientific knowledge must be developed. Replace consensus standards, to the extent feasible, with science-based standards. Review and update standards to reflect new knowledge, as it becomes available.

Potential priority topics for standards: Responsiveness to distinctive cultural values of diverse communities; self-care and maintenance of health-promoting activities; diagnosis and treatment of emotional and behavioral disorders and mental illness; provider screening; and prevention and early intervention in medical, psychiatric, behavioral, and oral health conditions for which individuals with MR are at heightened risk, such as premature aging, and for coexisting conditions, such as diabetes and mental illness.

Other potential priority topics: Recognition and treatment of emergency conditions, including sexual, physical, and psychological abuse and their sequelae; prevention, diagnosis, and treatment of substance abuse; development of plans of care, including self care, to achieve health goals of individuals and their families; development and revision of lifetime health plans for individuals with

MR; age-appropriateness of health services (including pediatric, adolescent, adult, geriatric, palliative, and end-of-life care); and age-related transitions, including pediatric-to-adult healthcare.

• ***Use:*** *Ensure that the practice, organization, and financing of health care services for individuals with MR promote improvement in their quality of care.*

Potential strategies: Determine whether and how existing standards for care of people with MR are used. Integrate standards of care for MR into the following: clinical practice guidelines; curricula for health professions training; guidance for individuals, their families, their other caregivers, and their primary and specialty care providers; organized health services (including managed care organizations, hospitals, community health centers, and others); and quality assessment and performance improvements in organized health services and individual provider practices.

Additional strategies: Explore methods of linking health care financing to appropriate standards of care for people with MR. Methods could include health care quality requirements in managed care contracts and oversight of such contracts by private and public purchasers, and projects to test such linkage in behavioral health, maternal and child health, family planning, oral health, and comprehensive health care services programs.

• ***Recognizing excellence:*** *Establish local, regional, and national awards that recognize excellence in providing health care to individuals with MR.*

Potential strategies: Work with individuals, their families and caregivers, academic institutions, medical, dental, and other health professions societies, and national associations and other interested parties and groups to recognize excellence in providing health care for individuals with MR. Recognition could include financial prizes and nonmonetary awards.

Goal 4: Train Health Care Providers in the Care of Adults and Children with Mental Retardation

> *The number one issue is lack of training to support healthy lifestyles [for individuals with MR] across the lifespan.*

The challenges and rewards of treating individuals with MR are rarely addressed in the training of physicians and other health care professionals. However, anecdotal evidence and limited data indicate that opportunities for clinical experiences with these patients, early in medical and other health professions training, increase the capacity of providers to value and accept these patients into their practices.

Action Steps

• ***Professional education:*** *Integrate didactic and clinical training in health care of individuals with MR into the basic and specialized education and training of all health care providers.*

Potential strategies: Evaluate existing health professions training curricula that address health and MR and disseminate those found to be efficacious. Partner with families and individuals with MR to develop and implement training modules. Use providers experienced in the care of individuals with MR and family members to mentor health professions students, residents, and fellows in the care of this population. Develop and implement criteria for accreditation and certification of health professions schools and training programs, based on inclusion of mental retardation in their curricula.

Potential curriculum topics: Dual diagnosis; health risks and expression, in people with MR, of age-related conditions found in other populations; direct interactions with these patients, such as history taking, including cultural practices, diagnosis, treatment, and counseling and supporting individuals in wellness and in adherence to treatment regimens; appropriate use of medications and alternative behavior management techniques; working with individuals and their families to develop and update goal-oriented health care plans, including lifetime plans and plans for transition points; and use of augmentative communications devices and other specialized equipment.

• ***Interdisciplinary education and training:*** *Support development and dissemination of effective training modules in interdisciplinary practice. Design modules to include social workers, family members, individuals with MR, and others, when relevant, such as teachers, personal care attendants, job counselors, and frontline office staff.*

• ***Provider competence:*** *Develop methods of evaluating and improving health provider competence in the health care of individuals with MR. These methods should be based on appropriate standards of care, including care that reflects understanding and respect for diverse cultures, and should be used to evaluate the competence of students and practicing providers, and to provide feedback and reevaluation of their performance.*

• ***Continuing education:*** *Develop, evaluate, and disseminate continuing education curricula for health care providers at all levels of practice in the care of individuals with MR. Such curricula should be based on appropriate standards of care and include training opportunities that reflect understanding and respect for diverse cultures.*

Goal 5: Ensure that Health Care Financing Produces Good Health Outcomes for Adults and Children with Mental Retardation

> *Let's develop reimbursement that is respectful of the diverse lifestyles of people with MR and their families and that is tied to outcomes they value, [but] be careful . . . that we don't develop policies that will cover more people, with more flexibility, without ensuring the basic level of care that we know our people need.*

High rates of poverty among adults and children with MR mean that a large proportion of them rely on publicly financed health care insurance, which is not always well adapted to serving their needs. People with MR find that many providers avoid the program, citing low reimbursement rates, administrative burden, and fear of being inundated with underfinanced patients. Providers who are committed to treating individuals with MR report that restrictive Medicaid rules on which services are covered, in which settings, can limit use of innovative service models. Families with private-sector coverage encounter gaps in coverage, unaffordable premium payments, and little flexibility in designing packages of services to meet their children's needs. Cost-avoidance and cost-shifting by both public and private payers force families to try to mediate between special education programs and third-party payers and between long-term and acute-care systems. Research and understanding of financing structures, to better accommodate service needs of individuals with MR, are hindered by lack of critical utilization and reimbursement data.

Action Steps

• ***Outcomes and financing:*** *Determine relationships among diverse financing mechanisms, service packages, and health outcomes for individuals with MR. Use findings to ensure accountability of flexible arrangements for financing services.*

Potential strategies: Test effects on health outcomes, for people with MR, of diverse models for providing health care services, service packages, and financing mechanisms. Identify factors in varying combinations that affect outcomes. Determine effects of adjunct services—including respite care, transportation, childcare, and case management, in combination with medical, dental, and other health services—on outcomes. Support longitudinal studies of portability of health services packages as educational, employment, and residential circumstances change. Develop methods of ensuring accountability for sufficiency and quality of health care services, including accountability for outcomes, in models for flexible health service financing.

• ***Definitions:*** *Use appropriate definitions of "effective," "cost-effective," and "health outcomes" in research, organization, and financing of health care for individuals with MR.*

Potential strategies: Explore expanding definitions of terms used in measuring the effects of health care financing and service models to include wellness, functionality, patient and family understanding of health maintenance and treatment regimens, capacity for consumer choice among services, and satisfaction and individualization of service packages. Calculate health care costs across all systems with responsibility for health care of individuals with MR, such as special education, and third-party payments for behavioral therapy. Support development of methods to determine cost-effectiveness of services over the lifespan, taking into consideration cost offsets among long-term, preventive, and acute care as well as other factors.

• ***Services:*** *Identify a package of health care services for individuals with MR that will produce good outcomes in terms of health maintenance, management of illness, functionality, and life goals across the individual's lifespan.*

Potential strategies: Review currently available public and private packages of health care and supportive services for cost, quality, and consumer satisfaction. Test models of comprehensive lifetime coverage to better meet the needs of persons throughout their lives and avoid age-related disruptions of financing and services. Assess the use of criteria, including acquiring and maintaining functionality for making decisions on coverage.

• *Leveraging: Evaluate models for leveraging health dollars to maximize purchasing power by and for individuals with MR. Ensure that individuals' coverage and access to primary and specialty health care and support services are not eroded by revisions in purchasing practices and policies.*

Potential strategies: Evaluate models for coordinated funding of pediatric, adolescent, adult, and geriatric care, including acute and long-term care, primary care, specialty services, and school-based services, through use of pooled funds, complementary financing from multiple funding streams, and other innovations. Evaluate models for tying funding mechanisms to good outcomes, as defined in the first action step. Evaluate models that enable individuals with MR and their families to choose needed health services on an individualized basis and to monitor outcomes and service utilization. Encourage third-party payers to reimburse for health care services in carefully monitored clinical trials and other studies at academic centers of excellence.

Additional potential strategies: Provide technical assistance to states, tribes, and health care programs and providers in using Medicaid authorities to finance innovative models for providing health care, and identify and eliminate financial disincentives for such models. For example, payer rules limiting reimbursements to one visit per patient per day may mean that families must make multiple appointments with multiple providers to complete multidisciplinary assessments. Evaluate and replicate the use of incentives, such as enhanced Medicaid reimbursement rates, to encourage states to develop and/or replicate effective models that meet the needs of individuals typically not covered.

• *Cost offsets: Explore strategies to offset financial costs to providers and health services programs that are associated with meeting specialized needs of patients with MR.*

Potential strategies: Assess the relationship between different rates of Medicaid and Medicare provider reimbursement and any impact on access to health care for individuals with MR. Identify sources and amounts of costs to providers that are associated with meeting specialized needs of individuals with MR. Assess the effect of offsetting such costs on provider acceptance of individuals with MR. Assess combined and separate effects of cost offsets and nonfinancial provider supports, described elsewhere in the blueprint, on provider acceptance.

Goal 6: Increase Sources of Health Care Services for Adults, Adolescents, and Children with Mental Retardation, Ensuring that Health Care is Easily Accessible for Them

> *Services can be wonderful and high quality, but if there aren't enough, or if you can't get to them, or if you don't know about them, [they're of] no help to you . . .*

Like other Americans, especially those who are poor and disabled, people with MR are confronted with a fragmented health care system in which primary and specialty sources of care are often poorly distributed, inadequate in number, and ill equipped to respond to their needs.

Action Steps

• *Diversity: Increase the number of physicians, dentists, clinical psychologists, and allied health care professionals who have appropriate training and experience in treating adults, adolescents, and children with MR, including those from socioeconomically and linguistically diverse communities.*

Potential strategies: Recruit students, residents and fellows, and practicing providers from diverse communities, and train them in providing health care to individuals with MR. Establish health professions curricula and continuing education modules in cultural competence in relating to patients with MR. Work with spiritual and other leaders who know the cultural and ethnic beliefs, values, and primary languages of individuals and families in diverse communities to plan and provide health care services, develop health profession training curricula, and otherwise ensure responsiveness to diverse ethnic, cultural, and linguistic needs in all aspects of health care for individuals with MR and their families.

• *Easier access: Make access to health care services less complicated for individuals with MR and their families and caregivers, whether in urban, rural, or remote communities.*

Potential strategies: Ensure that independent service coordinators who work on behalf of clients to locate and ensure access to and coordination of services are available for individuals with MR who wish such assistance. Co-locate primary and specialty medical, psychiatric/psychological, and dental services. Support multidisciplinary teams, including mobile teams to bring services to individuals' homes, schools, and other nonclinical sites. Ensure that individuals with MR receive assistance in care coordination and transportation to health care services. Ensure that individuals and families in various community settings receive usable information about available health care in their communities.

Additional strategies: Review eligibility to reduce the need for multiple applications and multiple determinations of eligibility for services. Promote the use of presumptive eligibility, once initial eligibility is established, for services through Medicare or Supplemental Security Insurance (SSI)/Medicaid.

• *Community-based care: Integrate health care services for individuals with MR into diverse community programs.*

Potential strategies: Incorporate preventive health education and interventions into early intervention and special education plans. Support development of protocols and dissemination for care of individuals with MR and coexisting conditions, at community and migrant health centers, community mental health services, addiction disorder services, family planning programs, rape/sexual abuse and family violence services, public health clinics, and other publicly funded, community-based health services and programs. Prohibit such programs and services from excluding individuals solely on the basis of IQ.

• *Health professionals: Expand the types of health professionals used in providing health care to individuals with MR, including geriatric, pediatric, and other nurse practitioners and nurses, physician assistants, dental hygienists, and behavioral therapists.*

Potential strategies: Identify and remove disincentives and barriers in Medicaid, Medicare, and private third-party payer reimbursements to expand the use of a wide variety of health professionals to care for persons with MR.

• *Supporting providers: Support supplementary services to help physicians, dentists, psychologists, and other providers and organized health services in providing care to individuals with MR.*

Potential strategies: Work with providers to identify nonfinancial "costs" in including individuals with MR in their practices and programs. Support needed services that could offset such "costs." Such services could include technical assistance with Medicaid and other types of claiming, case managers, preliminary health screening and referrals, completing informed consent procedures, and assembling complete and current medical and dental histories (including family histories) of individuals with MR. Explore the use of "health passports" (copies of up-to-date health histories, including family history) that "travel" to health services with individuals with MR.

• *Special equipment: Ensure that adaptive equipment and assistive technologies are available in urban, rural, and remote communities for use at clinical sites where individuals with MR receive health care.*

Potential strategies: Provide support to health care providers to finance the costs of purchasing and installing special equipment and modifications to practice sites, such as installation of automatic doors, specialized examining tables and chairs, and wheelchair-accessible bathrooms. Evaluate and support the use of overhead allowances, direct subsidies, cost- and time-sharing among providers, and other mechanisms for offsetting costs of acquiring (and, as necessary, training in the use of) specialized equipment.

• *Lifetime health: Ensure continuity of health care services throughout the life of an individual with MR.*

Potential strategies: Develop and implement state plans for providing age-appropriate, comprehensive, and continuous health services for individuals throughout their lives. Develop and disseminate models for individual lifetime health care plans, with periodic review and updates.

APPENDIX D
Research Issues Involving People with Intellectual Disability

Intellectual disability is frequently a criterion for exclusion from research studies. This exclusion historically is linked to concerns about protecting individuals who are vulnerable for research procedures that might have physical or psychological risk, but is also related to past misuse of persons with intellectual disability in research protocols and inappropriate experimentation that has occurred in the past. In addition, there has been a question about the ability to cooperate and consent in research studies. However, excluding individuals with intellectual disability from research interferes with the development of new knowledge in relation to intellectual disability. Recent advances in the neurosciences, genetic psychopharmacology, developmental neuropsychiatry, psychology and education show promise for improving the treatment of those with intellectual disability and developmental disabilities.

In recognition of the need for research that will benefit individuals with intellectual disability or provide new knowledge in understanding how intellectual disability syndromes may be applied to others, although not necessarily beneficial to those who participate, the Surgeon General recommended a research agenda for persons with intellectual disability. This report (U.S. Department of Health and Human Services, 2002) recommends the development of a national research agenda to identify gaps in existing scientific knowledge related to health and intellectual disability. This includes methodological challenges, priorities and time tables for achieving priority research. Strategies recommended by the Surgeon General's conference proposed developing specific agendas for basic clinical and translational research. Such studies may facilitate the efficacy of wellness and treatment services and examine service models for persons with intellectual disability. Research agendas must consider legal and ethical issues, health care financing and its relationship to outcomes, and other issues that are identified throughout the community. The Surgeon General recommended the implementation of the research agenda from the NIH Workshop on Emotional and Behavioral Health in Persons with Mental Retardation/Developmental Disabilities (National Institutes of Health [NIH] Workshop). Research activity should emphasize research collaboration across multiple research agendas and disciplines.

DATA COLLECTION FOR RESEARCH

Data on health status of persons with intellectual disability in relation to utilizing, organizing, and financing health services is needed. To do so, it is proposed that intellectual disability be added to population-based data collection on health status, health risk, health service utilization, and health care cost. It is necessary to test methods to identify patients with intellectual disability on Medicaid and other third-party payer claims for the purpose of collecting data. In doing so, it is essential to protect patient confidentiality.

RESEARCH SUBJECTS' PROTECTION

Ethical and legal rules for the protection of human research subjects as they relate to intellectual disability are critical. These rules are needed to facilitate the participation of persons with intellectual disability in clinical trials and other types of research. The goal in the research participation is full protection of autonomy, health, and safety. It is essential that individuals, families, and health care providers and advocates are engaged as full partners in evaluating and assessing these rules. To do so requires ensuring participation in institutional board reviews of research proposals related to intellectual disability.

TRANSLATIONAL RESEARCH: USING RESEARCH IN INTELLECTUAL DISABILITY

It is critical that individuals with intellectual disability and their families and health care professionals find, evaluate, and use research findings. Such research may be beneficial in prevention, diagnosis, and management of medical, psychiatric, psychological, and oral health and other health-related treatments. The Surgeon General's report proposed establishing and keeping current a national clearinghouse, a web site, and a list serve to guide users in identifying and evaluating research. These mechanisms may also facilitate communication and discussion about this information.

RESEARCH CAPACITY

In order to conduct research, it is necessary to increase the number of investigators who are trained in both physical and psychological aspects of intellectual disability research.

The Surgeon General proposed funding undergraduate training and postdoctoral research fellowships in medical, dental, and other health professional schools to specifically focus on issues related to intellectual disability. These proposals for research should be solicited from those engaged in the care and treatment of individuals with intellectual disability. To increase the number of investigators, it is critical that the visibility and the need for research for intellectually disabled people by enhanced.

CONSENT

In caring for individuals with intellectual disability, it is of utmost importance that health care professionals have their consent to participate, if they are able to provide it. Such consent shows respect for the right of individuals to determine what happens to their own bodies. Capacity to understand what is involved in research closely parallels an understanding of decisions about participation in evaluation and in treatment. For a person's consent to be valid, that individual must be (1) capable of making a particular decision, that is, competent to do so; (2) acting voluntarily and not under pressure from others; and (3) provided with enough information so they can make a decision (U.K. Department of Health, 2002). The process of seeking consent requires respect for the individual and is an ongoing process and not a one-time decision. The individual needs time and support to make a decision unless there is particular urgency. Moreover, individuals that give consent may change their mind and withdraw their consent at any point if they are competent and have the capacity to do so similarly. They may also change their minds and subsequently consent to an intervention that they had previously refused. It is important that they understand that they may change their minds in the future. If an individual objects or withdraws consent, the procedure should be stopped to clarify the individual's concerns. At times, an objection may reflect distress rather than withdrawal of consent so that reassurance may allow the individual to continue.

Questions about consent focus on whether the individual is competent to make informed decisions and, if they are competent, whether they should be allowed to make difficult choices in relation to medical procedures or research proposals (Alderson and Montgomery, 1996).

THE RIGHT TO PARTICIPATE IN HEALTH CARE DECISIONS

It is assumed that all people regardless of age and extent of handicap should be able to be appropriately informed about medical and treatment issues that pertain to them and be involved in decision making that deals with their care and treatment (Rutter, 2000). In some instances, the individual's level of understanding may be extremely limited so that effective communication about procedures is problematic. Thus, an individual who is profoundly intellectually disabled and whose language level is less than six months of age would not be able to engage in discussion of the treatment decision, yet that individual's responses could be gauged should the treatment be necessary, and sensitivity should be utilized in helping the child adapt to the treatment. For children with developmental disabilities who are higher functioning, at what chronological or mental age do they have sufficient understanding to engage in conversations about their treatment? Studies of young children's conversations at home indicate that three- and four-year-olds do discuss concerns and engage in decision making (Dunn, 1988). Verification about intellectually disabled individuals with mental ages at that level is needed. Still, the capacity to deal with complex issues is substantially less than that of older children and adults, but it is not absent. Thus, health care professionals should talk to individuals whose mental ages are in this age range about their treatment. This must be done so that the intellectually disabled person can understand. Patients should be provided with as much understanding as possible about issues that involve them and engage to the extent possible in decision making.

THE GROWTH OF UNDERSTANDING

Mental abilities, social understanding, and emotional competence increase during development. At a mental age of approximately two, children can appreciate inferences about the causes of events and may appreciate the psychological state of others (Kagan, 1981). Over the next several years, their ability to understand what other people are thinking gradually increases as they begin to appreciate others' intentions (Baron-Cohen, Tager-Flusberg, and Cohen, 1993). Still, thinking involving plans and goals does not become well established until later childhood or early adolescence (Kail, 1990). Moreover, there are marked individual differences in the extent to which children are suggestible. Younger children are more prone to be misled by leading questions. Those with lower mental ages and many individuals who are mentally retarded may also be misled by leading questions, and their decisions may be linked to wishes to please adults (Bruck and Ceci, 1999).

Mental abilities continue to develop throughout the teen years in normal development so that, in early adolescence, young people's thinking tends to be more abstract, more self-reflective, and more self-aware. At this age, individuals are able to hold in mind different aspects of a topic at the same time and to consider alternatives in their decision making. In addition, in normal adolescence, the ability to monitor one's thinking for inconsistency and for gaps in information continues to develop. There is also increased emotional introspection and a tendency to experience regret about past actions and to look forward to the future with understanding and perhaps with apprehension. Thus, in adolescence, long-term consequences of actions may be considered, and an appreciation of the effects of their behavior on others becomes more fully developed.

This gradual development from infancy through adolescence in intellectual abilities and emotional understanding may be linked to continuing brain development and to life experience. Yet, these changes are not simply the result of better information processing. New mental abilities reflect the knowledge attained, the ability to use that information, more sophisticated mental planning, and greater flexibility in information use (Sternberg and Powell, 1983). Yet understanding to make difficult decisions leading to a sense of competence is a complicated matter.

Making decisions requires both cognitive ability and emotional understanding. Cognitive and emotional abilities do not necessarily develop in parallel. Moreover, there is considerable individual variation in the time when a particular mental level is reached. Just as sexual maturity is reached at different ages, so also is cognitive maturity.

How should the skills involved in decision making be evaluated? One issue is that of general intelligence. Intelligence tests provide a guide to the extent that mental skills have been developed, but they must be interpreted individually.

Standardized tests of intelligence may underestimate what an individual can do in day-to-day life, for example, judgment to understand what others may be thinking. In addition, variations in mental performance are more striking when everyday experiences are different or unusual. There is evidence for context-specific knowledge in that people may be able to understand things if they are placed in context for them. Problem-solving also is better when the problem is familiar to the person than when the same problem is presented to them in an unfamiliar way. Moreover, failure on a mental task does not mean that the specific cognitive skill is not present. For example, children or those with cognitive impairment can be assisted in remembering aspects of a decision-making task by cueing. They also may use a different mental strategy from problem-solving and, in this way, solve problems that are unexpected for their age group (Gaswami, 1991).

In regard to emotional understanding, young children and intellectually disabled people with lower mental age may express mixed feelings. It is in the mental ages associated with middle childhood that insight into one's own emotional life is gained and emotional ambivalence appreciated. In addition, as children and those with cognitive impairments grow older, they learn various thinking techniques to control their emotions. However, this ability to control emotions is influenced by environmental circumstances. Therefore, both cognitive ability and emotional understanding must be considered in assessing individual competence to make a specific decision regarding medical care or treatment. The decision is based on how the individual deals with that specific decision, rather than simply focusing on standardized tests. Standardized tests are used to clarify the extent of cognitive impairment, however. Assessments must consider how the individual deals with the decision following the discussion and help with understanding it. Capacity must be considered then as a greater dimension and not as something that is either present or absent. Those with mental ages in the preschool range may have appreciation of what is involved in health care despite a limited capacity to appreciate long-term consequences and will be limited in their ability to balance various competing considerations in decision making.

After ascertaining the child's level of understanding, decision making should be shared in most cases. The children will not be the final arbiters of serious decisions but rather share in the decision with parents or guardians related to the issues discussed.

FURTHER CONSIDERATIONS IN CAPACITY TO CONSENT TO RESEARCH

The ability to understand is a graded one and not something that appears in a categorical way at a particular age. Young children can understand some of the issues, and it should be the expectation that efforts are made to help them appreciate what is asked of them and to join in decision making as much as possible. Secondly, with an individual child, level of understanding is not fixed. Level of understanding may be influenced by social-emotional context to the extent that past experiences weigh in on a particular decision. Such understanding can be enhanced by discussion, education, and through examples from the individual's familiar life. The ability to understand also may change over time with alterations in mental state, biological maturation, and new experiences. Thus, in research projects that go on over time, new understandings must be taken into account. In addition, because those with cognitive impairment understand to some extent, special justification is needed to override a clear and persistent objection to a research procedure that may carry any risk. Finally, those who are cognitively impaired are influenced by others who care about and care for them. Thus, they will be influenced by the attitudes of parents and guardians. Ordinarily, this is protective, but the investigator must take into account the person's best interest to make certain that the parent or guardian is representing the best interest.

THERAPEUTIC AND NONTHERAPEUTIC RESEARCH

Generally, a distinction is made in regard to whether the research on intellectually disabled persons is therapeutic or not therapeutic. People with intellectual disability have often been automatically excluded from participation in nontherapeutic research, yet supporters of normalization consider that this lack of participation may devalue the individual. Such exclusion may affect the representative nature of research when the research does not include those with lower level IQs. For example, the neurodevelopmental approach to schizophrenia is now considering individuals with cognitive disabilities and their inclusion in such research. Research participation should weigh the same benefits, discomforts, and risks for individuals with intellectual disability as for other groups. This applies to both therapeutic and nontherapeutic research (Frazier, 2000).

Individuals with intellectual disability have at times been excluded from survey research that does not affect their privacy due to uncertainty about their ability to give consent. What then justifies research in persons with intellectual disability? Frazier (2000) suggests that such research is appropriate when (1) its goal is to provide knowledge and treatment of individuals with a clinical condition; (2) it will not be carried out without their involvement; and (3) they are not exposed to more than negligible risks, that is, it is not unnecessarily invasive or restrictive and dose not interfere substantially with freedom and privacy.

EVALUATING CAPACITY

In adults with intellectual disability, the capacity of the person to make a decision includes the assistance of specialists for certain individuals who may help
with speech and language and in other deficits. To have the capacity to make a
decision, the individual should (1) comprehend and retain information pertinent
to the decision, which is especially important as to the consequences of participating or not participating; and (2) use this information in a decision-making
process. In assessing comprehension to use information and make a choice, one
might (1) explore the person's ability to paraphrase what was said, that is, repeating and using their own words to explain; (2) explore whether the individual
can compare alternatives or demonstrate thoughts on consequences other than
those discussed; and (3) explore whether the individual can apply the information to his or her own situation. These assessments are undertaken with support
from others who are close to the person, such as family members, caregivers,
guardians, or friends.

It must be borne in mind that some individuals have capacity to consent to
some interventions but not to others. Those with mild-to-moderate intellectual
disability may have a capacity to make straightforward decisions about their
own care and decisions to participate in certain aspects of research. It is never
to be assumed that these individuals can make no decisions because they have
been unable to make a decision previously. For example, an individual could
lack capacity to make a decision because of psychological problems, such as a
phobia (fear of blood drawing), but may have capacity to make other sorts of
decisions. Capacity is not to be confused with how reasonable a decision is.
Some individuals may make decisions based on their own religious beliefs or
value systems, although others might consider that decision not to be rational.
Seeking consent focuses on helping the person make his or her own informed
choice and appreciating that different people will come to different decisions.
Once a decision is made, it is important that the decision is communicated. That
communication between the professional and the individual may require the use
of interpreters, sign language, or other communication aids. A family member
who works closely with the individual, in addition to speech and language specialists, may be able to help with language difficulty.

INFORMATION THAT IS NEEDED FOR DECISION MAKING

Decisions should be based on (1) the discussion of benefits and risks of a proposed treatment, (2) what the treatment will involve, (3) the implications of not
having a treatment or not participating in research, (4) what alternatives are
available, and (5) the practical effects of participating or not participating. This
information needs to be presented in a way that the person can understand it.
This may require the use of pictures that explain what is involved in simple
terms and short sentences that may need to be reworded several times to clarify
understanding. Yes-no communication boards may also be helpful. Finally, the
way the information is presented is important. Information should be offered in

a respectful way and discussed in an appropriate and private setting, as it is confidential. It is critical to understand that a person's decision is truly his or her own decision. Individuals who help are important in discussing options, but the individual should not be coerced or forced into making decisions because of pressure from others or agreeing out of a desire to please or comply with someone in authority.

LACK OF CAPACITY

In assessing adults with intellectual disability, even though information is presented simply and clearly, some individuals will not be able to make decisions. This is likely in those with more severe degrees of intellectual disability. If a person is not capable of giving or refusing consent, one must take into account the person's best interest. This entails the involvement of family members to assist in decision making.

Two standards are generally considered: the best interest standard and the substituted judgment standard. The best interests are not limited to medical benefit but also include general well-being in relationships with those who are close to the individual and religious and spiritual welfare. Moreover, those who lack capacity to consent and refuse consent may still express willingness or unwillingness to cooperate with what is offered. These preferences must be considered as one considers the person's best interest. If an individual becomes quite distressed by a procedure, the distress is a factor in making the decision about proceeding. When deciding if a treatment is appropriate, it is the person's best interest that matters, not balancing those interests against the interests of the interests of health professionals or others in the community. Still, such interests will be intertwined, and a treatment decision must take into account family relations and support. Ordinarily, decisions will be made together with those closest to the person and health care professionals. In some instances, an agreement may not be reached and permission to proceed may not be obtained.

THERAPEUTIC AND NONTHERAPEUTIC RESEARCH

In any form of research, the individual who has the capacity to give or withhold consent decides for himself or herself whether or not to participate. In general, research is not carried out on individuals who cannot give their own consent if the research could be carried out on others who can give consent. An exception is made when participation may be in the person's own best interests or, in some instances, for nontherapeutic research in the interest of the class of individuals who have this disorder.

THERAPEUTIC RESEARCH

Therapeutic research may be conducted to develop new treatments or to evaluate the effectiveness of existing treatments. On occasion, it may be in the best interests of the person who lacks the capacity to consent to enter such a clinical trial of a new treatment. This might occur if the standard treatment is non-existent, has limited effectiveness, or has effectiveness in nonhandicapped in-dividuals but has not been appropriately evaluated in those who have a handi-capping condition. Any participation must be shown to be in the individual's best interest.

NONTHERAPEUTIC RESEARCH

In some instances, nontherapeutic research may be conducted that will not spe-cifically benefit the individual. If so, it is important that it is not against the interest of the individual.

RISK

In the U.S. federal regulation, there are guidelines for research in children in-volving minimal risk and minor increase over minimal risk (Field and Behrman, 2004, p. 102). These guidelines may be applied to children with intellectual disability and mental illness. However, the guidelines are specifically for children and their application to adults with intellectual disability requires consideration.

Minimal Risk

The common rule for protection of human subjects includes the following def-inition of minimal risk:

> Minimal risk means that the probability and magnitude of harm or discomfort anticipated in the research are not greater in and of themselves than those ordi-narily encountered in daily life during the performance of routine physical and psychological examinations or tests. (Field and Behrman, 2004, pp. 113–114)

With this rule, an institutional review board must determine that the level of risk is no greater than minimal, whether or not the research offers the prospect of benefit to the individual. There is some controversy and discussion about how to apply the minimal risk standard. The minimal risk generally is interpreted as risk associated with daily lives of normal and healthy and average children. Risk may include harms, discomforts, breaches of privacy, or embarrassment asso-ciated with the research. Using the minimal risk standard, a permissible level of risk in research is a socially allowable risk that parents generally permit their children to be exposed to when they are not engaged in research situations. Children do experience different levels of risk in their daily lives. Focusing on minimal risk in regard to socially allowable risks must take into account different risks experienced by children at different ages. At issue is the equivalence of risk and the definition whether the risk associated with the test or procedure is equivalent to or no greater than the risk of events ordinarily accounted for in the daily life of a normal, healthy child or socially allowable risk parents permit their normal, healthy children to take. In making these decisions, participation in research must be voluntary. Even if the research is minimal, there is no obligation for the person to participate. The person to be enrolled in research and their parents or guardian will determine together whether they choose to participate in a particular research study. The individual must be informed that, in this case, there is no prospect of benefit to the individual, that the assent and permission are voluntary and not coerced, with no obligation to be part of the research project even though the risk is minimal.

Minor Increase over Minimal Risk

Federal regulations of the United States covering research for children permit research that involves greater than minimal risk and no prospect of benefit if it is likely to yield generalizable knowledge about the child's or individual's disorder or condition under specific circumstances. Because of the seriousness of disorders associated with mental retardation, research may fall into this category for this group. The federal regulation is as follows:

> Research involving greater than minimal risk and no prospect of direct benefit to individual subjects but likely to yield generalizable knowledge about the subject's disorder or condition. (Field and Behrman, 2004, p. 102)

The Department of Health and Human Services, under this guideline, will conduct or fund research when the Institutional Review Board (IRB) finds that more than minimal risk to children is presented by an intervention or procedure but does not hold out the prospect of direct benefit for the individual subject, or by a monitoring procedure that is not likely to contribute to the well-being of a subject only if IRB finds that: (a) the risk represents a minor increase over minimal risk; (b) the intervention or procedure presents experiences to subjects that are reasonably commensurate with those inherent in their actual or expected medical, dental, psychological, social, or educational situations; (c) the intervention or procedure is likely to yield generalizable knowledge about the subject's disorder or condition that is of vital importance for the understanding or amelioration of a subject's disorder or condition; and (d) adequate provisions are made for soliciting the assent of children and permission of their parents or guardians as set forth in Section 46.408 (Field and Behrman, 2004).

This category regarding permissible research was initially proposed by the National Commission for the Protection of Human Subjects of Biomedical Research in its 1977 report (research involving children) and was integrated into final federal regulations in 1983. These regulations dealt with research of vital importance that would not otherwise be permissible concerning diseases, disorders, or conditions that affect children. The federal regulations impose a limit on the discretion of parents to permit the participation of children in research that entails more than minimal risk unless there is direct benefit. However, the regulations also permit important research for the long-term benefit of children. The decision is made by the institutional review board regarding the level of risk and what makes up a minor increment over minimal risk. Whereas minimal risk is indexed to risks encountered in the daily life of normal, healthy children, the level of risk that is permitted with a minor increase over minimal is more than that level and linked to the risks of interventions or procedures having been experienced or expected to be experienced for those children who have a specific disorder or condition. This allows the child and the parent to make decisions about assent and permission based on their disorder. The research investigator and the institutional review board consider whether the risk is justified to yield knowledge of vital importance for the understanding of a particular disorder or condition. The National Commission for the Protection of Human Subjects of Biomedical Research proposed a definition of disorder or condition. The word "condition" refers to situations that "jeopardize the health of children, interfere with optimal development, or adversely affect well-being in later years." The term "disorder or condition" refers to a group of potential individuals who might participate in research and suggests that this characteristic may be understood more broadly than a specific disease or diagnostic category. Consequently, prematurity, infancy, adolescence, poverty, living in a difficult physical environment, institutionalization, or having a genetic predisposition to future illness might be considered conditions that warrant research and present levels that are a minor increase over minimal without direct benefit.

References

Alderson, P., and Montgomery, J. (1996). *Health care choices: Making decisions with children.* Institute for Public Policy Research, London, UK.

Baron-Cohen, S., Tager-Flusberg, H., and Cohen, D. (1993). *Understanding other minds: Perspectives from autism.* Oxford University Press, Oxford.

Bruck, M., and Ceci, S.J. (1999). The suggestibility of children's memory. *Annual Review of Psychology,* 50:419–439.

Dunn, J. (1988). *The beginnings of social understanding.* Blackwell, Oxford, UK.

Field, M.J., and Behrman, R.E. (eds.). (2004). *Ethical conduct of research involving children.* The National Academies Press, Washington, DC.

Frazier, W.I. (2000). Appendix 3–Decision-making and assessment of competence in individuals with a learning disability. In *Guidelines for researchers and for research ethics committees on psychiatric research involving human participants.* Royal College of Psychiatrists' Working Party on Guidelines for Researchers and for Research Ethics Committees on Psychiatric Researching Involving Human Participants, London, UK.

Goswami, U. (1991). Analogical reasoning: What develops? A review of research and theory. *Child Development,* 62:1–22.

Kagan, J. (1981). *The second year: The emergence of self-awareness.* Harvard University Press, Cambridge, MA.

Kail, R.V. (1990). *Memory development in children,* 3rd ed. Freeman, San Francisco.

NIH Workshop. (2002). *Emotional and behavioral health in persons with mental retardation/developmental disabilities: Research challenges and opportunities.* November 29–December 1, 2001. Rockville, MD.

Rutter, M. (2000). Appendix 2–Children's level of understanding of medical decisions. In *Guidelines for researchers and for research ethics committees on psychiatric research involving human participants.* Royal College of Psychiatrists' Working Party on Guidelines for Researchers and for Research Ethics Committees on Psychiatric Researching Involving Human Participants, London, UK.

Sternberg, R.J., and Powell, J.A. (1983). The development of intelligence. In J.H. Flavell and E.M. Markman (eds.), *Cognitive development, Vol. 3, Mussen's handbook of child psychology,* 4th ed., pp. 341–419. Wiley, New York.

U.K. Department of Health. (2002). *Seeking consent: Working with people with learning disabilities.*

U.S. Department of Health and Human Services. (2002). *Report of the Surgeon General's conference on health disparities and mental retardation. Closing the gap: A national blueprint to improve the health of persons with mental retardation.* Office of the Surgeon General, Rockville, MD.

APPENDIX E
Emotional and Behavioral Health in Persons with Mental Retardation/ Developmental Disabilities: Research Challenges and Opportunities

SUMMARY

Individuals with intellectual disability or developmental disabilities are estimated to be three to four times more likely than those in the general population to experience an emotional or behavioral disorder. Recent advances in a number of fields and disciplines—including neuroscience, genetics, psychopharmacology, and behavioral psychology—show promise for improving the treatment and lives of those with intellectual disability. Despite advances in each of these areas, intellectual disability is frequently a criterion for exclusion from research studies. Enrollment of individuals with intellectual disability in research protocols addressing emotional and behavioral disorders has been rather limited, issues of informed consent persist, and more researchers with special interest in this population are needed.

To address these issues, a two-and-a-half-day workshop was convened by the National Institute of Neurological Disorders and Stroke (NINDS), the National Institute of Child Health and Human Development (NICHD), the National Institute of Mental Health (NIMH), the Office of Rare Diseases (ORD) and the Joseph P. Kennedy Jr. Foundation.

The workshop, entitled "Emotional and Behavioral Health in Persons with Mental Retardation/Developmental Disabilities: Research Challenges and Opportunities," drew more than 80 participants representing academic research institutions, government agencies, service providers, and consumer advocacy organizations.

The workshop was designed to address key questions that arise in the inclusion of people with intellectual disability and developmental disabilities in federally funded research in the United States. The goal was to define ways to include people with intellectual disability in research thus promoting evidenced-based treatments for this population.

The workshop was held several days prior to a scheduled Surgeon General's Conference on Health Disparities and Mental Retardation, December 5–6, 2001. Results of the workshop were expected to be presented publicly there for the first time. In the report, the term "mental retardation or developmental disability" (MR/DD) is used.

WORKING GROUP DISCUSSIONS

Each of the working groups met for one-half day to consider a number of questions, including:

- *Epidemiology*: What epidemiological evidence is needed to provide accurate estimates of the incidence and prevalence of emotional disorders among people with MR/DD? What are the barriers to obtaining it?
- *Diagnosis and Assessment*: What are the appropriate instruments needed to diagnose and formulate treatment for individuals with MR/DD? How can current diagnostic and assessment methods be made more applicable to individuals with MR/DD?
- *Ethical Considerations*: How should "assent" apply to research involving individuals with MR/DD, particularly research with no immediate therapeutic benefit? Should there be different standards for children and adults on the question of seeking consent from a guardian/legal decision maker?
- *Interventions Research*: What are the most pressing needs of people with MR/DD and co-occurring emotional and behavioral disturbances? How might interventions research be most effectively carried out in hospitals, schools, and community settings?
- *Research Design*: What are the most pertinent research designs for understanding the needs of people with MR/DD and co-occurring emotional and behavioral disturbances? What steps should be taken to adapt FDA guidelines for clinical medication trials in individuals with MR/DD?
- *Research Training Needs*: What are the best approaches to establishing new researchers with an interest in the emotional and behavioral health of people with MR/DD? Are there useful models from other areas of biomedical research that can be used?

WORKING GROUP RECOMMENDATIONS

Epidemiology

The working group on epidemiology stated that epidemiology is more than simply counting how many individuals are affected by an illness and measuring prevalence and demography. Epidemiology can delineate the nature and scope of MR/DD and the associated behavioral, emotional, and psychiatric problems. Modern experimental approaches allow for the study of causative processes, factors that influence the course of the disorder, and service needs. Epidemiological studies also can disclose individual developmental trajectories and the influences that shape those trajectories. Some of these influences promote risk; others provide protection and promote resiliency.

Critical Issues

- *There is a lack of adequate data on risk and protective factors for mental illness in people at different developmental stages, including preschool, school entry, school-to-work transition, and aging.*
- *New opportunities are available to study the interaction between genes and the environment.* It is expected that variations in the heritability of behavioral or cognitive traits will be observed across different social levels and environmental conditions.
- *Ensuring adequate sample sizes is paramount.* For example, many individuals with mild MR may be difficult to find beyond the school years. In addition, recruiting adequate numbers of individuals with more rare neurogenetic syndromes may be difficult.
- *There is a need to examine behavioral features, emotional problems, and psychiatric diagnoses in groups with specific neurodevelopmental syndromes, including Down syndrome, fragile X syndrome, and Prader-Willi syndrome.*
- *Systems research studies, including investigations focusing on state systems, residential units, group homes, supported living, and prison settings, are needed.* Understudied areas include the following: (1) factors leading to the success or failure of deinstitutionalization, and (2) the probable increase in use of medications during the last decade.

Recommendations

- *Conduct longitudinal studies to examine key life-stage transitions regarding risk and protective factors.* Comparisons should be made of such factors as time of diagnosis of the disorder, residential status, and family functioning. Although the working group focused primarily on concurrent longitudinal designs in its recommendations, the group also recognized the utility of case-control designs in behavioral genetics research and nonconcurrent longitudinal designs that make use of record linkages.
- *Use informative samples and innovative research designs for behavioral genetic research, including twin pairs studied from birth and informative family and sibling studies.*
- *Ensure that those with mild MR or rare neurogenetic disorders are sampled adequately.* Exploit opportunities to piggyback on existing surveys, such as the CDC's health risk behavior surveys and the National Health Interview Survey.
- *Conduct syndrome-specific cohort studies to ascertain specific vulnerabilities to common disorders, inform analysis of interactions between genes, brain, and behavior, and improve understanding of functioning.*
- *Consider convening another workshop to outline additional systems research studies.*

Diagnosis and Assessment

The Diagnosis and Assessment Working Group noted that a major impediment to treating psychiatric disorders in people with MR/DD is the inability to recognize mental health problems in these individuals. Assessment and diagnosis is particularly difficult due to intellectual, adaptive, and verbal impairments that limit reliability or reporting, as well as the presence of organic or environmental factors that may produce or exacerbate the pathologic behavior in question. In addition, receipt of services is frequently linked to the accurate diagnosis of a specific condition. As a consequence, individuals with MR/DD may not receive effective treatments, the treatment they receive may be harmful, and they may be denied important services.

Critical Needs

- *Research aimed at developing appropriate diagnostic procedures applicable to individuals with MR/DD.*
- *Investigations to evaluate the clinical utility of assessment procedures in treatment trials.*
- *Studies to identify the biological and environmental determinants of emotional and behavioral disorders in individuals with MR/DD.*
- *Research to determine whether differences in the expression of emotional disorders are due to cognitive or functional impairment.* The complex interrelationship between the expression of emotional disorders and cognitive and functional impairment places additional demands on the adequacy of assessment procedures.

Recommendations

- *Conduct research to assess the validity and reliability of adaptations of standard diagnostic and assessment strategies to accommodate people with developmental disability.*
- *Develop direct observation instruments to identify overt characteristics of emotional disturbance and their environmental correlates.*
- *Undertake studies to evaluate the tolerability of the diagnostic and assessment process for people with MR/DD and their families and care providers.*
- *Develop techniques to assess the impact of psychosocial stressors in the lives of people with MR/DD and to integrate this knowledge with diagnostic protocols, treatment strategies, and service systems.* It is equally important to determine protective factors and methods to quantify an individual's resilience.
- *Undertake efforts to characterize the phenotypic diversity of MR/DD.* Develop appropriate animal models to explore how genetic abnormalities give rise to mental retardation. In addition, complete neuropsychological assessments of MR/DD to determine the pattern of cognitive disabilities

and competencies and associated behavioral abnormalities present in various forms of MR/DD.

- *Conduct prospective studies to describe the developmental trajectory of behavior and skill acquisition in genetic disorders or syndromes associated with MR/DD.* While it is often assumed that the pattern of abilities and impairments will be maintained throughout development, available evidence suggests this is not so.
- *Carry out research aimed at uncovering how the manifestations of particular emotional and behavioral disorders and response to treatment may vary as a function of cognitive or functional disability or developmental level.*

Ethical Considerations

The Working Group on Ethical Considerations noted that there are a wide variety of ethical and legal issues surrounding the participation of people with MR/DD in research protocols. The members affirmed that it is in the interest of individuals with MR/DD to be included in nontherapeutic research that may offer information important to furthering the understanding of conditions affecting them. When there is no effective treatment, it is in the interest of people with MR/DD to participate in well-designed placebo controlled trials. The alternative is to get no treatment for disabling conditions, or to receive treatments where safety and efficacy have not been tested, often resulting in harm without compensating benefit. Any determinations about an individual's capacity to decide whether to participate in research should be based on his or her functional ability, not on IQ score or the simple label of MR/DD.

Critical Issues

- *The "Common Rule" governing the participation of human subjects in federally sponsored research does not adequately address the inclusion of individuals with MR/DD.* It remains unclear whether separate provisions are necessary for individuals with MR/DD, mental illness, or impaired decisional capacity.
- *The "minimal risk rule" guiding participation in nontherapeutic research is ambiguous and is being interpreted widely by IRBs.* Considerable variability in how IRBs determine the risk level in "ordinary" life, what medical tests are viewed as "routine," and whether such factors are indexed to people who are healthy or those who are ill is apparent.
- *Current understanding of informed consent and assent frequently does not take into consideration the varied capacities of individuals with MR/ DD to make decisions.* Decisional capacity in adults with MR/DD frequently is assumed to be global, across all decision-making tasks, which is contrary to available evidence.
- *Individuals with MR/DD may be more or less vulnerable to undue in-*

fluence and/or coercion depending on the residential setting or in the absence of an appropriate advocate.

- *Fear of federal sanctions is restraining IRB's from approving ethically acceptable research, particularly in vulnerable populations.* Similarly, IRB members and investigators express growing concerns about litigation. Punitive sanctions are frequently levied by federal oversight bodies for regulatory compliance infractions that do not harm research participants.
- *Lack of clarity in guidelines may impede genetic testing of individual with MR/DD.* One recent legal case raised the issue of whether family members should be considered research subjects if mentioned in the course of a genetic family history. The authority of surrogate decision makers to consent for genetic research with no direct therapeutic benefit to the patient remains unclear.

Recommendations

- *The Institute of Medicine should convene a meeting of all stakeholders to address deficiencies in the Common Rule with regard to individuals with MR/DD, mental illness, or impaired decisional capacity in federally sponsored research.*
- *A national workshop should be convened to help clarify the minimal risk rule as it applies to individuals with MR/DD who lack capacity to make decisions regarding research participation.* The workshop should also address the development of other federal guidelines, for example, clarifying whether taking a genetic family history necessarily makes a family member a "research subject" and when genetic testing for research purposes is permissible for individuals with MR/DD.
- *Further analysis is needed about issues of assent and dissent in individuals with MR/DD.* Individuals with MR/DD who have the capacity to consent should be given the widest latitude to consent or refuse to participate in research. If an individual with MR/DD appears unwilling to participate in research, dissent should generally be honored, even for procedures of minimal risk.
- *Appropriate tools for the assessment of decisional capacity in individuals with MR/DD need to be developed.* Further research on techniques to enhance the decision-making capabilities of individuals with MR/DD is needed.
- *Continued discussion on the legal authority of surrogate decision makers to authorize participation in research that does not offer the prospect of direct benefit to the patient is needed.* Because decisional capacity is situational in individuals with MR/DD, appointment of a surrogate for all decision making may be inappropriate. Absent state law to the contrary, a surrogate may authorize research that has the prospect of direct benefit to the person with MR/DD.

- *Additional discussion on the role of residential setting and associated factors in research protections is needed.* Issues of home ownership/control and contracting for services within the residential setting are a necessary part of the discussion.
- *Federal oversight bodies, such as the Office of Human Subjects Protection, should review the use of punitive sanctions for infractions that do not cause harm to research participants.*

Interventions Research

The Working Group on Interventions Research said that advances in the fields of genetics, neuroimaging, brain plasticity, behavioral sciences, and education show promise in generating effective interventions to improve the emotional and behavioral health of individuals with MR/DD. The group noted that a number of behavioral and psychosocial treatments have been well-researched in the general population but have not been tested for their efficacy in individuals with MR/DD. Similarly, newer and safer medications are available for a range of emotional and behavioral disorders, yet few rigorous tests of their efficacy in individuals with MR/DD have been performed. These and other challenges present critical opportunities for well-designed intervention studies in people with MR/DD.

Critical Opportunities

- *In genetics, characterization of specific behavioral phenotypes associated with varied genetic etiologies of MR/DD show promise in allowing researchers to craft and target interventions for specific disorders or behavioral disturbances.* Research identifying genes that code for new target proteins and the development of drugs that target those proteins could lead to better focused pharmacologic treatment strategies.
- *In neuroimaging, scientists have begun to document the effects of environment and experience on the brains of individuals with MR/DD using a variety of imaging techniques.*
- *Research on the plasticity of the brain, much of it accomplished in animal models, has illustrated the profound effects of early experience on brain development and development of aberrant behavior.* Research has shown that the consequences of central nervous system damage, even as a result of genetic mutations, can be ameliorated by complex environments. Evidence of is also accumulating that neural regeneration, in at least some areas of the brain, are possible across the life span.
- *In psychosocial research, functional analysis of behavior is essential for prescribing effective behavioral treatments for people with MR/DD who display severe behavior disorders.* Communication training has been shown to reduce the occurrence of emotional and behavioral problems. Intensive early educational interventions produce long-term gains in social and intellectual functioning in some at-risk populations.

Recommendations

- *In genetics, assess the differential effects of genetic polymorphism on treatment outcomes.* Develop psychotropic drugs selective for newly identified target proteins and test in animal models and controlled clinical trials. Tests the effects of experiential/behavioral manipulations on gene expression.
- *Use neuroimaging as a technique for assessing treatment outcome (along with behavioral and clinical outcomes).* Use neuroimaging to establish likely mechanisms of treatment effects.
- *In neuroplasticity research, test theory-based interventions for specific populations, using an array of new technologies to document central nervous system changes and behavioral outcomes.* Evaluate the importance of age, timing, and the intensity of intervention on neuroplasticity. Utilize appropriate animal models to test neuroplasticity associated with developmental insults to the central nervous system.
- *In psychosocial research, evaluate the impact of using functional analysis to test the efficacy of different treatment techniques and in a wider variety of emotional and behavioral disorders.* Test the efficacy of intensive early intervention and communication training to prevent or reduce emotional or behavioral disorders in children with MR/DD.
- *Assess the effects of combining pharmacological treatments with behavioral, psychosocial, and educational interventions and/or natural supports.*
- *Develop innovative research designs to address the potential confounds of ongoing treatments and co-occurring conditions.*
- *Urge revision of FDA drug approval standards to include alternative research designs.*
- *Engage consumers and family members in design, implementation, and evaluation of interventions.*
- *Create a federal task force to develop and implement an interdisciplinary clinical research network.* Fund meetings to create coalitions of researchers, advocates, and service providers.
- *Place funding priority on testing promising interventions.* Review portfolio of NIH funded studies that address prevention or treatment of emotional and behavioral disorders. Determine the feasibility of supplemental funding to add participants with MR/DD.

Research Design

The Working Group on Research Design noted that the primary purpose of research design is the production of unbiased and efficient data that can be used to serve the needs of all partners in the research enterprise. The group affirmed that while a multiplicity of research designs and analyses can be valid for addressing specific problems and questions in individuals with MR/DD, the randomized, controlled, blinded protocol remains the "gold standard" against which other research designs should be judged. The group noted that in current practice, research on individuals with MR/DD frequently relies on single-subject case reports, which do not uniformly produce optimal, valid answers. Through more informed decision making about research designs and their fit to research questions, the state of knowledge about the emotional and behavioral health of individuals with MR/DD can be improved.

Recommendations

- *It should be the normal expectation that individuals with MR/DD will be included in federally funded research.* The investigator must assume the responsibility for justifying any exclusion rules. Exclusions should be based on the functional and safety features of the experiments or interventions being studied, not sweeping criteria, such as "IQ less than 70," that frequently exclude many MR/DD individuals from research.
- *Research designs that emphasize our understanding of "for which person" and "under what circumstances" should be emphasized in research on MR/DD.* These research designs are preferred to models that only yield estimates of group means, such as ANOVA and regression models.
- *Multisite, multicollaborator designs should be the norm, not the exception.* These designs need to be utilized creatively and not limited to single protocols that are simply replicated at all sites.
- *Research designs used to assess the outcomes of interventions in individuals with MR/DD should include measures that assess functional and clinical improvement.* In general, a single variable, or a small number of variables, should be prespecified as the outcome variable of interest.
- *Longitudinal follow-up is critical for the full understanding the consequences of an intervention.* Longitudinal follow-up should be preplanned and examine both the primary outcome variable and other potential mediating variables.
- *Creating an archive of complete and well-documented data sets is essential for the development of cumulative science.* Federally supported researchers should expect to make their data available to the research community after an appropriate delay for publication of the study's primary outcomes.

Research Training Needs

The Working Group on Research Training Needs emphasized that the training of investigators in the emotional and behavioral health of individuals with MR/DD should necessarily be interdisciplinary and should draw on knowledge in a wide variety of disciplines. Efforts should be collaborative, emphasizing training, research, and clinical work, with a particular focus on translational research that bridges basic science and more applied investigations. Initiatives to train more researchers in this area face a number of impediments, including stigma (for example, the notion that MR/DD individuals are not "good patients"). Research in this area is frequently viewed as less prestigious or "real" compared with other fields, and disciplinary "silos" maintain barriers to the cross-disciplinary collaboration necessary in this research and essential to attracting new investigators to the field.

Critical Issues

- *There is no clear home for grants supporting research on the emotional and behavioral health in individuals with MR/DD.* Individual Research Career Development (K) awards may come too late in medical careers and provide insufficient research and salary support in the face of significant debt. Research into the emotional and behavioral health of people with MR/DD is not well regarded or understood by review groups.
- *Research training opportunities can come too late in clinical training.* Opportunities can be provided at the undergraduate level, during graduate/medical training, and during the residency/post-doc fellowship period. Junior faculty need forums to present their work, get feedback, and build networks. Trainees at all level lack sufficient exposure to individuals with MR/DD and emotional and behavioral problems.
- *Junior faculty face pressure to publish discrete inquiries in which they retain lead authorship.* Tenure committees frequently do not assign significant value to participation in large, interdisciplinary investigations characteristic of work in this area.
- *There is insufficient funding for seasoned investigators to mentor those in training or young investigators.* Not all mentors are "good" mentors; it is difficult to get good trainees to the right mentor.

Recommendations

- *Encourage a variety of training pathways and mechanisms for different individuals and disciplines.* Systematically evaluate all current research training mechanisms, seeking feedback from junior trainees who have successfully entered research careers and those who have chosen other career paths.
- *Consider which other disciplines should be at the table.* Special education; speech, language, and communication; social work; nursing; and occupational therapy are among the fields that could contribute to this discussion.
- *Look to program models in other areas to develop new training mechanisms.* Work group members highlighted NINDS's Neurological Sciences Academic Development Award and NICHD's Pediatric Scientist Development Training Program as examples
- *Augment existing support and seek new avenues to channel support.* Increase stipend and research dollar funding for training MD clinical investigators (NIH's T32 program). Add other training funds to University Affiliated Programs (UAPs) on Developmental Disabilities and other centers where MR/DD research is performed. Craft a specific RFA to encourage research on the emotional and behavioral health of people

with MR/DD. Develop new support for research training during medical residency and the postresidency fellowship years.

- *Create an NIH interinstitute coordinating group to promote research and training in MR/DD research and emotional and behavioral health.* Designate a program officer at each relevant institute to shepherd research in this area. Create special review groups for research training proposals and develop intramural programs for research on the emotional and behavioral health of individuals with MR/DD.
- *Create training centers of excellence in MR/DD research to promote the value of training efforts.*
- *Support and augment existing research training networks that could expand training of researchers in MR/DD.* These include the UAPs and the Mental Retardation Research Centers funded by NICHD, as well as the Leadership Education in Neurodevelopmental and Related Disabilities program (LEND) funded by the Maternal Child Health Bureau.
- *Create topical career development clubs for young investigators.* Use these as a vehicle to encourage early career mentoring and network building, and as a source of information about available funding opportunities.
- *Create new categories of special individual research career development awards ("Special K's") for investigators at various stages of their careers.* Craft a Special-K RFA for researchers interested in the emotional and behavioral health of people with MR/DD.
- *Seek private foundation partnerships.*
- *Develop a plan to monitor progress from the outside.* The Institute of Medicine represents one venue with experience in charting change and setting priorities.

References

Web site source for NIH Workshop recommendations: http://ord.aspensys.com/asp/workshops/search.asp

NIH research announcement: *Research on Psychopathology in Intellectual Disabilities* (PA-04–044) http://grants1.nih.gov/grants/guide/pa-files/PA-04-044.html

APPENDIX F
Keeping the Promises: National Goals, State of Knowledge, and Research Agenda for Persons with Intellectual and Developmental Disabilities

The United States has made important promises to its citizens with intellectual and developmental disabilities. We find them in the Developmental Disabilities Assistance and Bill of Rights Act, the Americans with Disabilities Act, Supreme Court decisions, the Individuals with Disabilities Education Act, the Rehabilitation Act, and President Bush's New Freedom Initiative. These are expressions of national values and commitments to people with intellectual and developmental disabilities. Among these promises are access to needed community services, individualized supports, and other forms of assistance that promote self-determination, independence, productivity, and integration and inclusion in all facets of community life. "Keeping the Promises" means that people with disabilities not only can participate in the community, but that people with disabilities have a place in the community.

In January 2003, nearly 250 invited participants came together to review the nation's goals for people with intellectual and developmental disabilities and the role of research in helping to achieve them. Participants were sponsored by more than 40 organizations, including nine federal agencies. Invited participants included national leaders in research, advocacy, policy, and program management. Family members and self-advocates with intellectual and developmental disabilities were well represented. Conference participants identified four general areas to improve progress toward national goals: (1) Improving Links between Current Knowledge and Public Policy; (2) Improving Relevance of Research for All Stakeholders; (3) Improving Translation of Research into Effective Common Practice; and (4) Improving Ways to Share Information with All Who Need It.

Twelve topical groups considered issues that arise throughout the life span and across social roles, from learning and development to work and community life. The topical groups were: (1) Early Development, (2) Education, (3) Transition to Adulthood, (4) Behavioral and Mental Health Supports, (5) Health Services, (6) Biomedical Research, (7) Integrated Employment, (8) Community Life, (9) Family Life, (10) Self-Determination and Self-Advocacy, (11) Technology, and (12) Aging.

A summary of the findings and recommendations was presented under the following headings: (1) The National Goals, (2) The State of Knowledge, (3) Knowledge Needed to Achieve National Goals, and (4) Emerging Issues. Conference findings and recommendations have been published by the AAMR. In the summary that follows, National Goals and Knowledge Needed to Achieve National Goals sections are listed; *asterisks mark recommendations that are considered particularly important by self-advocates.*

EARLY DEVELOPMENT

National Goals

- Children with or at-risk for developmental disabilities will be identified as early as possible so that they can access quality services.
- Measurable, cost-effective, and sound intervention strategies will be available to support the health and well-being of all children and to strengthen their ability to participate fully in family and community life.
- Families will be able to make informed decisions and partner effectively with professionals to achieve positive outcomes.
- All children and families will have access to community-based, coordinated systems of effective services from supportive and skilled personnel who value individual and cultural differences, provide continuity in supports, and promote community inclusion.

Knowledge Needed to Achieve National Goals

1. Early Identification

- What models of early identification are most effective and how can they best be organized to help more children and families?
- How can warning signs and early indicators of developmental delay or disability be used to identify children who need help more accurately and quicker?
- What are the short- and long-term benefits of earlier identification?

2. Measurable, Cost-Effective Strategies

- What outcomes for children and families best indicate successful early intervention?
- What intervention practices best promote the health, development, and well-being of young children? What variations on established practices respond most effectively to families with diverse needs and life circumstances?

- Are outcomes different for children raised by parents with disabilities than for children raised by parents without disabilities? What makes a difference in good and poor outcomes?*

3. Family and Professionals Partner

- How can the specific characteristics, preferences, and needs of specific families be effectively matched and accommodated with intervention practices to promote positive outcomes?
- How can professionals be better prepared and supported in their roles as partners with families (i.e., to share information, develop positive relationships, and communicate effectively)?
- What elements of intervention and support prepare families to feel more confident and competent to care and advocate for their children?
- How can information and resources be made more accessible to families with diverse needs and life circumstances?
- How can parents with disabilities better access information about community supports, parenting skills, child development, and school preparation?*
- How do parents' beliefs (religious, political, family, culture, ethnic background, race, sexual preference, and gender) affect their getting help for their children with disabilities? What alternative ways might be effective in reaching them?*
- How does engaging people with disabilities and family members in educating professionals (e.g., doctors, early intervention workers, genetic counselors) about the needs, goals, and expectations of individuals and families improve the quality of services, understanding, and relationships between professionals and the people to whom they provide supports?*

4. Community-Based, Coordinated System of Services

- What strategies (organizational, financing, etc.) are effective in creating and sustaining community-based, coordinated health, education, social services, and family supports for all children?
- To what extent do current federal programs impede or enhance the goal of community-based, coordinated systems of care and education?
- What approaches to education, training, and ongoing support of key personnel in health, education, and social services help promote evidence-based practices within a coordinated system of care?
- What approaches have been effective in promoting successful inclusion of children and families in the community?

EDUCATION

National Goals

- All children and youth with intellectual and developmental disabilities will receive an individually referenced, culturally relevant, effective education leading to valued post-school outcomes and provided in the least restrictive setting, such as education in the general education school and classroom.

- Parents and families and youth with intellectual and developmental disabilities will be full partners in determining what constitutes an effective education, as well as the least restrictive setting.
- Accountability standards and procedures will be sufficient to ensure that each child or youth with intellectual and developmental disabilities receives an effective education within the least restrictive setting.
- Children and youth with intellectual and developmental disabilities will have access to sufficient human and fiscal resources, supports, and services required for them to be effectively educated in the least restrictive setting.

Knowledge Needed to Achieve National Goals

- To what extent and under what conditions does the achievement of state standards by all students with intellectual and developmental disabilities, across the spectrum of needs, cultural and linguistic groups, and families at risk, lead to valued post-school outcomes?
- What educational practices, including teacher expectations, curricula and instruction, and settings are associated with positive academic and/or post-school achievement for persons with intellectual and developmental disabilities?
- What are the conditions (instructional techniques, curriculum, supplemental supports, school organization, staffing, class size, technology, experiences) under which all students with intellectual and developmental disabilities can participate in instructional and other school activities and can achieve state standards?
- What are the most effective strategies to support parent and caregiver involvement in the education of their children?
- What are the most effective practices and models to prepare all personnel, including special and regular educators, paraprofessionals, administrators and related professionals, to support all students with intellectual and developmental disabilities to achieve high standards and valued post-school outcomes in general education settings?

TRANSITION TO ADULTHOOD

National Goals

- Efforts will increase to promote self-determination and self-advocacy by students.
- Students with intellectual and developmental disabilities will have access to the general standards-based curriculum.
- Graduation rates of students with intellectual and developmental disabilities will increase.

- Schools will work with other appropriate agencies to ensure students' access to full participation in and support for post-secondary education, employment, and community living opportunities.
- Families will have informed participation in educational and life planning, decisionmaking and promotion of self-advocacy for their transition-aged children.
- Collaboration and cross-systems links will be created at all levels to support student self-determination, self-advocacy, and achievement of meaningful school, post-school, and adult role outcomes.
- A qualified workforce will be available to address the needs of youth with intellectual and developmental disabilities.
- All students with intellectual and developmental disabilities will have full, active participation in all aspects of social, recreational, and leisure community life.

Knowledge Needed to Achieve National Goals

- What policies and factors in policy implementation facilitate or inhibit effective processes and outcomes related to transition?
- What strategies can be identified through research and demonstration to "scale up" validated transition practices and systems to make "best practices" more common practices?
- What are the most valued post-school outcomes to serve as benchmarks to validate empirically effective transition practices on which consensus can be established and communicated in non-jargon to all who have a stake in monitoring transition program effectiveness?
- What are the most effective approaches to monitoring and enforcing transition policy, implementation, and outcomes?
- What are the differences in outcomes for students who have completed their educations who have stayed in the family home, lived on their own, or moved into the "provider world"?*
- In what ways and for what people does participating in special education and transition programs help achieve desired post-school outcomes?*

BEHAVIORAL AND MENTAL HEALTH SUPPORTS

National Goals

- Individuals with intellectual and developmental disabilities and problem behavior, and/or mental disorder, will have ongoing access to appropriate assessment that guides support practices, and that includes person-centered planning, mental health/medical evaluations, and functional behavioral assessment.
- Individuals with intellectual and developmental disabilities will have access to effective, positive, and evidence-based behavioral, mental health, medical, and social supports needed to (a) prevent and reduce problem

behaviors or mental disorders, (b) support social resilience, and (c) promote desired lifestyle outcomes.

- Individuals with intellectual and developmental disabilities and problem behavior (and/or mental disorders) will have access to ongoing monitoring of the extent to which behavior support plans (care plans) are implemented and are effective at both promoting desired lifestyle outcomes and reducing problem behaviors.
- Systems of care, including policy, organizational, and quality assurance variables, will be established for individuals with intellectual and developmental disabilities across the life span to enable the effective and sustained implementation of positive behavioral and mental health supports.
- Development of a comprehensive system of care that includes crisis prevention, intervention, and follow-up services. The services are designed to improve an understanding of problem behavior or mental disorder, reduce the rate or crisis contacts (defined as unplanned or emergency service use), prevent out-of-home placement, and maximize the effectiveness of social systems of support.
- A sufficient cadre of leadership, direct support, and support coordination personnel trained in the theory, practices, and systems of positive behavior and mental health supports will be available to self-advocates, families, schools, workplaces, and local communities.

Knowledge Needed to Achieve National Goals

1. Prevention and Support Practices

- What are the supportive contexts and personal competencies that prevent emergence of problem behaviors?
- How do environmental contexts and personal competencies interact in the development of problem behaviors?
- How can assessment better contribute to determining the need for medication as opposed to understanding problem behaviors as an intent to communicate anger and dissatisfaction about one's situation?*
- What differences exist in the types and amounts of problem behaviors between people who have and do not have counselors or peer support groups to help them express their feelings and emotions?*

2. Assessment

- What are the most appropriate and useful instruments and procedures to assess and design support and treatment?
- What approaches are the most useful and cost effective to assess treatment effects over time?
- How do people with disabilities, families, service providers, and policy makers perceive different labels and diagnoses? How do those perceptions affect attitudes, access to assistance, and expectations?

3. Systems of Care

- What are the core elements of effective, comprehensive systems of care to meet behavioral, mental health, and other support needs of people across the life span?
- What are the core services and features of effective crisis prevention and intervention service systems?

4. Skilled Personnel

- What are the core competencies and knowledge needed by systems of care staff to provide the needed assessments, treatment plans, and on-going supports?
- How does improved assessment and response to factors of personal history, context, and preferences help individuals reduce problem behaviors and achieve desired outcomes in their lives, e.g., find and keep jobs, live independently, have more friends?
- Who are the individuals and what are the roles that help individuals, across their life span, to limit problem behaviors and consistently achieve desired outcomes?
- What effective training and technical support approaches are available or need to be developed to provide basic training to primary caregivers, e.g., parents and direct support staff, with everyday roles in people's lives?

HEALTH SERVICES

National Goals

- People with intellectual and developmental disabilities will have access to high-quality health care that is appropriate, affordable, timely, comprehensive, and provided in their communities without regard to their ability to pay.
- The health care system for people with intellectual and developmental disabilities will promote their inclusion in the community.
- People with intellectual and developmental disabilities and their families will partner with health care providers to access and use health information to make choices and decisions about their own health care.
- People with intellectual and developmental disabilities will be treated with respect by health care providers who are well trained to respond to their general and specific health needs.
- People will have the opportunity to participate in the full range of health promotion and wellness activities available to other children and adults.
- People will have access to comprehensive mental health, behavioral, and other allied services and supports to meet their needs within the community.
- Knowledge about the health status of people with intellectual and developmental disabilities will be identified, evaluated, and expanded across the life span.

Knowledge Needed to Achieve National Goals

- What strategies effectively increase the knowledge and participation of people with intellectual and developmental disabilities in their own health promotion and health care decisions?
- What are the elements and impact of guidelines and standards on health outcomes and the utilization of health care services? How can the elements be validated and used to the best effects on the quality of outcomes and services?
- What is the impact of state funding variations and different models of health care financing on key health and functional outcomes of people with disabilities and on specific benefits and services?
- What information is still needed and what existing information needs wider dissemination to specific audiences to increase useful and appropriate information about health status and risks across the life span?
- What effective health care provider training methods (both pre- and in-service) result in a commitment to and positive attitudes about the knowledge and skills need to service people across the life span?
- How does people's dependence on Medicaid as a payer affect their access to and quality of care and what specific factors contribute to and need attention regarding limitations in access and quality?*
- Do alternative medicine approaches improve the health or well-being of some people with disabilities?*
- What are the results when genetic counselors introduce prospective families to a person who has the same disability that their child will have?*
- How does the health care provided by health professionals who are specifically trained to work with people with intellectual and developmental disabilities and families differ from those who have not received such training?*
- What are the most effective approaches to providing user-friendly health information to people with intellectual and developmental disabilities? Does providing this information lead to better health care choices and outcomes?*

BIOMEDICAL RESEARCH

National Goals

- New scientific techniques emerging from genetics, neurobiology, molecular biology, imaging, toxicology, behavioral/cognitive sciences, and related fields will be applied to specific mechanisms that interfere with development throughout the life span to reduce primary and secondary disability.
- Screening and diagnosis of conditions associated with intellectual and developmental disabilities will be employed to maximize opportunities for effective prevention or early intervention.

- Genetic, pharmacological, metabolic, and bioengineering advances will be employed to understand, treat, or cure intellectual and developmental disabilities throughout the life span.
- Access to screening, diagnosis, and treatment approaches will be provided without disparities in access or quality for individuals with intellectual and developmental disabilities.

Knowledge Needed to Achieve National Goals

(See also http://rtc.umn.edu/goals for a more complete listing of recommendations.)

1. Use new scientific techniques

Neurobiological Factors

- What breakthroughs might be achieved by establishing a national data warehouse and tissue bank to explore neurobiological causes of developmental disabilities?
- What might stem cell research reveal about how the human nervous system develops and the underlying causes of developmental disabilities?

Genetic Factors

- What might the study of single-gene and multiple-gene disorders associated with developmental disabilities, including both human and animal models, teach us about the causes and prevention of such disorders?
- What are the effects of gender on brain development and functioning over life span? Why do some developmental disabilities occur more in one gender (such as autism)?

Environmental Factors

- What might research reveal about secondary impairments associated with developmental disabilities, e.g., violent behavior, communication deficits, abnormal patterns of attention, depression, mood disorders, chronic pain, arthritis?
- What research would help us understand why some disabilities share such similar characteristics, e.g., autism and fragile X syndrome?

2. Enhance screening and diagnosis

- How can earlier, safer, and more reliable prenatal diagnosis and treatment be achieved and made readily available?
- How can identification and diagnosis of newborns with conditions associated with intellectual and developmental disabilities be improved and commonly practiced?
- How can screening tools for use in community settings, such as primary care, day care, and school, be improved and more commonly and effectively used to identify children with developmental delay?

3. Use new approaches in a variety of scientific fields

Molecular Genetics

- How can gene and protein therapy be used to prevent and treat genetic disorders associated with developmental disabilities?

Neurobiology

- What animal models and cellular research can be utilized to study neurobiological changes that occur with therapeutic interventions across the life span, including aging?
- What is the potential of stem cell therapies for developmental disabilities?

Pharmacology and Nutrition

- How can we utilize controlled trials to determine the effects of drugs, vitamins, and nutritional supplements on development, on the prevention/treatment of specific disorders, and on secondary medical/mental health problems associated with developmental disabilities?
- How can we develop and test new drugs to enhance memory, cognition, language, emotion, and behavior throughout the life span?

Behavioral and Educational

- How can we use clinical trials and longitudinal follow-up to determine the effects of early family-based and environmental interventions on development and behavior of infants and children at risk for developmental disabilities?
- How can we expand the use of biotechnology to improve cognition, sensory, motor, learning, language, vocational, and adaptive skills in individuals with developmental disabilities across the llife span?

4. Improve care without disparities

- How are specific developmental disabilities manifested across the life span, particularly during old age, e.g., autism, fragile X syndrome, Williams syndrome?
- How do age-related conditions like Alzheimer's disease, cardiovascular disease, diabetes, cancer, etc., affect individuals with various intellectual and developmental disabilities? How can we address the medical and management issues associated with these conditions?
- How can we ensure the inclusion of persons with intellectual and developmental disabilities in all federally funded biomedical research to assure that they are recipients of the potential benefits of this research?

5. Improve information and consent procedures

- How can informed consent procedures be improved through improved language use, pictures, and other means and then monitored to assure that individuals with intellectual and developmental disabilities understand their right to make choices about participating in and withdrawing from research when and as they choose?*

- Can sensitivity training about respect for people with disabilities included as part of the preparation of biomedical researchers improve the behavior of these researchers toward individuals with disabilities?*

INTEGRATED EMPLOYMENT

National Goals

- Access to adequately supported competitive employment, customized employment, self-employment, or other integrated work will be available to people with intellectual and developmental disabilities to permit their inclusion and productivity.
- Students will be involved in multiple paid integrated work experiences prior to leaving high school and will leave high school with a job or other work-related vocational plans.
- All federal and state funding programs, including Medicaid, will support integrated employment and full-day support in the community.
- Policy and funding emphasizing personal control of employment support resources will continue to grow and be available to all.
- Regard employers as partners and customers to increase employment and career opportunities.
- Individuals will have full and equal access to specialized and generic resources that provide job training and job placement/support as needed to support employment outcomes.
- Business ownership will be supported as a viable employment option by relevant federal agencies, such as the Small Business Administration.

Knowledge Needed to Achieve National Goals

- What are the best ways to enhance participation of self-advocates and families in the employment process?
- What strategies are effective in increasing business involvement in hiring, training, employment, and retention?
- What are the best sources of funding for small businesses and microenterprises?
- What are the best strategies to encourage states to fund integrated employment?
- What are the nation's training needs to prepare integrated employment service personnel?
- How much do families and self-advocates agree or disagree on vocational/life aspirations? What strategies work to ameliorate these differences?
- Compare existing traditional services (enclaves, workshops, Medicaid day services, supported work) versus new individualized, person-controlled work. What are people's levels of satisfaction? Are people doing the work they want? Do people have a career track and know that

they could have one? What kinds of supports do people need for their individualized employment situations and options?*

- What supports are available to people with disabilities in systems and programs that effectively help them find and keep jobs (help getting to work, types of support at work, training, technology, financial planning, help with personal organization, mentors, etc)?*

COMMUNITY LIFE

National Goals

- People with intellectual and developmental disabilities will live in and participate fully in their communities.
- People will choose the supports they need and want and exercise control in the selection of how those supports are provided.
- People will have access to stable, skilled support providers when and to the extent they are needed.
- People will have satisfying lives and valued social roles.
- People will be safe, have the assistance they need to manage life's risks, and be free from the exploitation of others.

Knowledge Needed to Achieve National Goals

1. Full community participation

- What efforts have "model" communities successfully undertaken to overcome barriers to people participating in community life (in transportation, social networks, jobs, emergency supports, communications, etc.)?
- To what extent do the country and individual states provide services and resources to assure people's right to live in and participate in the community?
- To what extent are national promises kept to different degrees in different states and for different groups of people? How can those who are not keeping the promises use information about these disparities effectively to stimulate improved response?
- How is community life different for people with intellectual and developmental disabilities when they are well supported to be included in the community? What are the factors associated with being included and feeling well supported?*
- What practices in the current "system" are associated with people developing community connections, such as housing options, employment status, family members, "benefactors," personal interests?*

2. Choose supports and control own resources

- How can the preferences and choices of people with the most severe disabilities be better understood and honored?
- When people exercise control over the resources to purchase services, what choices do they make, and what outcomes do they experience in

community participation and quality of life? How do these differ for persons in traditional community services and how does the public perceive these choices and outcomes?

- What changes in financing practices, at the federal and/or state level, would support choice, control, and expanding connections?

3. Support providers

- What kinds of workplace culture and organization support a quality and stable workforce?
- What characteristics for staff and staffing patterns help support quality-of-life outcomes?

4. Satisfying lives and valued social roles

- What similarities and/or differences are found in measures of life satisfaction between people with intellectual and developmental disabilities and the general population?
- What factors, experiences and circumstances are most directly associated with general life satisfaction?
- What community supports enable people to have valued social roles?
- As efforts are made to engage people with intellectual and developmental disabilities as respondents in surveys about the quality of their services and daily lives, what survey practices are most effective in obtaining reliable and stable responses from persons with more significant intellectual disabilities?

5. Safety and support to manage life's risks

- How big is the problem of abuse, neglect, and exploitation within families and between consumers? Does it differ for people with different skills or across settings?
- How can we address the problem of abuse, neglect, and exploitation? What works? What are the challenges?

FAMILY LIFE

National Goals

- The overarching goal is to support the caregiving efforts and to enhance the quality of life of all families so that families will remain the core unit of American society. (This goal subsumes six associated goals, each of which has the same priority and importance as each other one.)
- The first associated goal is to ensure that family-professional partnerships are used in research, policy making, and the planning and delivery of supports and services so that families will control their own destinies with due regard to the autonomy of adult family members with disabilities to control their own lives.
- The second associated goal is to ensure that families fully participate in communities of their choice so that they will have comprehensive, in-

clusive, neighborhood-based, and culturally responsive supports and services.

- The third associated goal is to ensure that services and supports for all families are available, accessible, appropriate, affordable, and accountable.
- The fourth associated goal is to ensure that sufficient public and private funding will be available to implement these goals and that all families will participate in directing the use of public funds authorized and appropriated for their benefit.
- The fifth associated goal is to ensure that families and professionals have full access to state-of-the-art knowledge and best practices so that they can collaborate in using them.
- The sixth associated goal is to ensure that sibling perspectives are included in all research and policy.

Knowledge Needed to Achieve National Goals

- What do (a) periodic national or subnational assessments of family, including siblings, needs for supports and services and (b) periodic policy and fiscal analyses reveal relative to helping to ensure that federal and state family support policies and services remain relevant and responsive to family needs and outcomes?
- What do families expect the outcomes of services to be, across all domains of all family life and across family life spans? How can those outcomes be implemented to ensure program accountability, develop cost-benefit analyses of family support policies and programs, and develop more family-responsive policies and programs?
- What can be determined from research and demonstration project evaluations related to the desirability and means to convert traditional agency-based services to effective and flexible family-driven supports and services and to take demonstration programs involving "converted" services to scale?
- What does research reveal about the effectiveness of family-professional and family–policy maker partnerships in developing policy, conducting research, and planning and using family supports and services? Among these approaches must be those that are sometimes called "Participatory Action Research." This term includes partnerships among researchers, family members, practitioners, and policy leaders to design, execute, interpret, share, and use research and demonstration data.
- What are the most effective strategies for enhancing research, policy making, and service delivery partnerships with all families but especially with traditionally underserved and nontraditional families?
- What federal and state policies best advance family support policy and practice, including the promotion of timely distribution and use of research findings and increasing funding for family support and services?
- What are the criteria for determining effective family support policies

and programs and ensuring that best practices are available to families and practitioners?

- What are the domains of family quality of life across the life span of families, and what new models of supports and services are valid for ethnically and racially diverse families?
- What is the most effective way to provide training to self-advocates and families related to such legal instruments as advance directives, last wills and testaments, trusts, guardianship procedures, and other means of support?
- How do Medicaid rules influence the use of guardianship for people living in institutions and other segregated places? What are the characteristics and duties of guardians? How do guardians advance or impede the independence, integration, and productivity of their wards?

SELF-DETERMINATION AND SELF-ADVOCACY

National Goals

- People with disabilities are equal partners in research.
- People shall make informed decisions about their lives.
- People with disabilities shall have the opportunity to build their capacities, such as their knowledge, skill, and resources, to control their lives and contribute to their communities.
- People with disabilities shall have control over their resources, such as funding and supports.
- People with disabilities shall have meaningful opportunity and support to advocate for themselves and to demonstrate leadership.
- People with disabilities shall have the freedom and opportunity to participate in social activities and have the social relationships that they desire.

Knowledge Needed to Achieve National Goals

1. Equal partners

- What opportunities do individuals with developmental disabilities have to conduct research?
- How many and what types of current projects involve people with developmental disabilities as co-principal and/or principal investigators?
- What opportunities are currently available for individuals with disabilities to learn about research, e.g., read RFPs; write, review, or manage grants; design studies; gather, analyze, or interpret data; write and edit manuscripts; disseminate findings; promote the use of findings by policy makers and other groups?
- How can participatory action research be designed and conducted to involve individuals with intellectual and developmental disabilities? What are the most effective ways for researchers with and without disabilities to work together?

2. Informed decisions

- How and to what extent do individuals with intellectual and developmental disabilities have opportunities to make decisions about their lives (e.g., where to go to school, live, and work; friendships and relationships; how to spend personal and service money; what services and supports are needed and how they are provided)?
- How do opportunities for informed decision making vary by factors such as setting (community, employment, home), circle of support, severity of disability, guardianship, involvement in the service system, and race and ethnicity?
- What successful strategies have changed attitudes and practice of systems, policy makers, and family members in assuring that people are provided opportunities to make informed choices?

3. Build own capacities

- To what extent are people with disabilities able to make informed decisions about their lives?
- What information, resources, skills, and supports do people need to be able to make informed choices and create their future?
- How does the service system support and hinder opportunities for people to take charge of their own lives?
- Study community volunteerism among self-advocates and self- advocacy organizations.*
- Do college and junior college degree programs for adult learners allow self-advocates to get college credits from their experiences?*

4. Control own resources

- What control do people really have over their resources, such as their funding and supports from the person's, the family's, the guardian's, or the professional's perspective?
- Analyze changes that have occurred within service systems that have implemented essential elements of self-determination.
- What are effective practices for promoting control over resources by people with diverse disabilities, cultural backgrounds, and support networks?

5. Self-advocacy

- How does involvement in self-advocacy impact people's lives in the areas of personal development, social connection and treatment by others, access to supports and resources, safety, quality of life, etc.?
- What experiences and effective practices do self-advocates report in their work to change and develop policies?
- What are the leadership development needs of self-advocates, and to what extent are leadership development opportunities available?
- What are the relationships between self-advocacy leaders and their sup-

porters or advisors? What barriers exist in these relationships and what strategies promote their success?

- Has the mandate for self-advocacy in the Developmental Disabilities Act made a difference across the states and territories?*

6. Social activities

- To what extent are people with intellectual and developmental disabilities becoming involved in their communities, establishing friendships, marrying and raising children?
- How, and to what extent, are friendships supported outside the "program" setting?
- What practices and policies can be effectively used to support community belonging, friendship, and love by people with developmental disabilities?
- What are the best experiences of families supporting people in:
  - Developing friendships with people with and without disabilities
  - Making connections and enjoying hospitality
  - Getting around their communities
  - Understanding sexuality
  - Supporting marriage and parenthood

TECHNOLOGY

National Goals

- Expand research on the application of existing technologies for people with intellectual and developmental disabilities.
- Promote research on the application of emerging technologies for persons with intellectual and developmental disabilities.
- Develop a national network of research centers on cognitive disability and technology.
- Establish training based on fundamental competencies and skills; promote the initiation of undergraduate and graduate training programs in technology for persons with cognitive disabilities based on these "core competencies."
- Ensure information regarding technology is accessible to self-advocates, their families, and support networks.

Knowledge Needed to Achieve National Goals

- What is the need for assistive technologies for persons with intellectual and developmental disabilities in the states?
- How many persons with intellectual and developmental disabilities in the states have access to appropriate technology devices and services?
- Do people with physical disabilities have different access than those with

intellectual or developmental disabilities to the technological devices and supports that they need? If so, what explains the differences?*
- What are the principal components of "accessibility" as this term pertains to people with intellectual and developmental disabilities and their use of information technology?
- How can access to information on technology for persons with cognitive disabilities be increased?*
- How can the digital divide between persons with intellectual and developmental disabilities and the general population be reduced?
- What are the benefits of technology use by persons with intellectual and developmental disabilities?
- What are the costs of providing technology to persons with intellectual and developmental disabilities in each of the states?
- How can common technologies available to the general public be adapted for use by persons with intellectual and developmental disabilities?
- How can technologies found to be beneficial to persons with other disabilities (such as physical disabilities, Alzheimer's disease, traumatic brain injury, stroke) be adapted for use by persons with intellectual and developmental disabilities?
- What effective training practices for technology access, use and outcomes exist?
- What funding sources are available for people to purchase the technology they need to live in the community?

AGING

National Goals

- Communities will be "aging and disability friendly" by instituting universal design, environmental modifications, and technologies that make communities fully accessible to people with disabilities as they age.
  - Transportation, moving about, safety
  - Accessing goods, services, supports
  - Information access
  - Collaboration between aging and disability networks
  - Universal design, signage, and "visitability"
  - A focus on changing community environment: residential, service, health care
- Family and other caregivers of older adults with intellectual and developmental disabilities will receive sufficient economic, social, and emotional supports to provide caregiving in the later life of the individuals with intellectual and developmental disabilities or their caregivers. This includes tax credits, better training and education, and special attention to underserved communities.

- Older adults with intellectual and developmental disabilities will live in community settings of their choice. Those settings will provide sufficient supports and material security to support aging in place and to maximize their independence and interdependence, including remaining in their "home community," aging in place, transportation and safety, personal assistance, and economic security.
- Older adults with intellectual and developmental disabilities will have opportunities for valued social roles and full participation in community life. This includes lifelong learning, self-determination, life activity, friendships and meaningful relationships, and developing and maintaining strong social networks across the life span.
- Adults with intellectual and developmental disabilities will have increased longevity with improved mental and physical health. This requires reducing health disparities; advancing knowledge of age-related secondary conditions; adopting a "life-span approach" and improving access to health care.

Knowledge Needed to Achieve National Goals

- What are the new technologies, user-friendly interfaces, and environmental strategies that promote "aging and disability friendly" communities?
- How do we support caregiver capacity and transition planning in later life?
- How do we support "aging in place" for older individuals with intellectual and developmental disabilities?
- What are the contributions of lifelong learning, self-determination, meaningful life activity, friendships, and strong social networks on aging well?
- How do we predict, diagnose or prevent emerging secondary age-related physical and mental health compromises in older individuals with intellectual and developmental disabilities?
- What supports or programs help individuals with disabilities who live at home with their elderly parent(s) become part of their community after their parents die?*
- What choices do older people with disabilities who live in nursing homes have compared to their peers who live in the community, e.g., retiring from work, age-appropriate leisure and recreation, transportation, and choice of living arrangement?

APPENDIX G
The President's Committee for People with Intellectual Disabilities (PCPID)

The President's Committee for People with Intellectual Disabilities (PCPID), formerly known as the President's Committee on Mental Retardation, was initially organized as a blue ribbon panel by President John F. Kennedy in 1961 and formally established as a committee by President Lyndon B. Johnson in 1966 under an executive order. Eight years later, in 1974, new goals for the committee focusing on deinstitutionalization, prevention, and legal rights were established by President Nixon. In 1990, President George Bush supported landmark legislation for protecting the rights of people with disabilities. The Americans with Disabilities Act (ADA) set forth standards of equal opportunity in the areas of employment, transportation, telecommunications, public accommodations, and community- and home-based services. In 1996, a new set of goals for the committee encouraging full community inclusion and citizens' rights were created by President William J. Clinton. In 2001, President George W. Bush introduced the New Freedom Initiative to promote community integration and issued an executive order for tearing down barriers for people with disabilities. Support for the ADA and the Olmstead Decision for community inclusion was emphasized. On July 25, 2003, he signed the executive order renaming the President's Committee on Mental Retardation to the President's Committee for People with Intellectual Disabilities.

Much has changed for people with intellectual disabilities since the 1960s owing to advances in medicine, technology, research, education, and public understanding. It is the purpose of the PCPID to advise the president on the achievements, continuing needs, and emerging issues in this dynamic field. PCPID evaluates the adequacy of current practices and programs and reviews federal agency activities impacting on people with intellectual disabilities. The committee highlights the need for appropriate changes and encourages research, education, services, and supports relating to people with intellectual disabilities.

As opportunities may present themselves, the committee collaborates with other federal agencies and national organizations in convening conferences and forums and disseminating information to the public on issues and accomplishments of people with intellectual disabilities.

The members of the PCPID have taken the New Freedom Initiative and built their work around the same basic categories: expanding educational opportunities, increasing access to technology, improving individual and family support, increasing employment and economic independence, and promoting access and integration into community life.

COMPOSITION OF THE PCPID

The committee consists of 21 citizen members and 13 ex officio (federal government) members designated by the president. These 21 members consist of individuals who represent a broad spectrum of perspectives, experience, and expertise on intellectual disabilities, and include self-advocates with intellectual disabilities and members of families with a child or adult with intellectual disabilities and persons employed in either the public or the private sector. Except as the president may from time to time otherwise direct, appointees under this paragraph have two-year terms, except that an appointment made to fill a vacancy occurring before the expiration of a term shall be made for the balance of the unexpired term.

The president shall designate the Chair of the President's Committee for People with Intellectual Disabilities from the 21 citizen members. The chair shall advise and counsel the committee and represent the committee on appropriate occasions.

The Department of Health and Human Services, to the extent permitted by law, provides the PCPID with necessary staff, administrative services, facilities, and funding.

The 13 ex officio members include the Secretary of Health and Human Services, Secretary of Education, Secretary of Labor, Secretary of Housing and Urban Development, Secretary of Commerce, Secretary of Transportation, Secretary of Interior, Secretary of Homeland Security, the Attorney General, the President and CEO of the Corporation for National and Community Service, the Chair of the Equal Employment Opportunity Commission, the Chair of the National Council on Disabilities, and the Commissioner of the Social Security Administration. The ex officio members undertake committee duties in addition to their daily occupations

MISSION

It is estimated that between 7 and 8 million Americans of all ages, or three percent of the general population, experience intellectual disability. Nearly 30 million, or 1 in 10 families in the United States, are directly affected by a person with intellectual disabilities at some point in their lifetime. Intellectual disabilities present a major challenge to the social, educational, health, and economic systems within the United States. The PCPID focuses on this critical subject of national concern.

The committee acts in an advisory capacity to the president and the Secretary of the Department of Health and Human Services on matters relating to programs and services for persons with intellectual disabilities. Since 1966, the committee has fostered state planning, stimulated development of strategies, policies, and programs, and advanced the concept of community participation in the field of intellectual disabilities.

To continue to best fulfill its purpose, the president has adopted several national goals to better recognize and uphold the right of all people with intellectual disabilities to enjoy a quality of life that promotes independence, self-determination, and participation as productive members of society. These goals include the assurance of full citizenship rights of people with intellectual disabilities, the provision of all necessary supports to individuals and families, the reduction of the occurrence and severity of intellectual disabilities, and the promotion of the widest dissemination of information of models, programs, and services within the field of intellectual disabilities.

FUNCTION

The PCPID provides such advice and assistance in the area of intellectual disabilities, as the president or Secretary of Health and Human Services may request, and particularly advises with respect to the following areas:

1. evaluating and monitoring the national effort to establish appropriate policies and supports for people with intellectual disabilities;
2. providing suggestions for improvement in the delivery of services to people with intellectual disabilities, including preventive services, the promulgation of effective and humane policies, and the provision of necessary supports;
3. identifying the extent to which various federal and state programs achieve the national goals for people with intellectual disabilities described in the preamble of the Executive Order for the President's Committee for People with Intellectual Disabilities so as to have a positive impact on the lives of people with intellectual disabilities;
4. facilitating liaison among federal, state, and local governments, foundations, nonprofit organizations, other private organizations, and citizens concerning people with intellectual disabilities;
5. developing and disseminating such information as will tend to reduce the incidence and severity of intellectual disabilities; and
6. promoting the concept of community participation and development of community supports for citizens with intellectual disabilities.

To assist the PCPID in providing advice to the president, federal departments and agencies requested to do so by the committee designate liaison officers to the committee. Such officers, on request by the committee, and to the extent permitted by law, provide the committee with information on department and agency programs that do contribute to or could contribute to achievement of the President's goals in the field of intellectual disabilities.

Index

Note: page numbers followed by *t* and *f* indicate tables and figures.